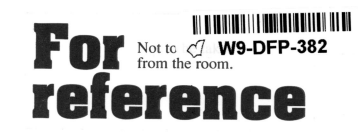

DATE DUE

THE NETTER COLLECTION
OF MEDICAL ILLUSTRATIONS

VOLUME 8 • PART III

The Netter Collection of Medical Illustrations
Musculoskeletal System Volume 8: **Part III:** Trauma, Evaluation, and Management
Prepared by
Frank H. Netter, M.D.

See page 222 for a complete list of The Netter Collection of Medical Illustrations

Published by Icon Learning Systems, LLC, a subsidiary of Medimedia USA, Inc.

First Printing, 1993
Second Printing, 1997
Third Printing, 2002

ISBN 0-914168-79-7
Library of Congress Catalog No.: 97-76569
Printed in Canada

Printed by Friesens.
"Original Printing by Avanti/Case-Hoyt Corporation"
Film Prep by PAGE Imaging, Inc., Pittsburgh, PA

THE NETTER COLLECTION OF MEDICAL ILLUSTRATIONS

VOLUME 8

A Compilation of Paintings on the
Normal and Pathologic Anatomy of the

MUSCULOSKELETAL SYSTEM

PART III

TRAUMA, EVALUATION, AND MANAGEMENT

Prepared by

FRANK H. NETTER, M.D.

Consulting Editor

JAMES D. HECKMAN, M.D.

Managing Editor

REGINA V. DINGLE

WITH A FOREWORD BY HENRY J. MANKIN, M.D.,

Edith M. Ashley Professor of Orthopaedic Surgery, Harvard Medical School

Commissioned and published by

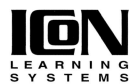

ICON
LEARNING
SYSTEMS

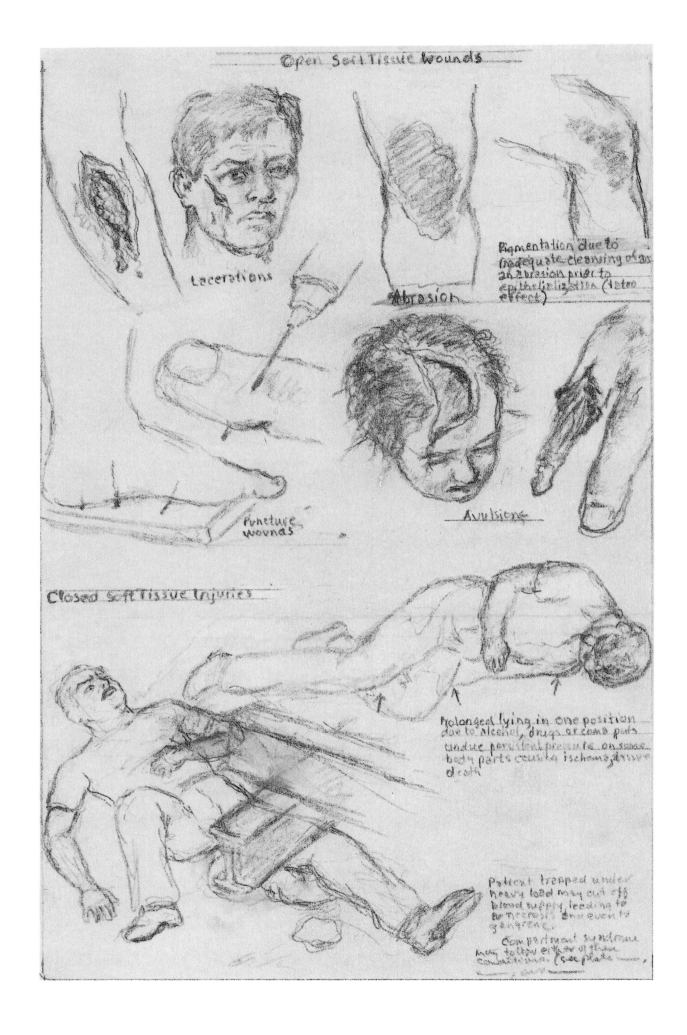

Open Soft Tissue Wounds

Lacerations

Abrasion

Pigmentation due to inadequate cleansing of an abrasion prior to epithelization (tatoo effect)

Puncture wounds

Avulsions

Closed Soft Tissue Injuries

Prolonged lying in one position due to alcohol, drugs or coma puts undue persistent pressure on some body parts causing ischemia, tissue death

Patient trapped under heavy load may cut off blood supply, leading to tissue necrosis and even to gangrene.

Compartment syndrome may follow either of these conditions (see plate ___)

Foreword

In 1953, as an intern at the University of Chicago, I obtained a copy of the very first of the now world-famous CIBA COLLECTION masterpieces by Frank Netter, M.D. The subject was the *Nervous System* that, after an amazing thirteen printings, is now in its third printing of a revised edition. My colleagues and I at that time and all subsequent generations of physicians over the last 35 years marveled at the artistry and extraordinary clarity of those illustrations; and how remarkably, when coupled with the short but well-written text, they provided such a clear definition of complex three-dimensional structures and confusing relationships that we had struggled sometimes in vain to comprehend. There was little doubt in our minds that we were looking at the works of a genius—not only because he saw so much and so clearly, but because he could make us see it with equal clarity. We waited, as did the world, for subsequent volumes and were not disappointed with any of the next six. The *Reproductive System*, published in 1954, the *Digestive System* in 1957, the *Endocrine System* in 1965, the *Heart* in 1969, the *Kidneys, Ureters, and Urinary Bladder* in 1973, and the *Respiratory System* in 1979 all showed the same remarkable ability to portray the anatomy and embryology, physiology, pathology, and clinical states with such extraordinary clarity and in sufficient detail as to become, for each of these disciplines, major teaching and reference texts. I wonder how many times in these past 35 years a Netter illustration has been used for a lecture or demonstration in a medical school or residency classroom, and how many copies have been made of the figures to subsequently reside in teaching collections throughout the world? Surely the number must be exceeded only by the number of physicians who hold the volumes as cherished possessions and have read them over and over in a quest for knowledge or as part of a scholarly pursuit.

Having said that, I must express a degree of disappointment on behalf of my colleagues in Orthopaedics, Rheumatology, Physiatry, and the sciences associated with connective tissue diseases, with the evident fact that with the exception of some of the plates in Volumes 1 and 4 there were few of these teaching atlases that had any relevance to our rather sizable corner of the world of medicine. It is therefore with great enthusiasm and unbridled pleasure that our specialties now greet *Volume 8: Musculoskeletal System*. Furthermore, after consideration of the contents and study of the magnificent plates and text, I conclude that not only was the product worth waiting for but in my opinion the three parts comprising this latest work are the author's finest! Frank Netter, M.D., has not only "done it again" but he's done it better than he ever did it before!

The *Musculoskeletal System* is one of Dr. Netter's most ambitious projects. Any of the subjects covered would seem to require a separate volume, and perhaps one of the major aspects of the genius of the artist is deciding what to include. Realizing that each plate contains several main themes and multiple facts (all nicely tied together by the artistry of the author), it is not surprising that anatomy and physiology (including metabolic disorders) are included in the 214 plates that comprise Part I; and that congenital and developmental disorders can be depicted in 111 plates, neoplasms in 34, rheumatic disorders in 73, and joint replacement surgery in another 28, all in Part II. Part III on injuries (155 plates), infections (18 plates), amputations (11 plates), and rehabilitation (17 plates) completes the set. If one totals these plates, the number exceeds 660 (what a fantastic effort even for Dr. Netter!), and with the text supplied by the numerous contributors, the three parts of Volume 8 should rapidly become classic teaching texts for our specialties.

One may wonder why Volume 8 required so many plates and so much text as compared with the other disciplines, and upon consideration, I believe the answer is self-evident. The musculoskeletal system comprises most of the body's supportive and protective elements and provides movement and prehension. The tissues included vary from the undifferentiated fibrous supporting membranes to the remarkably complex organ systems of the bones and joints, and the anatomic structures are as different as the big toe and the first cervical vertebra. While trauma is almost exclusively related to the bones and joints, metabolic bone disease involves the endocrine and renal systems; genetic disorders, other multiple organ systems; arthritis, the sciences of immunology and internal metabolism; and neoplasms, the entire field of oncology. What brings these fields together in this remarkable volume and in the scientific world is the anatomic structures and, perhaps more relevantly, the entire background framework of connective tissue chemistry, mechanical engineering, and materials science, which Dr. Netter has woven so beautifully and understandably into every section.

The students, scholars, and practitioners who deal with the musculoskeletal system have been waiting along with me since 1953 for Frank Netter's Volume 8. I don't think they will be disappointed.

HENRY J. MANKIN, M.D.
Boston, July 1987

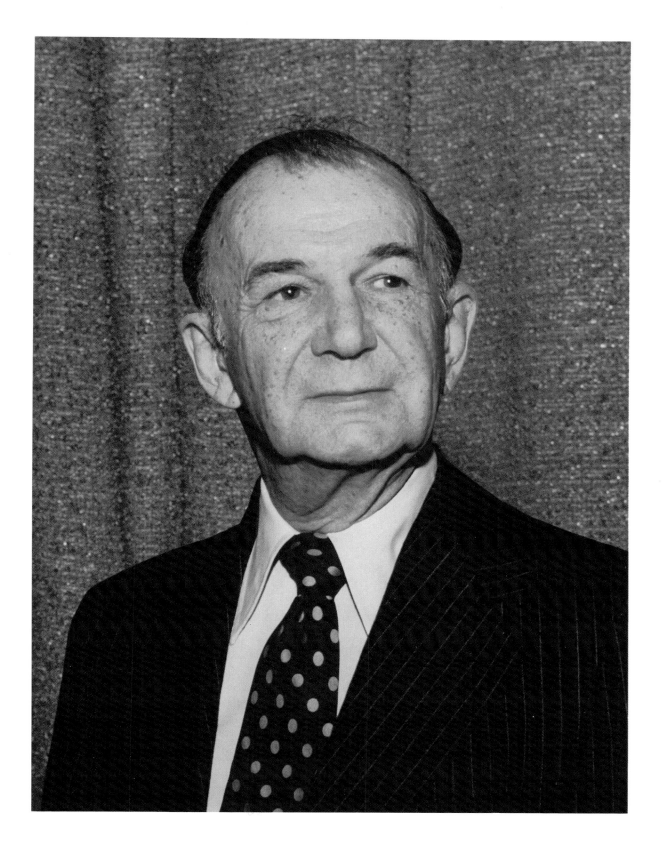

FRANK H. NETTER, M.D.
1906–1991

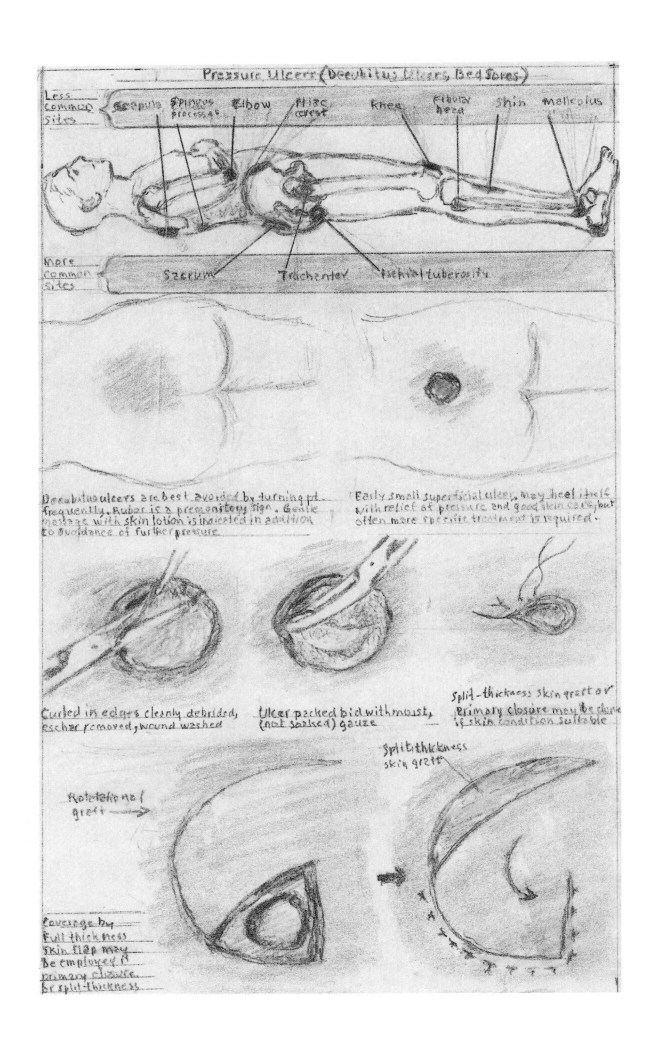

Pressure Ulcers (Decubitus Ulcers, Bed Sores)

Less common sites: Scapula, Spinous processes, Elbow, Iliac crest, Knee, Fibular head, Shin, Malleolus

More common sites: Sacrum, Trochanter, Ischial tuberosity

Decubitus ulcers are best avoided by turning pt. frequently. Rubor is a premonitory sign. Gentle massage with skin lotion is indicated in addition to avoidance of further pressure.

Early small superficial ulcer may heal itself with relief of pressure and good skin care, but often more specific treatment is required.

Curled in edges cleanly debrided, eschar removed, wound washed

Ulcer packed bid with moist, (not soaked) gauze

Split-thickness skin graft or primary closure may be done if skin condition suitable

Rotation flap graft

Split-thickness skin graft

Coverage by full thickness skin flap may be employed if primary closure or split-thickness

Introduction

With great pride but also with great sadness, I write this introduction to Part III of Volume 8 of the CIBA COLLECTION. The pride stems from 10 years of planning and eventually seeing come to fruition a unique compendium on musculoskeletal injury and disease. The sadness results from the fact that the creator of this marvelous work is no longer here to share in the joy of its publication. As we were in the final phases of production in September of 1991, Dr. Netter passed away after a long illness. During the 8 years before his death, and indeed right up until the time of his final illness, we, the authors, had the joy of seeing our vague ideas become lifelike and clearly defined through Dr. Netter's hand. The opportunity to work with him in the development of this atlas will always be one of the highlights of my career, and I know I speak for all the other contributors as I express thanks and a most fond farewell to Frank. Dr. Netter died before all of the illustrations were painted, and two of his sketches are printed as he left them, to help all of us appreciate his marvelous skills.

Many individuals contributed substantially to the creation of this volume. Many former and present members of the faculty at the Department of Orthopaedics, The University of Texas Health Science Center at San Antonio—Fred G. Corley, Jr., Peter L.J. McGanity, Franklin J. Dzida, Michael J. Hanley, Praveen K. Reddy, and Harry A. Snowdy—collaborated on the section on musculoskeletal injury. The rehabilitation section was developed and coordinated by Nicolas E. Walsh, chairman of the Department of Rehabilitation Medicine, with the collaboration of Daniel Dumitru and Leslie D. Porter.

We also sought the specialized expertise of renowned authorities at other institutions to address particular subjects: Basil A. Pruitt, Jr., burns; Ronald L. Linscheid, infection; Carl T. Brighton, R. Bruce Heppenstall, and Frederick S. Kaplan, fracture healing and nonunion; Harold E. Kleinert, Anthony C. Berger, and Steven J. McCabe, replantation; and Scott J. Mubarak, compartment syndrome.

This talented group of experts provided clear and concise discussions as a counterpoint to the artistic expertise of Dr. Netter, and I am grateful to all for their patience and perseverance.

Coordination of the project from start to finish was the responsibility of Colleen Mann and Anne Little at our office and Gina Dingle at Ciba. Without their unflagging dedication, extraordinary editorial skills, good humor, and tolerance, our work would not have been published. I extend to each one my gratitude for, and appreciation of, a job well done.

I hope that this collection of illustrations will be a useful resource for orthopaedic educators, an inspiration to all of our students, and—most important—an appropriate tribute to the prodigious, majestic, and lifelong achievements of Frank H. Netter, M.D., medical illustrator extraordinaire.

JAMES D. HECKMAN, M.D.
San Antonio

Contributors and Consultants

Anthony C. Berger, M.B.B.S., F.R.A.C.S.

Hand Surgeon, Plastic and Reconstructive Surgery Unit; Senior Research Fellow, Microsurgery Research Center, St. Vincent's Hospital, Melbourne, Victoria, Australia

Carl T. Brighton, M.D., Ph.D.

Paul B. Magnuson Professor of Bone and Joint Surgery, Department of Orthopaedic Surgery, University of Pennsylvania School of Medicine, Philadelphia, Pennsylvania

Fred G. Corley, Jr., M.D.

Associate Professor, Department of Orthopaedics, The University of Texas Health Science Center at San Antonio, San Antonio, Texas

Daniel Dumitru, M.D.

Associate Professor and Deputy Chair, Department of Rehabilitation Medicine, The University of Texas Health Science Center at San Antonio, San Antonio, Texas

Franklin J. Dzida, M.D.

Greater Los Angeles Orthopedic Medical Group, Downey Community Hospital, Downey, California

Michael J. Hanley, M.D.

Orthopaedic Surgeon, Palestine, Texas

James D. Heckman, M.D.

Professor and Chairman, John J. Hinchey, M.D. Chair, Department of Orthopaedics, The University of Texas Health Science Center at San Antonio, San Antonio, Texas

R. Bruce Heppenstall, M.D.

Professor and Chief of Orthopaedic Surgery, Hospital of the University of Pennsylvania, Philadelphia, Pennsylvania

Frederick S. Kaplan, M.D.

Associate Professor of Orthopaedic Surgery and Medicine; Chief, Division of Metabolic Bone Diseases, University of Pennsylvania School of Medicine, Philadelphia, Pennsylvania

Harold E. Kleinert, M.D.

Clinical Professor of Surgery, University of Louisville School of Medicine, Louisville, Kentucky; Clinical Professor of Surgery, Indiana University–Purdue University of Medicine, Indianapolis, Indiana

Ronald L. Linscheid, M.D.

Professor of Orthopaedic Surgery, Mayo Medical School; Consultant, Department of Orthopaedic Surgery, Division of Hand Surgery, Mayo Clinic, Rochester, Minnesota

Steven J. McCabe, M.D.

Christine M. Kleinert Institute for Hand and Micro Surgery, Inc., Louisville, Kentucky

Peter L. J. McGanity, M.D.

Associate Professor of Orthopaedics, The University of Texas Health Science Center at San Antonio, San Antonio, Texas

Scott J. Mubarak, M.D.

Clinical Professor, Department of Orthopedics, University of California; Director, Orthopedic Institute, Children's Hospital, San Diego, California

Leslie D. Porter, M.D.

Medical Director, Baylor Institute for Rehabilitation; Staff Physician, Baylor University Medical Center; Clinical Assistant Professor, The University of Texas Southwestern Medical School, Department of Physical Medicine and Rehabilitation, Dallas, Texas

Basil A. Pruitt, Jr., M.D.

Commander and Director, U.S. Army Institute of Surgical Research; Professor of Surgery, Uniformed Services University of the Health Sciences; Clinical Professor of Surgery, The University of Texas Health Science Center at San Antonio, San Antonio, Texas

Praveen K. Reddy, M.D.

Chief Resident, Department of Orthopaedics, The University of Texas Health Science Center at San Antonio, San Antonio, Texas

Harry A. Snowdy, M.D.

Clinical Associate Professor of Surgery, Department of Surgery, Section of Orthopaedic Surgery, The Medical College of Georgia; Orthopaedic Surgeon, St. Joseph Hospital, Augusta, Georgia

Nicolas E. Walsh, M.D.

Professor and Chairman, Department of Rehabilitation Medicine, The University of Texas Health Science Center at San Antonio, San Antonio, Texas

Contents

Section I

Injury

Frank H. Netter, M.D.

in collaboration with

Carl T. Brighton, M.D., Ph.D. *Plates 152–155*

Fred G. Corley, Jr., M.D. *Plates 41–68*

Franklin J. Dzida, M.D. *Plates 94–104*

Michael J. Hanley, M.D. *Plates 33–40*

James D. Heckman, M.D. *Plates 1–4, 17–22, 26–32, 107–116, 127–151*

Frederick S. Kaplan, M.D. and R. Bruce Heppenstall, M.D. *Plates 23–25*

Harold E. Kleinert, M.D., Anthony C. Berger, M.D.,
  and Steven J. McCabe, M.D. *Plates 117–126*

Peter L. J. McGanity, M.D. *Plates 79–93, 105–106*

Scott J. Mubarak, M.D. *Plates 11–16*

Basil A. Pruitt, Jr., M.D. *Plates 5–10*

Harry A. Snowdy, M.D. and Praveen K. Reddy, M.D. *Plates 69–78*

Closed Soft Tissue Injuries

Injury to Soft Tissue

Three basic mechanisms cause soft tissue injuries: blunt trauma, crushing injury, and penetrating trauma. Blunt and crushing traumas are called closed injuries because they do not penetrate the overlying skin. Penetrating (open) injuries violate the protective skin layer, contaminating the wound and thus producing open injuries.

Closed Soft Tissue Injury

Closed injuries are characterized by variable degrees of damage to skin and underlying tissue (Plate 1). Blood vessels are most vulnerable to injury; thus, closed soft tissue injuries usually produce bleeding and swelling beneath the skin. Bleeding results from disruption of the blood vessels, and swelling results from damage to the endothelial lining of the blood vessels, which allows plasma to leak into the soft tissue spaces.

The most common soft tissue injury is a contusion (bruise) caused by blunt trauma that damages blood vessels and results in bleeding or swelling into the soft tissues. Usually, the blood and the edema fluid dissect between the cells of the soft tissues, causing localized swelling. Bleeding produces the typical black-and-blue discoloration of a contusion. If large vessels are disrupted, the pressure of the escaping blood can induce separation of tissue planes, leading to the accumulation of a large hematoma beneath the skin or between the deeper layers of soft tissue.

Contusion and hematoma formation may accompany more serious injuries of the limbs, such as fractures, dislocations, and sprains. The clinical examination of a patient with a painful contusion must rule out more serious underlying problems. A simple contusion or hematoma is treated with the immediate application of ice, a gentle compression dressing, and elevation of the injured part. Temporary restriction of activity—voluntary or with the application of a compression dressing or splint—facilitates the body's ability to repair a soft tissue injury. The simple mnemonic *ICES* (*I*ce, *C*ompression, *E*levation, and *S*plinting) can be used to remember the principles of treatment. Because soft tissue injuries rarely cause significant disruption of important soft tissue structures, the body reabsorbs the extravasated blood and edema fluid within a few days, allowing gradual return of function. A large hematoma may take several weeks to resolve, however.

Although a hematoma or contusion results from the *sudden* application of a blunt force, soft tissues can also be damaged by the continuous application of force over relatively long periods of time (hours or days). This mechanism of injury, called a crushing injury, causes damage by direct force and also by impairment of circulation to the tissues. Continuous pressure that is in excess of the

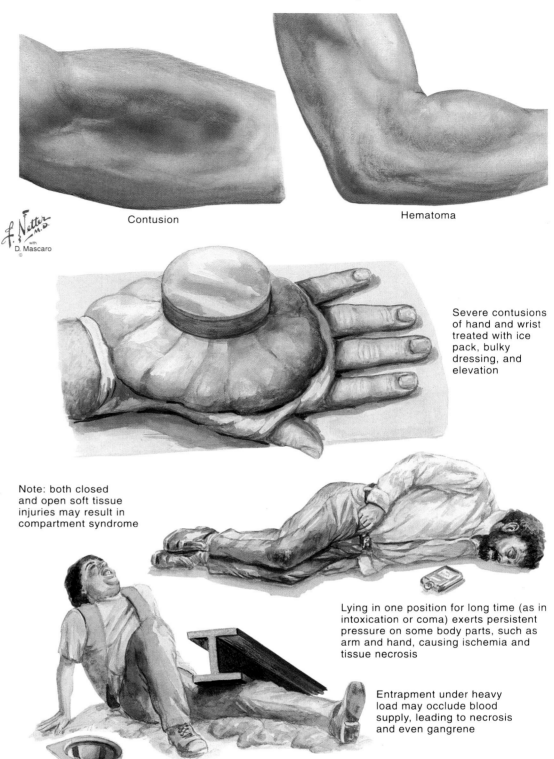

Contusion

Hematoma

Severe contusions of hand and wrist treated with ice pack, bulky dressing, and elevation

Note: both closed and open soft tissue injuries may result in compartment syndrome

Lying in one position for long time (as in intoxication or coma) exerts persistent pressure on some body parts, such as arm and hand, causing ischemia and tissue necrosis

Entrapment under heavy load may occlude blood supply, leading to necrosis and even gangrene

capillary filling pressure causes the compressed soft tissue to become ischemic and die.

Crushing injury takes many forms. One of the most vulnerable soft tissues is the skin; continuous pressure applied for more than 2 hours can result in ischemia and the development of a pressure sore. Pressure ulcers are particularly likely to develop in skin that overlies a bony prominence and is compressed against a firm surface such as a cast, a rigid shoe or brace, or even a firm mattress. Although the initial lesion is closed, when the skin dies, it sloughs, and the lesion may become infected.

Another type of crushing injury occurs when a heavy load falls on a limb, rendering it immobile

and obstructing the blood flow (venous, arterial, or both) for several hours. The result is a compartment syndrome. If the resulting ischemia lasts for more than 2 hours, it often causes the death of muscle tissue, with associated permanent loss of function. When blood flow is restored to a crushed limb, the necrotic muscle releases myoglobin into the venous circulation. The myoglobin may sludge in the kidneys, producing acute renal failure. The risk of this complication may be minimized by adequate hydration of the patient following a crush injury. Ischemia that persists for a long time leads to gangrene of the entire crushed limb.

Injury to Soft Tissue
(Continued)

Open Soft Tissue Injury

Open soft tissue injuries are, by definition, contaminated (Plate 2). The many different types of open soft tissue injuries—abrasion, laceration, avulsion, puncture, and amputation—are caused by a variety of mechanisms. Regardless of the particular pattern of injury, the common denominators are penetration of the skin and bacterial contamination of the deeper tissues, which establish the potential for infection. Blood loss in open wounds is usually greater than in closed injuries, because the bleeding is not limited by the tamponade effect created by the encompassing soft tissues.

Treatment of open wounds initially focuses on controlling the bleeding and contamination. Compression dressings must be applied to the wound at once to stop bleeding, and tetanus prophylaxis must be confirmed or provided. After the bleeding is controlled, all open wounds must be thoroughly debrided to remove as much contaminating material as possible. Whenever the adequacy of the initial debridement is in doubt, wound closure should be delayed until the surgeon is confident that no deep contaminants persist and there is no sign of active wound infection. In patients with severe contamination, antibiotics can be used to help control the onset of infection but should never be used as a substitute for surgical debridement. Excellent cosmetic and functional results can be obtained by debriding the wound, packing it open with a sterile compression dressing, and repeating the debridement at 48 to 72 hours. Delayed primary closure is carried out at this time.

With the exception of certain nerve injuries, all soft tissues heal by the formation of collagenous scar tissue. Prompt, careful, and anatomic reapproximation of injured tendon, muscle, and skin provides the best basis for a functional and satisfactory result. Failure to achieve repair of an injured tendon often results in significant functional loss.

Effective repair of a lacerated tendon remains a great surgical challenge because tendons often heal with an excess of scar tissue and loss of their natural gliding function. The principles of tendon repair therefore include thorough debridement of the wound, precise anatomic reapproximation, and protected active range of motion during healing to help maintain the mobility essential for normal function. The range of motion allowed following repair is limited by the particular tendon injured, the location of the laceration along the course of the tendon, and the strength of the surgical repair.

Open Soft Tissue Wounds

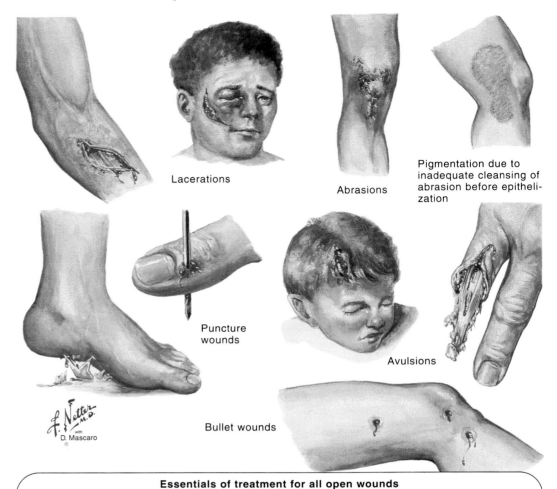

Lacerations

Abrasions

Pigmentation due to inadequate cleansing of abrasion before epithelization

Puncture wounds

Avulsions

Bullet wounds

Essentials of treatment for all open wounds

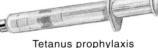

Cleansing
Debridement of nonviable tissue
Antibiotics (local or systemic)
Control of bleeding with local pressure
Tetanus prophylaxis

Methods of wound closure

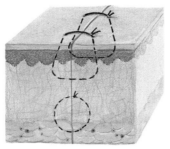

Simple suture. Deep part of suture longer than superficial part to slightly evert wound edges. Deep sutures used to close dead space

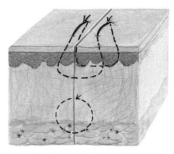

Mattress suture

Half-buried mattress suture

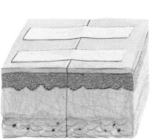

Some superficial wounds may be closed with adhesive strips rather than sutures

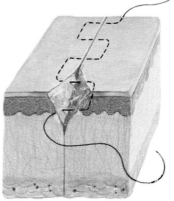

Subcuticular running stitch (Halsted)

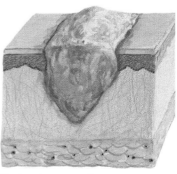

Obviously contaminated wounds are best debrided, packed open for 48–72 hours, debrided again, and delayed primary closure done

Injury to Soft Tissue
(Continued)

Laceration of a peripheral nerve disrupts the axons that normally carry impulses to and from the central nervous system, and restoration of nerve function depends on the effective repair of these axons. The nerve cell retains its ability to regenerate an axon from the point of transection distally. Satisfactory repair of the nerve sheath allows axons to grow across the site of injury and down the sheath to the motor end plate or to the skin to restore motor function or sensation. The principles of peripheral nerve repair include adequate debridement, careful anatomic reapproximation of the perineurium, and often microsurgical repair of the epineurium of individual nerve fascicles. Failure to achieve satisfactory repair of a lacerated peripheral nerve results in permanent loss of its function and often produces a painful neuroma at the injury site.

Pressure Ulcers

Pressure ulcers are localized areas of necrosis involving both skin and deep tissue (Plates 3–4). They develop when the soft tissue is compressed for long periods of time between a bony prominence and a rigid or firm surface. Pressure ulcers are common complications of immobilization. Elderly patients are particularly at risk, and in patients more than 70 years of age, pressure ulcers increase the risk of death up to four times. Pressure ulcers, formerly called decubitus ulcers and bedsores, can occur anywhere, but the most common sites are over the heel, sacrum, greater trochanter, and ischial tuberosity. Pressure ulcers are classified into four stages: stage 1, nonblanchable erythema of intact skin; stage 2, partial-thickness skin loss involving the epidermis or dermis; stage 3, full-thickness skin loss involving subcutaneous tissue but superficial to the underlying fascia; and stage 4, deeper, full-thickness lesions extending into muscle or bone.

Pressure in excess of 30 mmHg impedes capillary blood flow, resulting in ischemia of the soft tissues. The resulting interstitial edema and localized hemorrhage eventually lead to necrosis of the epidermis and dermis. Necrotic tissue is highly susceptible to bacterial infection, which contributes to further necrosis and destruction of both soft tissue and bone. Other factors that contribute to the development of pressure ulcers, particularly in elderly patients, are impaired circulation, poor nutrition, and possibly impaired immune response. Maceration of the skin, usually due to incontinence, also significantly increases the risk of ulceration. Bedridden and wheelchair-bound patients are particularly vulnerable to the development of pressure ulcers.

A pressure ulcer requires intensive and costly long-term treatment. Therefore, aggressive intervention programs are essential to prevent or abort their formation, particularly in high-risk patients.

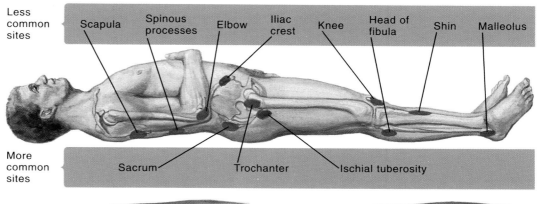

Pressure Ulcer

Less common sites: Scapula, Spinous processes, Elbow, Iliac crest, Knee, Head of fibula, Shin, Malleolus

More common sites: Sacrum, Trochanter, Ischial tuberosity

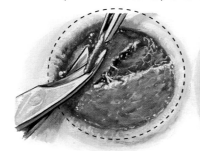

Pressure ulcers prevented by turning patient often, gentle massage with skin lotion, and avoidance of further pressure. Rubor a premonitory sign

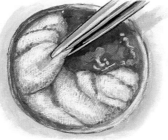

Early, small superficial ulcer may heal itself with relief from pressure and good skin care. More often, specific treatment necessary

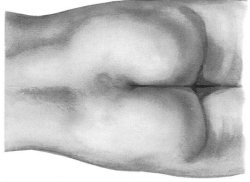

Curled-in edges cleanly debrided, eschar removed, and wound washed

Ulcer packed with moist (not soaked) gauze twice a day

Split-thickness skin grafting or primary closure done if skin condition adequate

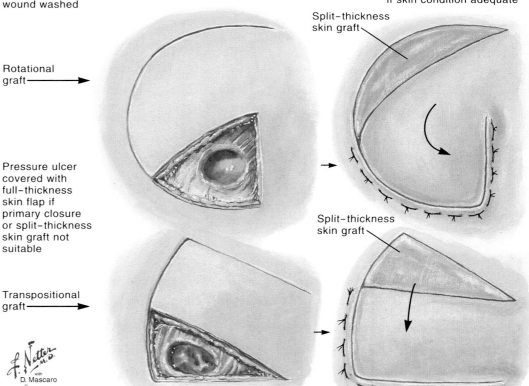

Rotational graft

Pressure ulcer covered with full-thickness skin flap if primary closure or split-thickness skin graft not suitable

Transpositional graft

Split-thickness skin graft

Split-thickness skin graft

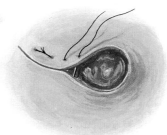

Excision of Deep Pressure Ulcer

Injury to Soft Tissue
(Continued)

The most effective means of prevention is the frequent repositioning of patients who are confined in bed, chair, or wheelchair. Position changes must occur every 2 hours to avoid continued excessive pressure over any single bony prominence. Vulnerable skin areas must be monitored frequently, and pressure on stage 1 lesions must be avoided to prevent further progression. For patients at risk for pressure ulcers, passive cushioning devices such as supersoft mattresses and wheelchair cushions should be used; patients who are severely immobilized require active pressure-relieving devices such as an alternating pressure mattress. Sedation should be avoided, incontinence controlled, and any nutritional deficiencies corrected in all immobile patients. Several studies have shown that aggressive intervention applied by an effective multidisciplinary team can greatly reduce the incidence of pressure ulcers in hospitalized patients.

Treatment

Treatment of an established pressure ulcer must be aggressive and persistent. Pressure-relieving strategies are essential during the entire course of treatment to facilitate healing. The first step in management is to assess the extent, depth, and stage of the lesion. Local treatment of a specific ulcer begins with removing the source of pressure. Second, any necrotic tissue is removed. Debridement of necrotic and infected tissue is accomplished with frequent changes of wet-to-dry dressings or with surgical excision of the infected necrotic tissue followed by the application of wet-to-dry dressings. The use of topical disinfectants and antibiotics is controversial. Although such medications effectively decrease the local bacterial count, many also have the disadvantage of causing local tissue necrosis of the ulcer bed. Dilute noncytotoxic solutions of povidone-iodine or sodium hypochlorite may help to decrease the bacterial count without causing tissue necrosis.

Once the ulcer is clean and a granulation tissue bed well established, the lesion should be kept moist at all times to allow for further development of granulation tissue and eventual epithelialization. Small, superficial ulcers heal by secondary intention as long as pressure is kept off the affected area. Larger lesions can be treated surgically with split-thickness skin grafting; occasionally, primary skin closure is accomplished by mobilization of adjacent skin flaps. Large ulcers, especially ulcers occurring over the greater trochanter or the ischial tuberosity, occasionally require full-thickness coverage with a local full-thickness rotational skin flap. At the time of flap rotation, the underlying bony prominences are removed or remodeled to reduce the potential for recurrent pressure ulcers. In areas that are particularly vulnerable to recurrence, rotation of a myocutaneous flap to provide greater padding over the bony prominence should be considered. □

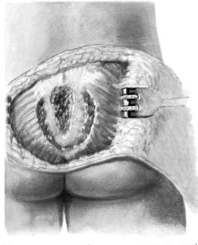

Deep pressure ulcer over sacrum excised, and crests of sacrum removed with wide osteotome. Split–thickness skin graft used to complete coverage of donor site

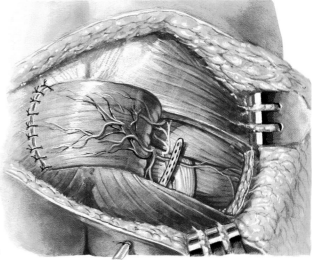

Flap of gluteus maximus muscle formed, turned over defect, and sutured in place. Drain passed through puncture wound

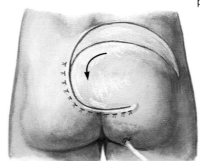

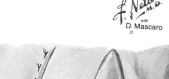

Full–thickness skin flap rotated to cover sacral defect, and split–thickness skin graft applied to cover residual donor site defect

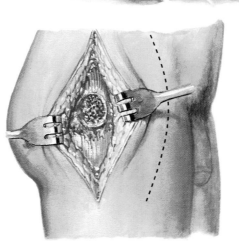

Deep pressure ulcer over trochanter widely excised with sinus tracts and trochanter. Broken line indicates skin–relaxing incision

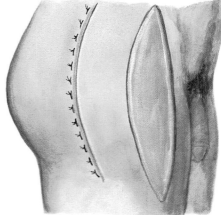

Bipedicle flap of skin and subcutaneous tissue pulled over and sutured to cover defect. Donor site closed with split–thickness skin graft

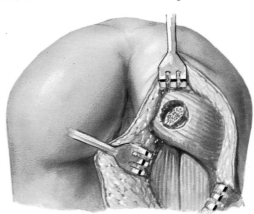

Ischial pressure ulcer removed completely along with ischial prominence

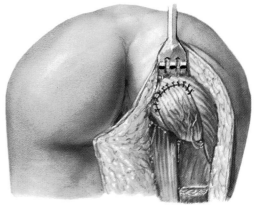

Biceps femoris muscle divided, turned up, and sutured over defect. Skin closed with direct sutures plus skin graft, if needed

Classification of Burns

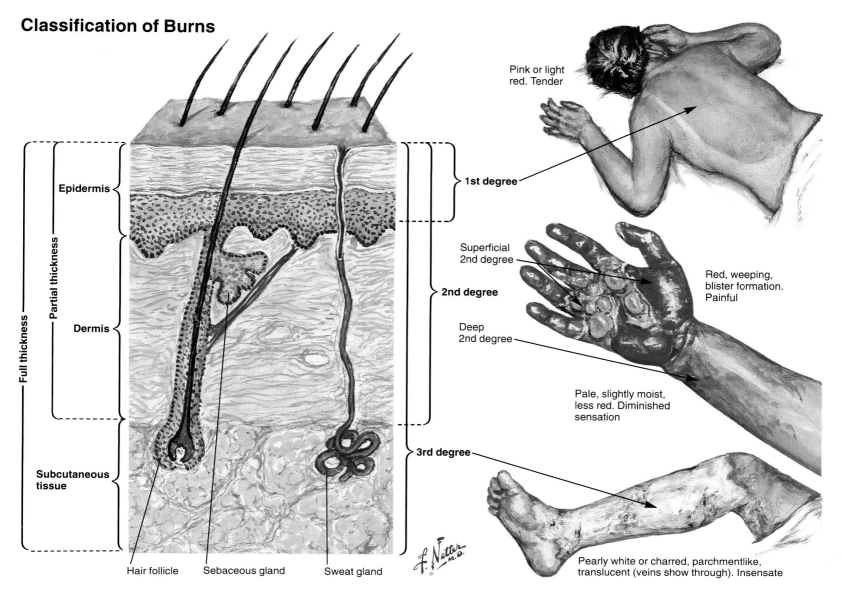

Epidermis

Full thickness

Partial thickness

Dermis

Subcutaneous tissue

Hair follicle   Sebaceous gland   Sweat gland

1st degree — Pink or light red. Tender

Superficial 2nd degree

2nd degree

Deep 2nd degree — Red, weeping, blister formation. Painful

Pale, slightly moist, less red. Diminished sensation

3rd degree — Pearly white or charred, parchmentlike, translucent (veins show through). Insensate

f. Netter M.D.

Burns

Classification

More than 2 million people in the United States are burned every year. The severity of tissue damage due to heat is related to both the temperature and the duration of exposure. The local effects of a burn, the wound care required, and the ultimate functional and cosmetic results are determined by the depth of cell injury. The outer layer of the skin, the epidermis, is made up of stratified epithelial cells that arise by proliferation of the basal layer and become progressively keratinized as they are slowly elevated to the surface, where they desquamate (Plate 5). The dermis is the inner layer of vascularized and variably dense connective tissue in which arise the skin appendages (hair follicles, sebaceous glands, and sweat glands). Beneath the dermis lies a layer of fatty, loose areolar connective tissue.

Heat of sufficient intensity and duration causes coagulation necrosis and cell death, but the cell damage due to heat of lesser intensity is potentially reversible. The region of immediate cell death caused by a burn is the *zone of coagulation*. Areas of progressively less damaging cell injury are the *zone of stasis*, in which the initially compromised blood flow improves with time, and the *zone of hyperemia*, in which there is marked increase in blood flow as a consequence of burn-induced inflammation. In a full-thickness (third-degree) burn, the zone of coagulation comprises the entire thickness of the dermis. In a partial-thickness (second-degree) burn, a variable portion of the dermis is involved, and in a first-degree burn, only the epidermis is affected.

Partial-Thickness Burns. A *first-degree burn* is the most superficial form of a partial-thickness burn, sunburn being the most common. The skin is pink or light red; the surface is usually dry, although small blisters may form. The skin remains soft with minimal edema, with subsequent exfoliation of the superficial epidermis. Such injuries are hypersensitive but heal in 3 to 6 days. They require little treatment other than administration of analgesics and oral acetylsalicylic acid (aspirin) to minimize inflammation. Cool showers help lessen postural hypotension and provide some pain relief. At the time of exfoliation, antipruritic treatment may be necessary.

Second-degree burns, also partial-thickness injuries, can be subdivided into superficial second-degree burns, which heal within 21 days, and deep second-degree burns, which take longer to heal. Second-degree burns are caused by limited exposure to a hot liquid, flash, flame, or chemical agent. Superficial second-degree burns appear pink or bright red with profuse serous exudation from the surface or into bullae. These injuries are hyperesthetic—even a draft of air can cause pain. The surface of a deep second-degree burn is moist and mottled in various hues of red. Sensation to pinprick is reduced but pressure sensation remains intact. If protected from infection, these injuries heal spontaneously in 4 to 6 weeks, although often with scarring.

Full-Thickness Burns. Third-degree burns result from prolonged exposure to a flame, hot object, or chemical agent or from contact with high-voltage electricity. The surface of the burn appears pearly white, charred, translucent, or parchment-like; thrombosed superficial vessels are often visible. In young children, the initial appearance of third-degree burns can be misleading: the initially dark red, slightly moist, and pliable wound desiccates and becomes unpliable and dark reddish brown. Strong acid burns produce deep tanning of the skin, which may be confused with suntan. High-voltage electric injury typically causes loss of tissue and dense charring at contact sites. Exposure to strong alkali may result in soapy tissue necrosis. The wound surface of all full-thickness burns is insensate and always requires skin grafting for closure.

Causes and Clinical Types of Burns

Burns

(Continued)

Causes and Clinical Types

The incidence and causes of burn injury are related to age, occupation, and economic circumstances, with the economically disadvantaged, the elderly, and the very young at greatest risk of both burn injury and death from that injury (Plate 6).

Flame Burns and Scalds. Flame burns are the most common burns in adults. They are usually caused by the mishandling of flammable liquids, ignition of clothing, and house fires and result in an injury of variable thickness: charred, leathery full-thickness burns are intermixed with areas of partial-thickness injury. Sometimes, focal areas of uninjured skin in the axilla, groin, antecubital space, and palm are found within the burn. In children less than 5 years of age, spill scalds are the most common form of burn injury.

Electric Burns. The risk of high-voltage electric injury is greatest in electricians, construction workers, farm workers who move irrigation pipes, oil field workers, truck drivers, and antenna installers. The damage to the tissue is due to heat produced by the resistance of tissue to the passage of electric current. The cell damage is greatest at the site of cutaneous contact but also includes the subcutaneous tissues and organs in the path of the electric current flow. Extensive devitalization of muscle may occur beneath deceivingly small cutaneous lesions. Current arcing also causes severe cutaneous injury at the flexor surfaces of joints, such as the wrist, elbow, and axilla. Claw hand deformity with inability to extend the fingers indicates severe and irreversible damage to the tissues of the hand and forearm and commonly predicts the need for amputation.

Formation of edema beneath the investing fascia of injured tissue may result in impaired blood supply to the distal unburned tissue, necessitating a fasciotomy to reduce the fluid pressure in tissue and prevent ischemic necrosis of unburned tissue.

Chemical Burns. Chemical agents cause exothermic reactions, dehydration, liquefaction necrosis (alkalis), and delipidation in tissue. The severity of a chemical burn is related to the concentration of the chemical and the amount and duration of contact with tissue. In patients with chemical injury, immediate wound care is the priority, unlike treatment of all other burn patients, in whom systemic support takes precedence. All contaminated clothing should be removed immediately and copious water lavage begun to dilute the chemical agent and reduce the heat in the injured tissue. Strong acids may produce profound tanning of the skin, and strong alkalis penetrate tissue rapidly, causing characteristic liquefaction necrosis of soft tissue.

Formation of edema in the burn area is the result of increased vascular permeability and alterations in the relationships of transvascular pressure. Effects of edema are particularly marked in the loose areolar tissues of the face and oropharynx.

Extensive full-thickness flame burn. Appears charred and leathery. Note sparing of axilla

High-voltage electric burn (after fasciotomy). Typical, claw hand deformity and accentuation of burn at wrist and antecubital fossa due to arcing of current

Penetrating chemical burn caused by strong alkali. Characteristic dissolution of soft tissues

Severe facial burn. Eyebrows and eyelashes singed, lids closed by edema, tongue swollen and protruding owing to involvement of oropharynx. Oropharyngeal edema necessitated nasotracheal intubation to ensure airway patency

Head 9%

Upper limbs (each) 9%

Trunk Front 18% Back 18% 9%

18% 18%

Lower limbs (each)

Rule of nines for estimating percentage of body surface involved

The eyelids swell rapidly and may obstruct vision, even though the globe is typically protected by the blink reflex. Swelling of the tongue and other oropharyngeal tissues may compromise the supraglottic airway, necessitating endotracheal intubation to ensure adequate ventilation.

The magnitude and duration of physiologic changes are proportional to the extent of second- and third-degree burns, expressed as a percentage of the body surface. The extent of the burn can be most easily estimated using the rule of nines. In the adult, the surface area of specific anatomic parts represents 9% or a multiple thereof of the total body surface: head and neck, 9%; each upper limb, 9%; each lower limb, 18%; anterior trunk, 18%; posterior trunk, 18%; and genitalia, 1%.

Burns

(Continued)

Escharotomy

Formation of edema beneath the unyielding leathery eschar of a circumferential third-degree burn on a limb or on the trunk can compromise circulation and ventilation (Plate 7). As the edema increases, tissue pressure rises to exceed venous pressure and approach arteriolar pressure, impairing blood flow to underlying unburned tissues. In the distal unburned tissue, edema and coolness to touch normally accompany thermal injury. Clinical signs of impaired circulation are cyanosis and delayed capillary refilling of distal unburned skin, as well as neurologic change, particularly progressive paresthesias and unrelenting deep pain. Neurologic change is the most reliable of the clinical signs that predict the need for escharotomy, but an absence of pulsatile blood flow or progressive diminution of flow detected with serial assessments using an ultrasonic flowmeter is a far more reliable indicator. The palmar arch vessels in the upper limb and the posterior tibial vessels in the lower limb are used for the assessment. Since hypovolemia and vasoconstriction can attenuate the flowmeter signal, assessment of blood flow should be made only in patients whose hemodynamic stability has been restored with the administration of resuscitation fluid.

Direct measurement of tissue pressure in muscle compartments using a slit or wick catheter is also useful in determining if escharotomy and fasciotomy are needed (Plate 14). However, use of a catheter increases the risk of infection of the muscle because the catheter must traverse the invariably contaminated burn wound.

Evidence of vascular embarrassment mandates immediate escharotomy, which is performed at bedside using either a scalpel or an electrocautery device. Anesthesia is not required since the incisions are made in an insensate third-degree burn. The escharotomy incision is placed in the midmedial or midlateral line of the involved limb and must extend from the distal margin to the proximal margin of the encircling eschar. The incision is carried through the eschar and the immediately subjacent superficial fascia only to the depth necessary to permit the cut edges of the eschar to separate. Bleeding, which is minimal in a properly performed escharotomy, is readily controlled with electrocautery or brief application of external pressure. The escharotomy incisions must be carried across involved joints, where there is the least amount of subcutaneous padding and the vessels and nerves are most easily compressed by the edema-generated pressure.

If a midlateral escharotomy does not restore circulation to a circumferentially burned limb, a second incision is placed in the midmedial line. If the circulation remains impaired following the second escharotomy, fasciotomy must be considered. Rarely, encircling burns of the neck require escharotomy in the line of the anterior margin of

Escharotomy for Burns

Escharotomy incision on midlateral aspect of forearm for circumferential 3rd-degree burn

Escharotomy incision on midmedial aspect of upper limb for circumferential 3rd-degree burn

Medial and lateral escharotomy incisions for circumferential 3rd-degree burns of lower limbs

Preferred sites for escharotomy incisions (lines shown thicker over joints to emphasize importance of carrying incisions across involved joints)

Escharotomy incisions for circumferential 3rd-degree burns of lower limbs and trunk in severely burned patient

the sternocleidomastoid muscle, and a circumferentially burned penis may require escharotomy in the middorsal line.

If edema formation beneath an encircling third-degree burn on the trunk impairs the ventilatory excursion of the chest wall, mild hypoxemia may develop, and increased pressure may be needed to ventilate the patient. Bilateral escharotomy

incisions extending from the clavicle to the costal margin should be made in the anterior axillary line. If the burn involves a significant portion of the anterior abdominal wall, the anterior axillary incisions should be connected by an incision at the costal margin. All escharotomy incisions must be protected by a generous application of a topical chemotherapeutic agent.

Prevention of Infection in Burn Wounds

Burns
(Continued)

Prevention of Infection

If a burn wound is not protected by topical chemotherapeutic agents, the originally sparse, predominantly gram-positive surface flora proliferates and changes with time, until gram-negative microorganisms predominate (Plate 8). These organisms penetrate the full-thickness of the eschar and multiply in the subeschar space (the interface between nonviable and viable tissue). If host resistance to microbial invasion is inadequate, the microorganisms penetrate viable tissue to a variable depth. Systemic spread may occur when *Pseudomonas* organisms invade the microvasculature and spread by lymphatic and hematogenous routes to remote tissues and organs.

After resuscitation of the patient, management focuses on wound care to limit microbial proliferation and prevent invasive infection of unburned underlying tissue. Initial care of burn wounds includes gentle cleansing with a surgical detergent disinfectant, debriding all loose nonviable tissue, and shaving all body hair from the burn and a 3- to 4-cm margin of unburned skin. A topical antimicrobial agent is then applied. Three effective topical agents are mafenide acetate burn cream, silver sulfadiazine burn cream, and 0.5% silver nitrate solution. Mafenide acetate cream is applied to the surface of the burn wound in a layer ⅛-inch thick; the wound is left exposed. Silver sulfadiazine cream is applied in a similar way but may be covered with a light occlusive gauze. The burn cream of choice is reapplied 12 hours later. Silver nitrate soaks, applied as a multilayered dressing, are changed two or three times a day and kept moist by periodic instillation of the dilute silver nitrate solution. When applied immediately after burning, all three agents effectively control the bacterial density of the burn wound, but silver sulfadiazine burn cream and silver nitrate soaks have a limited ability to penetrate the eschar. Only mafenide acetate cream, which contains a water-soluble active component, can freely diffuse into the eschar and establish an effective antimicrobial concentration in the burned tissue.

None of the available topical agents sterilize the burn wound; therefore, protection from invasive infection is not complete. During daily wound cleansing or dressing change, when all of the topical agent has been removed, the physician must examine the entire wound to ascertain the adequacy of microbial control and identify local signs of burn wound infection. Common color changes that signal an infection are focal, multifocal, or generalized dark brown, black, or violet discoloration. The most reliable sign of invasive infection is the conversion of an area of partial-thickness burn to full-thickness necrosis. Other local signs include hemorrhagic discoloration of subeschar tissue; unexpectedly rapid separation of the eschar

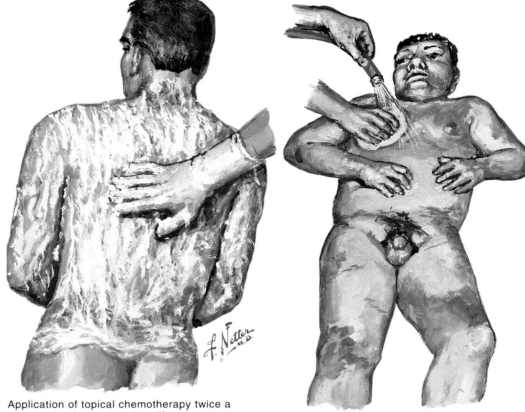

Application of topical chemotherapy twice a day to minimize bacterial proliferation

Daily cleansing of burned area with surgical detergent disinfectant

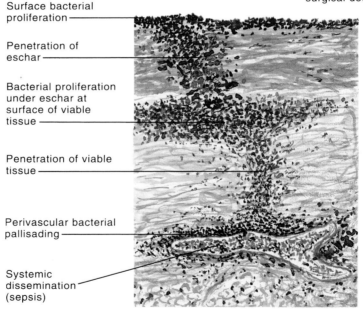

Surface bacterial proliferation

Penetration of eschar

Bacterial proliferation under eschar at surface of viable tissue

Penetration of viable tissue

Perivascular bacterial pallisading

Systemic dissemination (sepsis)

Schematic section shows bacterial penetration of burn wound

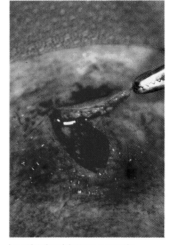

Lenticular biopsy sample elevated from burn wound, which is insensate. Specimen must include both burned and unburned tissue

(most commonly due to fungal infection); green pigment visible in the subcutaneous fat; edema or violet discoloration, or both, of unburned skin at the margin of the wound; and rapidly expanding ischemic necrosis.

Since factors other than infection, such as minor local trauma, can induce similar color and physical changes in the burn wound, identification of these signs necessitates assessment of the microbial status of the wound. A 500-mg lenticular biopsy sample is harvested from the area that shows the most marked changes. The tissue sample must include the eschar and underlying unburned tissue so the pathologist can examine

the nonviable-viable tissue interface at which invasive infection begins. One-half of the specimen is cultured, and the other half is sent for histologic examination.

On histologic verification of the presence of microorganisms in unburned viable tissue, local and systemic therapy is begun immediately. Treatment comprises application of mafenide acetate burn cream, if another topical agent has been used; subeschar injection of a broad-spectrum penicillin solution into the areas of infection, followed by surgical excision of the infected tissue; and systemic administration of an antibiotic to which the invading organism is sensitive.

Metabolic and Systemic Effects of Burns

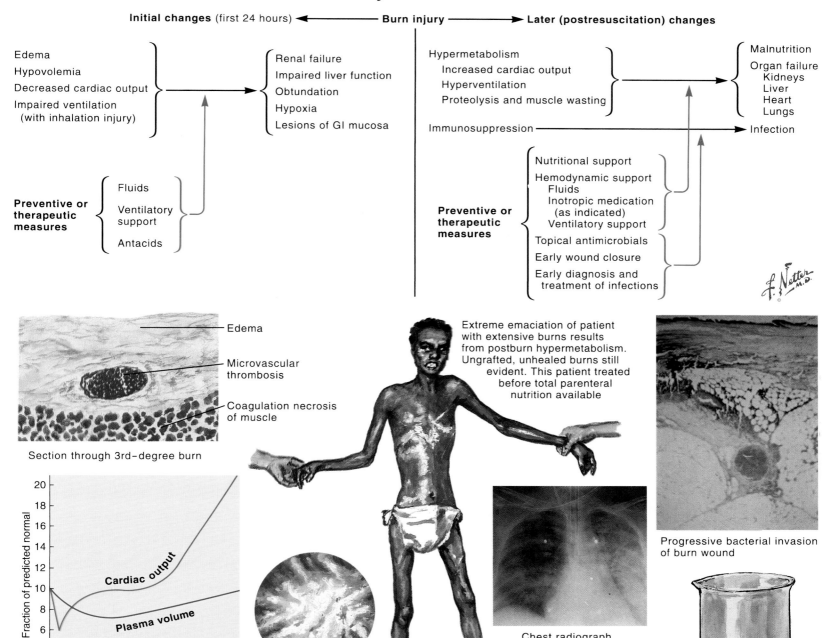

Initial changes (first 24 hours) ◄——— Burn injury ———► Later (postresuscitation) changes

Edema
Hypovolemia
Decreased cardiac output
Impaired ventilation
(with inhalation injury)

Renal failure
Impaired liver function
Obtundation
Hypoxia
Lesions of GI mucosa

Hypermetabolism
　Increased cardiac output
　Hyperventilation
　Proteolysis and muscle wasting

Immunosuppression

Malnutrition
Organ failure
　Kidneys
　Liver
　Heart
　Lungs
Infection

Preventive or therapeutic measures
Fluids
Ventilatory support
Antacids

Preventive or therapeutic measures
Nutritional support
Hemodynamic support
　Fluids
　Inotropic medication
　　(as indicated)
　Ventilatory support
Topical antimicrobials
Early wound closure
Early diagnosis and treatment of infections

Edema
Microvascular thrombosis
Coagulation necrosis of muscle

Section through 3rd–degree burn

Extreme emaciation of patient with extensive burns results from postburn hypermetabolism. Ungrafted, unhealed burns still evident. This patient treated before total parenteral nutrition available

Progressive bacterial invasion of burn wound

Fraction of predicted normal

Cardiac output

Plasma volume

20 18 16 14 12 10 8 6 4 2

6 12 18 24 30 36 42 48 54 60
Time postburn (hours)

Endoscopic view of focal ischemic changes in gastric mucosa 3–5 hours after severe burn

Chest radiograph shows evidence of adult respiratory distress syndrome

Diminished (or absent) urine output following severe burn (renal failure)

Burns

(Continued)

Metabolic and Systemic Effects

The deleterious effects of burn injuries on every organ system are proportional to the extent of the thermal injury. The prominence and clinical importance of the various systemic effects are time related. Some systemic effects are evident immediately, whereas others develop only after resuscitation or even far into the convalescent period. The initial and later (postresuscitation) changes and appropriate preventive or therapeutic measures are shown on the illustration (Plate 9).

During the first 24 hours, hemodynamic and pulmonary dysfunctions predominate and require therapeutic intervention to minimize complications. During the second 24 hours, functional capillary integrity is restored, plasma volume is reconstituted by continued administration of resuscitation fluid, and cardiac output rises to supranormal levels—the first manifestation of postinjury hypermetabolism.

Metabolic and immunologic changes due to the burn injury itself can all be aggravated by superimposed complications, particularly infection and sepsis. Early diagnosis and prompt treatment of infections that do develop minimize the occurrence of sepsis-related kidney, liver, heart, and lung failure. Pulmonary insufficiency due to sepsis predisposes the patient to pneumonia, the most common fatal complication, and may also impair oxygenation of peripheral tissues and increase susceptibility to invasive wound infection. Failure to meet the patient's markedly elevated nutritional needs not only permits erosion of lean body mass but is associated with delayed healing, impaired take of skin grafts, exaggeration of immunologic deficits, increased risk of infection, and delayed convalescence.

Maintaining pulmonary and cardiac functions to provide adequate tissue blood flow and oxygenation ameliorates the incidence and severity of the complications of these late metabolic and immunologic changes, thereby optimizing the resistance of the burn wound and other tissues to infection. Total metabolic support entails maintenance of fluid balance, mechanical ventilatory support, use of topical antimicrobial creams, nutritional support, and early wound closure.

Excision and Grafting for Burns

Burns
(Continued)

Excision and Grafting

Surgical excision of burn wounds should be performed as soon after resuscitation as the patient's hemodynamics and pulmonary status permit (Plate 10). Surgical removal of the necrotic tissue contributes to minimizing the risk of infection and the degree and duration of physiologic stress.

Deep, unequivocally full-thickness burns may be excised to the level of the investing fascia using a scalpel, an electrocautery device, or even a laser. The excised wound must be covered with a skin graft to prevent desiccation of the exposed tissue and to effect definitive closure.

Tangential excision is commonly employed in the treatment of partial-thickness burns. Successive thin layers of nonviable tissue are removed until a wound bed of viable tissue, characterized by uniformly dense capillary bleeding, is developed. If the full thickness of the skin is involved, the excision should extend until normal fatty tissue is encountered. The wound is closed with a split-thickness skin graft. Blood loss associated with tangential excision, which can be prodigious, can be minimized by the application of gauzes soaked in a thrombin solution; by subcutaneous injection of ornithine vasopressin; or, if the burn is on a limb, by use of a tourniquet.

In patients with extensive burns but limited donor sites, the use of meshed grafts increases the area of burn wound that can be covered with skin harvested from a donor site of given size. Although the expansion ratio of meshed grafts can be as great as 9:1, such large grafts are associated with a prolonged time of epithelization of the interstices and increased scarring. Therefore, expansion should be limited to the commonly used ratios of 2:1 or 3:1. When donor sites are inadequate because of extensive burns, any of several biologic dressings can be used for temporary coverage of the wound. Viable cutaneous allograft is the gold standard of biologic dressings. However, limited supply and risk of disease transmission have promoted the use of other biologic dressings, such as cutaneous xenografts (commonly porcine), amniotic membrane, and collagen-based bilaminate skin substitutes.

The benefits of burn wound excision are realized at specific physiologic costs: blood loss, pulmonary effects of anesthesia and surgery, and sacrifice of any partial-thickness burn within the area of a full-thickness burn. Along with physiologic fluid resuscitation, improved ventilatory support, and effective control of infection, excision has greatly helped survival in burn patients over the past 4 decades. The survival of even patients with extensive burns has increased significantly, and, in young adults, the size of a burn that causes a 50% death rate has increased from 43% of body surface to 76%. Improvements in functional and cosmetic therapies further facilitate rehabilitation of patients. □

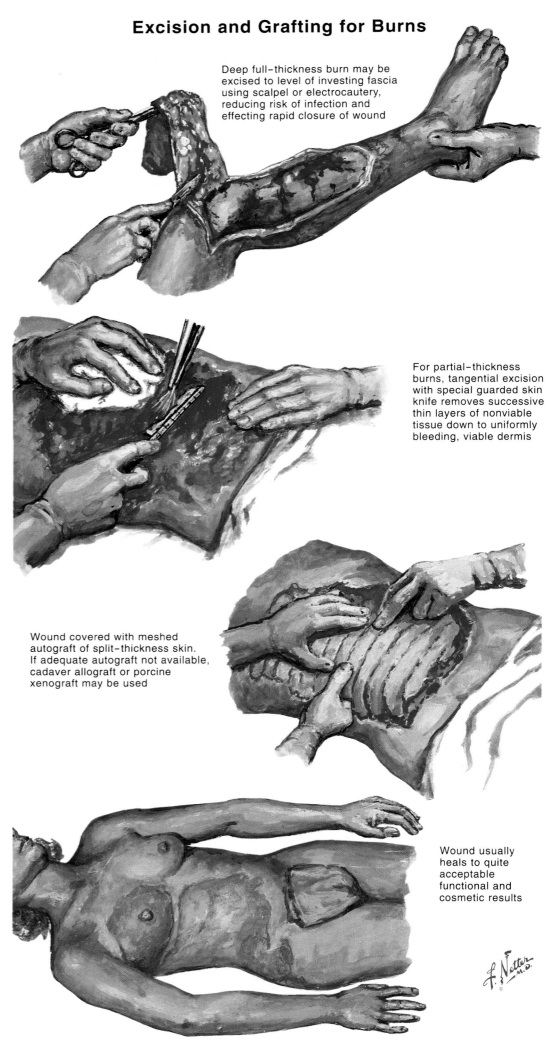

Deep full-thickness burn may be excised to level of investing fascia using scalpel or electrocautery, reducing risk of infection and effecting rapid closure of wound

For partial-thickness burns, tangential excision with special guarded skin knife removes successive thin layers of nonviable tissue down to uniformly bleeding, viable dermis

Wound covered with meshed autograft of split-thickness skin. If adequate autograft not available, cadaver allograft or porcine xenograft may be used

Wound usually heals to quite acceptable functional and cosmetic results

Compartment Syndrome

Etiology

Compartment syndrome results when fluid accumulates at high pressure within a closed fascial space (muscle compartment), reducing capillary perfusion below the level necessary for tissue viability. Volkmann contracture is the residual limb deformity that follows untreated acute compartment syndrome or ischemia due to arterial injury. The term "Volkmann ischemia" should not be used because it does not define the cause of the ischemia. Compartment syndromes remain poorly understood and are frequently misdiagnosed or poorly managed. However, prompt diagnosis and early and effective treatment can result in a limb with normal function.

The three main causes of compartment syndrome are increased accumulation of fluid, decreased volume (compartment constriction), and restricted volume expansion secondary to external compression (Plate 11). Although compartment syndrome develops most frequently in the four compartments of the leg, it can also occur in the forearm, hand, arm, shoulder, foot, thigh, buttocks, and back.

Increased Accumulation of Fluid. The most common mechanism of compartment syndrome is increased fluid content in the compartment. The most common cause is a fracture, with the tibia the most often fractured bone. Compartment syndrome may also be noted after open fractures (particularly of the tibia) or after severe contusion of the limb with no fracture.

Injury to a major blood vessel may produce compartment syndrome by three mechanisms: (1) bleeding into the compartment, (2) partial occlusion of the artery secondary to spasm or intimal tear with inadequate collateral circulation, and (3) postischemia swelling after circulation is restored. Postischemia swelling and compartment syndrome result if repair of the artery and restoration of the circulation are delayed more than 6 hours.

Extreme exertion may initiate acute or chronic compartment syndrome. The more common chronic form is a mild, recurrent compartment syndrome associated with exertional pain in the anterior compartment of the leg and frequently a muscle hernia. Symptoms abate when the excessive exercise is discontinued.

Thermal injuries (burns), in addition to decreasing compartment space, are associated with massive edema. Measurement of intramuscular pressure is needed to document the underlying compartment tamponade and the need for treatment with decompressive escharotomy.

Another cause of fluid accumulation is hemorrhage in patients who are receiving anticoagulant therapy following arterial puncture and in patients who have a bleeding diastasis such as hemophilia. Infiltration of exogenous intravenous fluid into the compartment and venomous snakebites may also produce compartment syndrome.

Constriction of Compartment. Compartment syndrome may also result from surgical closure of a fascial defect. For example, a high-performance

Etiology of Compartment Syndrome

Constriction of compartment

Closure of fascial defect

Scarring and contraction of skin or fascia, or both, due to burns

Increased fluid content in compartment

Fracture

Intracompartmental hemorrhage

Direct arterial trauma

Fluid from capillaries (edema) secondary to bone or soft tissue trauma, burns, toxins, venous or lymphatic obstruction

Muscle swelling due to overexertion

Burns

Infiltration of exogenous fluid (intravenous needle slipped out of vein)

External compression

Excessive or prolonged inflation of air splint

Tight cast or dressing

Prolonged compression of limb (as in alcohol- or drug-induced, metabolic, or traumatic coma)

runner may develop a muscle hernia and fascial defect. The hernias are usually bilateral and develop in the lower third of the leg overlying the anterior and lateral compartments, causing pain on exertion and often numbness. Unfortunately, some hernias are treated with surgical closure of the fascial defects, which decreases the volume of the compartment and increases intracompartmental pressure. The disastrous result is an acute compartment syndrome. The treatment of choice for a runner with exertional leg pain and muscle hernia is fascial release, not fascial closure.

Another cause of compartment volume is circumferential full-thickness (third-degree) burns.

This injury decreases compartment size and coalesces the skin, subcutaneous tissue, and fascia into one tight, constricting eschar that requires immediate decompression.

External Compression. Unconsciousness following drug overdose can precipitate not only multiple compartment syndromes but also the crush syndrome if the unconscious person lies with the limbs trapped beneath the torso or head. Compression of the forearm or leg produces persistent elevation of intracompartmental pressure, which often is greater than 50 mmHg. Prolonged inflation of air splints and incorrect application of circumferential casts may also produce external

Pathophysiology of Compartment and Crush Syndromes

Compartment Syndrome
(*Continued*)

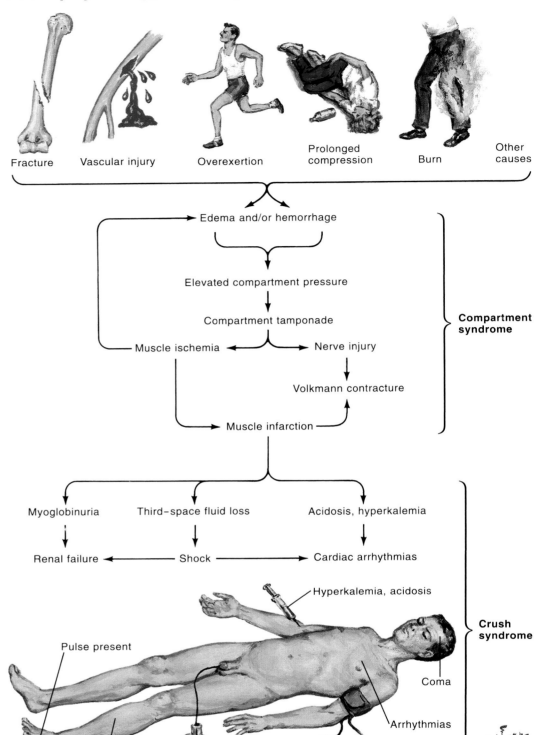

Fracture   Vascular injury   Overexertion   Prolonged compression   Burn   Other causes

Edema and/or hemorrhage

Elevated compartment pressure

Compartment tamponade

Muscle ischemia ← → Nerve injury

Volkmann contracture

Muscle infarction

Compartment syndrome

Myoglobinuria   Third–space fluid loss   Acidosis, hyperkalemia

Renal failure ← Shock → Cardiac arrhythmias

Hyperkalemia, acidosis

Pulse present

Coma

Arrhythmias

Hypotension

Swollen, tense limb   Renal failure

Crush syndrome

compression that limits compartment swelling. Deflating the splint and splitting the cast quickly decrease the compressive pressure. Usually, neither device causes compartment syndrome unless there is an underlying injury such as fracture or contusion.

Pathophysiology

Compartment Syndrome. A compartment syndrome may be initiated by a variety of conditions such as fracture, vascular injury, burns, exertion, prolonged limb compression, or contusions. These traumatic events cause hemorrhage or edema, or both, in a muscle compartment enclosed in relatively noncompliant osseofascial boundaries (Plate 12). Pressure then builds up within the compartment, producing compartment tamponade. If the pressure remains sufficiently high for several hours, normal function of muscle and nerves is jeopardized. The resulting ischemia produces further edema and the self-perpetuating cycle of a compartment syndrome. Left to its natural course, the resulting nerve injury and muscle infarction lead to the sequelae of Volkmann contracture. Prompt diagnosis and decompression with a fasciotomy, which allows the muscles to expand out of their fascial enclosure, are therefore essential to restore circulation and prevent irreversible changes.

Crush Syndrome. This condition can result if multiple compartments are involved and a significant amount of muscle infarction is present. Crush syndrome refers to the systemic effects of myonecrosis on the renal and cardiovascular systems. Although the exact pathogenesis of myoglobinuric renal failure is not completely understood, it is known that myoglobin is deposited in the distal convoluted tubules, ultimately occluding them. This occlusion precipitates renal failure, although toxicity of the renal tubules and hypotension appear to be contributing factors. Third-space fluid loss occurs rapidly, leading to further hypotension and shock. The myonecrosis causes acidosis and hyperkalemia. Since the excessive potassium released from the damaged muscle is not excreted in the presence of renal failure, cardiac arrhythmias may occur.

The most common cause of crush syndrome is prolonged compression of a limb (> 12 hours) following alcohol or drug intoxication and stupor. Occasionally, trauma resulting from entrapment in debris produces the same effects. The presenting signs are hyperkalemia, acidosis, disorientation or coma, possibly cardiac arrhythmias, hypotension, renal failure, and swollen, tense limbs with pressure sores. Results of laboratory studies are typically very abnormal. Concentration of creatinine phosphokinase is usually greater than 10,000 IU, and serum levels of creatinine, blood urea nitrogen, and potassium are also elevated. The finding of myoglobinuria confirms the diagnosis. Treatment consists of managing the coma, shock, respiratory depression, renal failure, and

hyperkalemia, as well as prompt decompression of the involved compartments.

Acute Compartment Syndrome

Clinical Manifestations. The most important symptom of an impending compartment syndrome is pain that is out of proportion to the primary problem or injury. However, *pain may be absent* if there is a superimposed deficit of the central or peripheral nervous system. Other early symptoms are best remembered by the *six Ps* of a compartment syndrome (Plate 13).

Pressure. The earliest finding is a swollen, palpably tense compartment. Palpation is a crude

method of detecting increased intracompartmental pressure and is difficult to quantify. Furthermore, significant subcutaneous edema may mask the underlying pressure. Direct pressure measurement is needed to confirm the clinical finding.

Pain on stretch. Passive movement of the digits may produce pain in the involved ischemic muscles. However, stretch pain is a subjective sensation and depends on the patient's reliability and pain threshold. It is difficult to differentiate pain caused by ischemic muscle from pain caused by fracture; later, with a sensory deficit, the pain associated with the compartment syndrome may be absent.

Compartment Syndrome
(Continued)

Paresis. Muscle weakness may be due to primary nerve involvement, muscle ischemia, or guarding secondary to pain.

Paresthesia or anesthesia. The most reliable physical finding in a conscious and cooperative patient is a sensory deficit. Initially, the sensory deficit may manifest as paresthesia but may progress to hypesthesia and anesthesia if treatment is delayed. Careful sensory examination helps determine the compartments involved.

Pulses present and Pink color. Unless there is a major arterial injury or disease, peripheral pulses are palpable, and capillary refill is routinely present. Although compartment pressures are occasionally high enough to occlude a major artery, in more than 90% of patients, the pulses are intact or can be confirmed with Doppler ultrasonography.

Differential Diagnosis. In patients with limb injuries and neurovascular deficits, the differential diagnosis is limited primarily to compartment syndrome, arterial injury, and nerve injury. Identification of the problem is important because the treatments differ: a compartment syndrome requires immediate decompression; an arterial injury requires immediate restoration of the circulation (either by repair of the artery or by removal of a thrombus); a nerve injury associated with a fracture or contusion (most commonly neurapraxia) is usually treated with observation.

Compartment syndrome, arterial injury, and nerve injury frequently coexist, and the clinical findings overlap. Each condition may have associated motor and sensory deficit and pain. Arterial injury usually results in absent pulses, poor skin color, and decreased skin temperature, but a pseudoaneurysm and adequate collateral circulation may allow for a distal pulse. In contrast, in compartment syndrome, peripheral pulses are nearly always intact. Nerve injuries usually cause little pain, but the pain caused by antecedent trauma may be difficult to differentiate from ischemia pain. Diagnosis of neurapraxia is by exclusion of the other two entities. Doppler ultrasonography and arteriography are useful in diagnosing an arterial injury, and measurement of intracompartmental pressure is frequently required to detect compartment syndrome.

Measurement of Intracompartmental Pressure

Several techniques are used to measure intracompartmental pressure (Plate 14). The needle technique, first described in 1884, was popularized in the United States in the 1970s by Reneman and Whitesides. A variation of the needle technique employs continuous infusion of saline for long-term pressure monitoring.

Wick Catheter Technique. In 1973, Mubarak and associates were the first to use the wick catheter to diagnose compartment syndrome. This technique does not require the injection or continuous infusion of saline solution to measure equilibrium pressure. The wick catheter was designed to prevent the catheter tip from being blocked by soft tissue and to maximize the surface area

Acute Anterior Compartment Syndrome

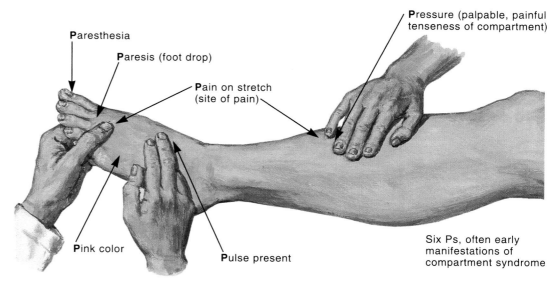

Six Ps, often early manifestations of compartment syndrome

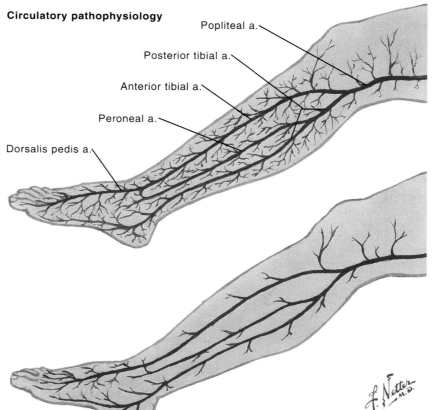

Normally, pressure of tissue fluid is less than 30 mmHg, which permits blood to flow freely through large arteries, smaller arterioles, and capillaries to nourish and oxygenate tissues

When pressure of tissue fluid rises above 30 mmHg, as in compartment syndrome, small nutrient arterioles and capillaries compressed. Flow in larger, more resistant arteries persists. Pulse may therefore be palpable despite tissue ischemia, giving false impression of adequate circulation

Differential diagnosis			
	Compartment syndrome	Arterial occlusion	Neurapraxia
Pressure increased in compartment	+	−	−
Pain on stretch	+	+	−
Paresthesia or anesthesia	+	+	+
Paresis or paralysis	+	+	+
Pulses intact	+	−	+

between the saline in the catheter and the fluids in the soft tissue. The fully automated, fluid-filled wick catheter system is connected to a pressure transducer and to a recording device for constant measurement of tissue pressure.

Slit Catheter Technique. This method combines accuracy, reproducibility, large surface area, immediate measurement of equilibrium pressure, and continuous monitoring of pressure during muscle contraction and exercise. The slit catheter

Measurement of Intracompartmental Pressure

Compartment Syndrome
(Continued)

system is less likely to induce coagulation during long-term measurements, has a faster response time during exercise studies, and is more easily manufactured than the wick catheter. Currently, several devices allow rapid measurement of intracompartmental pressure at bedside using either a wick or a slit catheter.

Indications. Measurement of intracompartmental pressure is recommended whenever clinical symptoms and signs are absent or confusing and is particularly valuable in three groups of patients. (1) Uncooperative or unreliable patients: interpretation of clinical findings may be difficult or not possible in adults with alcohol or drug intoxication. Frequently, children with fractures may be so frightened that careful neurologic evaluation is not possible. (2) Unresponsive patients: clinical evaluation of patients who are unconscious because of head injuries or drug overdose is not possible. The only reliable physical finding may be a swollen leg, making confirmation of the intracompartmental pressure mandatory. (3) Patients with associated neurovascular injury: it is often difficult to differentiate a nerve deficit associated with neurapraxia or with arterial injury from a compartment syndrome without measuring the intracompartmental pressure.

Pressure Threshold for Fasciotomy

The pressure threshold at which fasciotomy should be performed remains controversial, but studies suggest that decompression should be considered when the intracompartmental pressure reaches 30 mmHg. Frequently, the duration of the increased pressure is not known, and treatment must be based on the patient's systemic blood pressure, peripheral perfusion, overall condition, progression of symptoms and signs, cooperation and reliability, and type of injury, as well as intracompartmental pressure. In borderline cases, it is more prudent to decompress the compartment earlier rather than later.

Decompression of Compartment Syndrome

There are no satisfactory nonsurgical methods for treating compartment syndromes. Therefore, surgical decompression, which allows the volume of the compartments to increase, is the primary means of relieving pressure. Each of the surrounding envelopes of the compartment may play a role in limiting compartment volume and must be considered, including volume-restricting plaster casts and circular dressings. Splitting and spreading a plaster cast may result in a 65% decrease in intracompartmental pressure. However, if symptoms of neurologic deficit persist more than 1 hour after cast splitting, the top half of the cast and all circular dressings must be removed and the limb examined. At this time, measurement of intracompartmental pressure is diagnostic. The skin may be a limiting envelope if, for example, there is significant subcutaneous edema or thermal injuries that have merged skin

Wick catheter technique

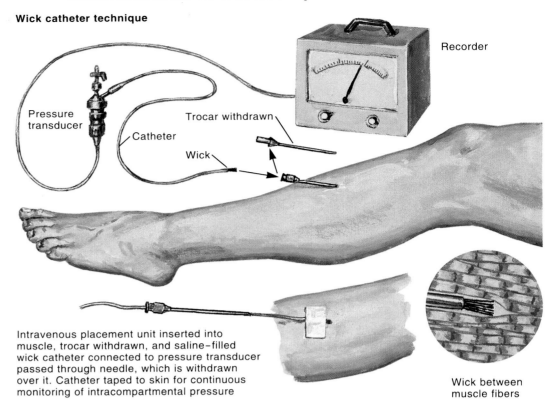

Recorder

Pressure transducer

Catheter

Trocar withdrawn

Wick

Intravenous placement unit inserted into muscle, trocar withdrawn, and saline-filled wick catheter connected to pressure transducer passed through needle, which is withdrawn over it. Catheter taped to skin for continuous monitoring of intracompartmental pressure

Wick between muscle fibers

Slit catheter technique

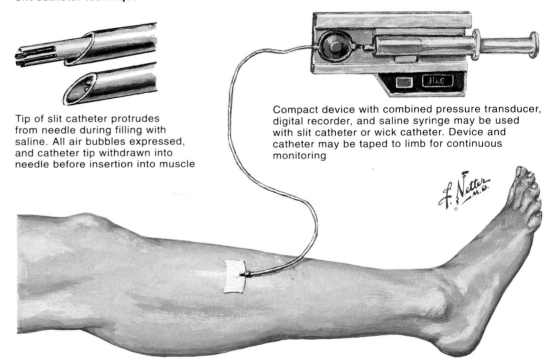

Tip of slit catheter protrudes from needle during filling with saline. All air bubbles expressed, and catheter tip withdrawn into needle before insertion into muscle

Compact device with combined pressure transducer, digital recorder, and saline syringe may be used with slit catheter or wick catheter. Device and catheter may be taped to limb for continuous monitoring

and fascia. In these cases, adequate decompression is achieved with a long dermatomy and fasciotomy.

Incisions for Forearm and Hand. The primary approaches for decompression of the forearm are the straight dorsal and the curvilinear volar incisions (Plate 15). Both approaches lower pressures in the volar compartment, and in about one-half of patients, also lower pressures in the dorsal compartment. The curvilinear volar incision is preferred because it allows exposure of all major nerves, arteries, and the mobile wad. The advantage of the dorsal ulnar incision is a better skin coverage over the neurovascular bundles and tendons after decompression.

The curvilinear volar incision begins proximal to the antecubital fossa and extends to the middle of the palm. It is gently curved medially until it reaches the midline at the junction of the middle and distal thirds of the forearm and is continued straight distally to the proximal wrist crease, just ulnar to the palmaris longus tendon. The forearm incision is extended across the volar wrist crease to aid release of the carpal tunnel. It is carried no farther radially than the midaxis of the ring finger to avoid injury to the superficial palmar branch of the median nerve.

Median nerve neuropathy, in addition to carpal tunnel release, requires exploration of the nerve

Compartment Syndrome
(Continued)

in the proximal forearm. The three main areas of potential nerve compression are the bicipital aponeurosis (lacertus fibrosis), the proximal edge of the pronator teres muscle, and the proximal edge of the flexor digitorum superficialis muscle.

Following the volar fasciotomy, which is made in the same line as the skin incision, compartment pressure is checked to ascertain that all the deep flexor muscles have been decompressed. After volar decompression, pressure measurements of the volar compartment, mobile wad, and dorsal compartments are repeated. If the pressures in the mobile wad and dorsal compartments are greater than 15 mmHg, these compartments should also be decompressed. The mobile wad can be approached through the volar curvilinear incision by lifting up the volar flap over that area. The dorsal compartment is approached through a longitudinal incision that is approximately one-third the length of the forearm. Through this incision, the fasciotomy is performed and final pressure measurements made. The skin incisions for all wounds are not closed at the time of fasciotomy but are loosely pulled together with rubber bands. If the diagnosis was delayed or some muscle appears necrotic, superficial debridement is carried out and more definitive debridement performed 4 to 7 days later, when muscle viability can be determined more accurately.

Postoperative care of the forearm includes a bulky dressing and splinting. The dressing is changed in 3 to 4 days, in the operating room. Split-thickness skin grafts are almost always required, but skin grafting and closure are postponed until all necrotic tissue has been debrided and quantitative cultures indicate that the underlying wounds are appropriate for skin grafting. Active and active-assisted range-of-motion exercises for the hand are started immediately after surgery. The bulky dressing is usually removed at 3 weeks, and volar splints are then used until full motion is restored.

Compartment syndromes of the forearm associated with fracture of the distal humerus, radius, or ulna are usually treated with internal reduction and fixation. Treatment of an associated arterial injury must be individualized.

Decompression of the hand may be required after crushing injuries. Diagnosis is based on the increased pressure in the interosseous compartments. Dorsal decompression is performed through longitudinal incisions in the intermetacarpal spaces, and the adductor muscles of the thumb are decompressed via an incision over the dorsal web space. Decompression of the arm and shoulder uses longitudinal incisions over the involved muscles. With involvement of the deltoid muscle, where fascia and epimysium form one layer, multiple incisions in the fascia are necessary.

Incisions for Leg. Current treatment of compartment syndromes of the leg is decompression that avoids fibulectomy. The most frequently used approach is the double-incision technique described by Mubarak and Owen (Plate 16). This

Incisions for Compartment Syndrome of Forearm and Hand

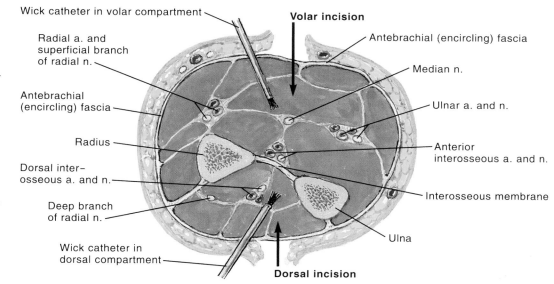

Wick catheter in volar compartment — Volar incision

Radial a. and superficial branch of radial n.

Antebrachial (encircling) fascia

Median n.

Antebrachial (encircling) fascia

Ulnar a. and n.

Radius

Anterior interosseous a. and n.

Dorsal interosseous a. and n.

Interosseous membrane

Deep branch of radial n.

Wick catheter in dorsal compartment

Ulna

Dorsal incision

Section through midforearm

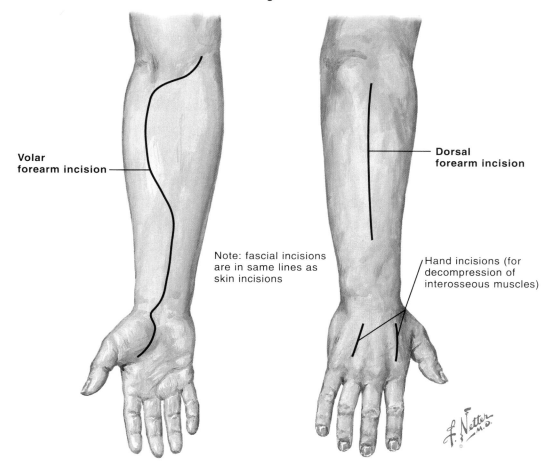

Volar forearm incision

Dorsal forearm incision

Note: fascial incisions are in same lines as skin incisions

Hand incisions (for decompression of interosseous muscles)

technique is simple, requires minimal dissection, and can be performed, using local anesthesia, at the bedside of the patient who is very sick and a poor risk for general anesthesia. This technique is faster and safer than other techniques because the fascial incisions are all superficial and avoid the deep neurovascular structures. The fibula is left intact, and any of the four compartments of the leg can be decompressed. The two skin incisions can be shorter (approximately one-third the length of the leg) if intraoperative pressure monitoring is performed.

Decompression of the anterior and lateral compartments is performed through an incision placed

halfway between the shaft of the fibula and the tibial crest. The incision is made approximately over the intermuscular septum dividing the anterior and lateral compartments, allowing easy access to both. When a slightly shorter incision is used, it is extremely important to undermine the skin incisions proximally and distally to allow wide exposure of the fascia. A transverse incision is made just through the fascia to identify the anterior intermuscular septum that separates the anterior and lateral compartments; this is important because the superficial peroneal nerve that lies in the lateral compartment next to the septum must be located. Fasciotomy of the lateral compartment

Incisions for Compartment Syndrome of Leg

Compartment Syndrome
(Continued)

is made in line with the shaft of the fibula posterior to the anterior intermuscular septum.

The posteromedial approach is used for decompression of the superficial and deep posterior compartments. This incision is made slightly distal to the anterolateral incision and 2 cm posterior to the posterior margin of the tibia to avoid injuring the saphenous nerve and vein located in this area. The skin edges are undermined and the saphenous nerve and vein retracted anteriorly. A transverse fascial incision allows identification of the septum between the deep and superficial posterior compartments. The tendon of the flexor digitorum longus muscle in the deep posterior compartment and the Achilles (calcaneal) tendon in the superficial posterior compartment are identified. Usually, it is easier to decompress the superficial posterior compartment first. The fasciotomy is extended proximally as far as possible and then distally behind the medial malleolus. The deep posterior compartment is released distally and then proximally under the bridge of the soleus muscle. If the soleus muscle attaches to the tibia in the distal third, it should be released initially to allow visualization of the deep posterior compartment and to aid decompression.

Following the four-compartment fasciotomy, intraoperative monitoring of intracompartmental pressure should be performed to document the decompression. Very little muscle should be debrided at the time of initial decompression, as it is difficult to differentiate an infarcted muscle from an ischemic but recoverable muscle.

Postoperative care of leg wounds is similar to that of forearm wounds, but in compartment syndrome without associated fractures, closure in a week is often possible without skin grafting. Necrotic muscle is debrided once or twice a week until a satisfactory granulation bed is present. Skin grafting or closure prior to this may lead to infection and the need for subsequent amputation. To prevent the insidious development of contractures, the ankle is splinted posteriorly in neutral position.

Compartment syndrome associated with fractures of the tibia should be treated with internal fixation, using either intramedullary rods or plates, but open fractures may require external fixation. A major disadvantage of the external fixation device is that mobilization of skin for delayed primary closure is not feasible, and skin grafting is nearly always required.

Prophylactic decompression of the leg should be carried out following tibial osteotomy or use of the tibia as the donor site of a bone graft. During debridement of an open fracture of the tibia, compartments accessible through the exposed wound should also be opened if the anatomy is not distorted by the fracture and the location of the superficial nerves is apparent. Arterial injury, thrombosis, and arterial bypass surgery also predispose to compartment syndromes. If the period of ischemia lasts longer than 6 hours, prophylactic decompression of the four compartments of the leg should be considered.

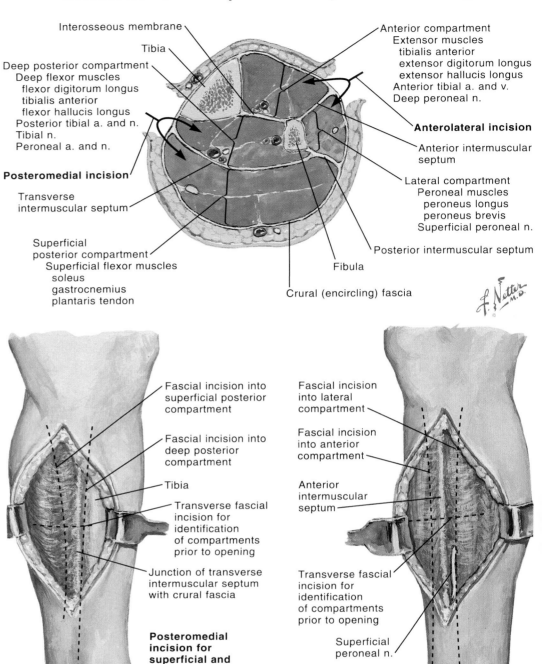

Incisions for Thigh, Buttock, and Foot. Compartment syndrome of the thigh and gluteus muscles is not common but may progress to a crush syndrome because of the large bulk of muscle involved. Longitudinal incisions are made over the thigh to decompress the adductor, quadriceps, or hamstring muscles. Measurement of pressure is very helpful in the diagnosis of compartment syndromes in these areas because sensory deficits are rare. Gluteus compartment syndromes, most often due to limb compression following drug overdose, involve three separate compartments: the gluteus maximus, gluteus medius–gluteus minimus, and tensor fasciae latae

muscles. The Gibson posterolateral incision allows exposure of all three gluteus compartments. The fascia superficial to the gluteus maximus muscle is relatively thin and blends with the epimysium, which sends septa into the muscle, forming multiple subdivisions. For adequate decompression, multiple incisions in this fascia-epimysium are required.

In the foot, the interosseous compartments are released via longitudinal incisions over the dorsum, and the medial plantar structures are released using a medial incision. Again, measurement of intracompartmental pressure is helpful to ascertain the need for decompression. □

Healing of Soft Tissue

Healing of Incised, Sutured Skin Wound

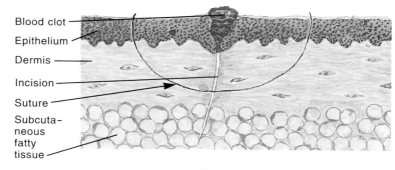

Blood clot
Epithelium
Dermis
Incision
Suture
Subcutaneous fatty tissue

Immediately after incision
Blood clot with fine fibrin network forms in wound. Epithelium thickens at wound edges

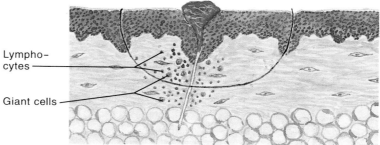

Lymphocytes
Giant cells

24–48 hours
Epithelium begins to grow down along cut edges and along suture tract. Leukocyte infiltration, chiefly round cells (lymphocytes) with few giant cells, occurs and removes bacteria and necrotic tissue

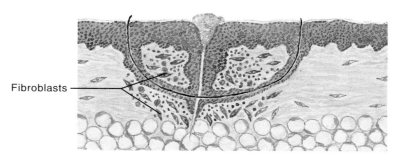

Fibroblasts

5–8 days
Epithelial downgrowth advances. Fibroblasts grow in from deeper tissues and add collagen precursors and glycoproteins to matrix. Cellular infiltration progresses

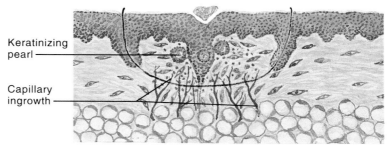

Keratinizing pearl
Capillary ingrowth

10–15 days
Capillaries grow in from subcutaneous tissue, forming granulation tissue. Epithelium bridges incision; epithelial downgrowths regress, leaving keratinizing pearls behind. Fibrosed clot (scab) being pushed out. Collagen formation progresses and cellular infiltration abates

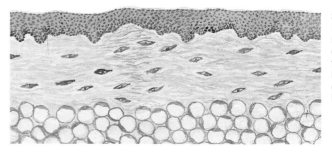

3 weeks–9 months
Epithelium thinned to near normal. Tensile strength of tissue increased owing to production and cross-linking of collagen fibers; elastic fibers reappear later

Healing of Incised, Sutured Skin Wound

The healing of a typical incised wound can be divided into three phases: the lag (or latent) phase, the fibroblastic proliferation phase, and the maturation phase (Plate 17).

The first step in the *lag phase* is the formation of a blood clot, which controls bleeding and forms a thin fibrin network, bridging the wound margins. Simultaneously, an intense inflammatory reaction develops, with the arrival of a large number of leukocytes that remove bacteria, necrotic tissue, and other debris from the wound. Almost immediately after injury, fibroblasts begin to mobilize from the deeper dermal structures and migrate toward the wound edges. Simultaneously, the cut epithelial edges begin to proliferate, with new epithelial cells accumulating at the cut edges.

The second phase, *fibroblastic proliferation*, begins 48 to 72 hours after injury. The epithelial surface is usually resurfaced with new cells by 48 hours after injury. The epithelial cells continue to divide, thickening the new epithelial layer. New capillaries form, bringing oxygen and nutrients to the proliferating cells and a characteristic red color to the tissue. After approximately 5 days, the fibroblasts are synthesizing collagen precursors as well as mucopolysaccharides and other glycoproteins to form the wound matrix. Collagen is secreted into this matrix and quickly polymerizes to begin to add tensile strength to the wound. The production of collagen continues for approximately 2 weeks. During this time, there is further fibroblastic proliferation into the depths of the wound.

The third phase of the healing of an incised wound is the *phase of maturation*, which begins

Healing of Soft Tissue
(Continued)

Healing of Excised Skin Wound

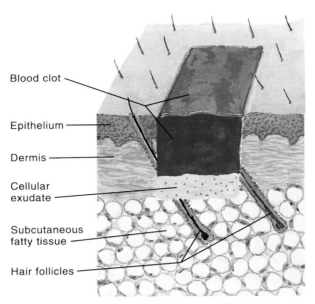

Blood clot
Epithelium
Dermis
Cellular exudate
Subcutaneous fatty tissue
Hair follicles

Immediately after excision. Wound gap filled with blood clot

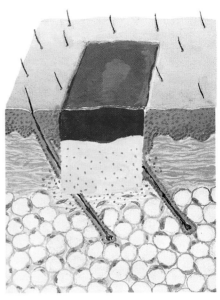

2–3 days after excision. Clot retracted somewhat, and cellular exudate beneath it increased. Surface epithelium begins to grow down along wound edges. Fibroblasts proliferate at base of wound

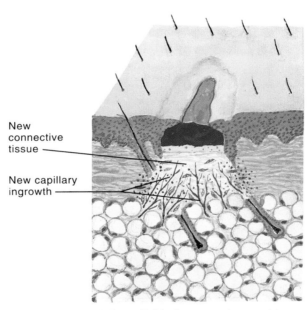

New connective tissue
New capillary ingrowth

6 days. Epithelium at surface and from severed skin appendages has grown partially across gap. Connective tissue at base increases, and new capillaries grow into it to form granulation tissue

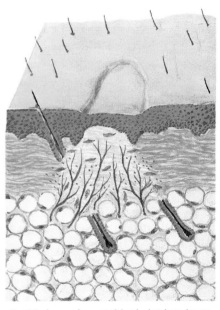

8–10 days. Any residual clot has been cast off or resorbed and epithelium grown completely across defect, which is being narrowed by contraction of surrounding connective tissue and filled by deposition of new tissue that is vascularized and collagen rich. Eventually, granulation tissue replaced with collagenous scar tissue devoid of skin appendages

about 3 weeks after injury and lasts as long as 9 months after injury. During this phase, the tensile strength of the wound continues to increase owing to the further cross-linking of collagen fibers combined with the remodeling of collagen fibers along the lines of mechanical stress, producing a stronger and more durable matrix.

Healing of Excised Skin Wound

The healing process of the excised wound is very similar to that of the incised wound (Plate 18). A large blood clot immediately fills the excised defect. At the edges of the wound, epithelial cells rapidly proliferate and migrate downward into the edges of the wound. In 2 to

3 days after injury, the clot retracts somewhat and a large cellular exudate, composed mostly of leukocytes, begins to develop beneath the clot. Epithelium continues to advance from the edges of the wound as well as from any transected skin appendages such as hair follicles.

Fibroblasts begin to proliferate in the base of the wound. The fibroblastic proliferation is followed immediately by the development of new capillaries bringing nutrients and oxygen to the newly formed tissues.

The blood clot is gradually elevated by the cellular exudate beneath it, allowing epithelial cells to grow across the base of the wound. Active contraction of the wound begins about 8 to 10 days after injury as more collagen-rich connective tissue is laid down in the base of the wound. Eventually, the highly vascular granulation tissue disappears, and a dense collagenous scar tissue persists underneath the new layer of epithelium. The new epithelium is devoid of normal skin appendages. □

Types of Joint Injury

Fractures, Dislocations, and Sprains

Injury to the musculoskeletal system takes many different forms, depending on the mechanism of injury, the amount of deforming force applied to the skeleton, and the location at which the force is applied. Many terms and classification systems are used to define the various patterns of musculo-skeletal injury, including eponyms and colorful descriptions that are often misleading and incor-rectly applied. The best and most accurate way to describe patterns of injury to the musculo-skeletal system is to use specific and objectively definable terminology, which facilitates commu-nication among health care providers and thus improves patient care.

Types of Joint Injury

A *dislocation* is a complete and persistent dis-placement of the articular surfaces of the bones that make up a joint, with disruption of at least part of the supporting joint capsule and some of its ligaments (Plate 19). Following a dislocation, a muscle spasm locks the two displaced bone ends in an abnormal position, usually creating an obvi-ous and significant deformity.

A *subluxation* is a partial dislocation of a joint; that is, the bone ends are partially separated from each other and the articular surfaces are no longer congruent. Although not as severe as dislocations, subluxations usually also damage part of the joint capsule and some of the supporting ligaments. Following subluxation, the patient may still be able to move the joint to some degree. Failure to recognize and treat a subluxation may result in persistent ligament laxity and joint incongruity. Joint injuries are often a combination of a frac-ture and a dislocation. In a *fracture dislocation* or *fracture subluxation*, the joint surfaces are no longer congruent, and segments of the bone adjacent to the joint are pulled off or knocked off as the dis-location occurs. A bimalleolar fracture of the ankle is a good example of a fracture subluxation. In this condition, fractures of the medial and lateral malleoli create instability of the ankle joint, result-ing in subluxation of the tibiotalar articulation.

A *sprain* is a temporary subluxation of a joint in which the articular surfaces subsequently return to their normal alignment. Even though the

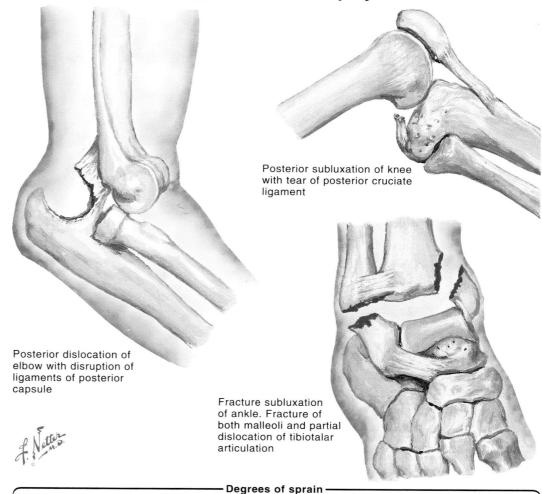

Posterior subluxation of knee with tear of posterior cruciate ligament

Posterior dislocation of elbow with disruption of ligaments of posterior capsule

Fracture subluxation of ankle. Fracture of both malleoli and partial dislocation of tibiotalar articulation

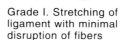

— Degrees of sprain —

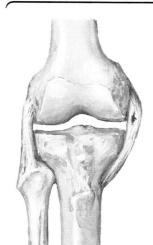

Grade I. Stretching of ligament with minimal disruption of fibers

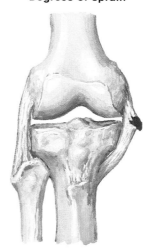

Grade II. Tearing of up to 50% of ligament fibers; small hematoma. Hemarthrosis may be present

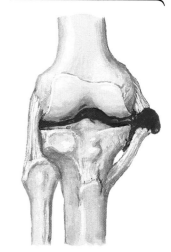

Grade III. Complete tear of liga-ment and separation of ends, hematoma, and hemarthrosis

displacement is transient, significant damage may occur to the joint capsule and ligaments. Except for swelling, sprains cause no serious deformity. Joint movement is limited only by pain and not by joint incongruity. A sprain should not be con-fused with a *strain*, which is the stretching injury of a musculotendinous unit.

Sprains are graded into three categories accord-ing to the severity of damage to the joint capsule and some of the supporting ligaments. A grade I (mild) sprain is characterized as a slight stretch-ing of the capsule and some of the supporting ligaments. Grade I sprains usually heal in 3 to 4 weeks without significant loss of function. A grade

II (moderate) sprain describes a partial disruption of the supporting ligaments and capsule. Most grade II sprains also heal in 3 to 4 weeks if the injured structures are protected from excessive loads or stretching. A grade III (severe) sprain refers to a complete rupture of the capsule and supporting ligaments. A grade III sprain is as severe an injury as a complete dislocation. The only difference between a grade III sprain and a dislocation is that in the sprain, the articular sur-faces spontaneously return to their normal posi-tions. In severe sprains, surgery is often required to repair the completely torn ligaments and capsule.

Fractures, Dislocations, and Sprains

(Continued)

Classification of Fracture

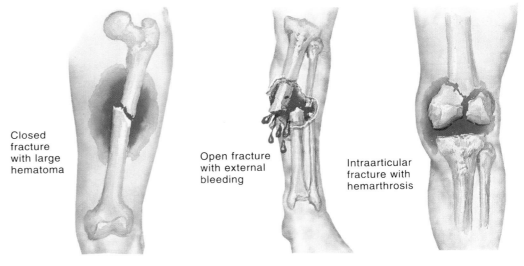

Closed fracture with large hematoma

Open fracture with external bleeding

Intraarticular fracture with hemarthrosis

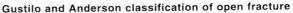
Gustilo and Anderson classification of open fracture

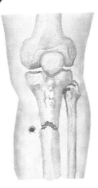 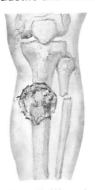 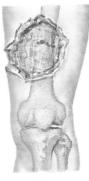 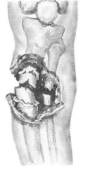 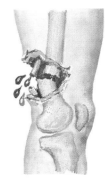

Type I. Wound <1 cm long. No evidence of deep contamination

Type II. Wound >1 cm long. No extensive soft tissue damage

Type IIIA. Large wound. Good soft tissue coverage

Type IIIB. Large wound. Exposed bone fragments, extensive stripping of periosteum

Type IIIC. Large wound with major arterial injury

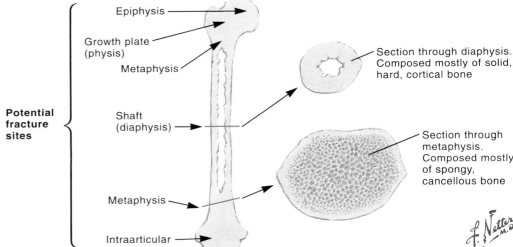

Epiphysis

Growth plate (physis)

Metaphysis

Potential fracture sites

Shaft (diaphysis)

Metaphysis

Intraarticular

Section through diaphysis. Composed mostly of solid, hard, cortical bone

Section through metaphysis. Composed mostly of spongy, cancellous bone

Classification of Fracture

A fracture is a break in the surface of the bone, either across its cortex or through its articular surface. Fractures range in severity from a simple crack to a complete disruption of bone architecture. A fracture through the cortex of a bone disturbs the normal load-bearing function of the bone. In addition, at the time of fracture, the overlying periosteum is torn, bleeding at the fracture site produces a hematoma, and electric and biochemical signals initiate the fracture healing process.

Proper management of all fractures and dislocations—regardless of location, extent, or severity—is based on three criteria: the integrity of the overlying skin and soft tissues (ie, open or closed fracture), the specific location of the fracture within the bone, and the degree of displacement of the injured parts. Therefore, the initial evaluation must describe the musculoskeletal injury in terms of these three variables.

Open and Closed Fracture. In a *closed* fracture, the overlying skin remains intact; in an *open* fracture, the integrity of the overlying skin and soft tissues has been violated (Plate 20). Disruption of this envelope of soft tissue around the fracture site substantially increases the risk of complications. Open fractures result in greater blood loss, decreased healing rate, and increased risk of infection.

Bleeding occurs with every fracture because, at the time of injury, the periosteal vessels and the vessels supplying the soft tissues surrounding the fracture are disrupted, which leads to the formation of a large hematoma. In a closed fracture, the increased interstitial pressure within the hematoma compresses the blood vessels, limiting the accumulation of blood and thus the size of the hematoma. Nevertheless, the amount of bleeding in closed fractures remains substantial. For example, a closed fracture of the femoral shaft may result in a blood loss of as much as 1 liter before

the increased pressure within the hematoma tamponades the bleeding vessels. However, since the tamponade effect is lost in an open fracture, blood loss is even greater and may be life threatening.

Any open fracture can become infected because the hematoma that forms around the open fracture site is contaminated by contact with the external environment. The risk of infection is directly related to the severity of soft tissue damage. An infection that becomes established at a fracture site is much more resistant to treatment than a soft tissue infection and may be impossible to eradicate. Chronic purulent drainage from the fracture site may persist for the rest of the patient's

life. This chronic infection of the bone, called posttraumatic osteomyelitis, often cannot be cured or even controlled in spite of repeated and aggressive surgical debridement and appropriate antibiotic therapy (see Section II, Plate 16).

Because of the devastating nature of chronic posttraumatic osteomyelitis, all open fractures must be identified immediately and prompt treatment instituted to prevent infection in the fracture hematoma. The best means of managing the contaminated fracture is through prompt and thorough surgical debridement combined with intravenous administration of broad-spectrum antibiotics immediately following the injury

Fractures, Dislocations, and Sprains
(Continued)

Types of Displacement

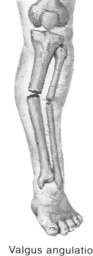
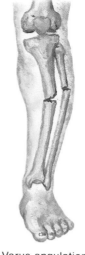
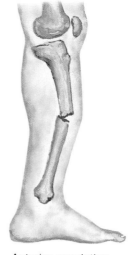
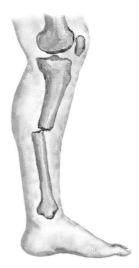

Valgus angulation   Varus angulation   Anterior angulation   Posterior angulation

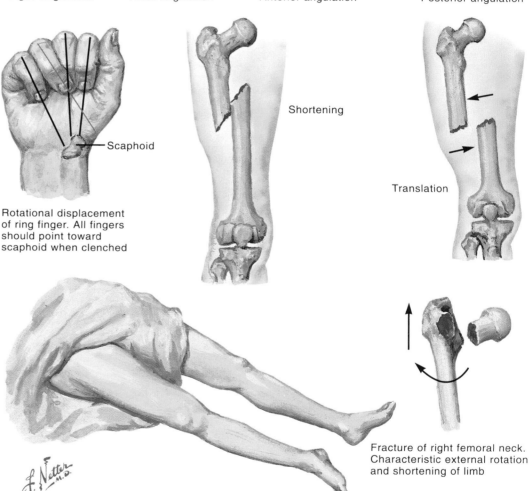

Rotational displacement of ring finger. All fingers should point toward scaphoid when clenched

Scaphoid

Shortening

Translation

Fracture of right femoral neck. Characteristic external rotation and shortening of limb

(Plate 143). Debridement is usually repeated in the first few days after injury. Primary closure of the wound is delayed until there is no evidence of residual contamination at the fracture site.

Gustilo and Anderson Classification

This useful classification grades open fractures according to several factors, including the severity of soft tissue damage (Plate 20). In a type I open fracture, the wound is less than 1 cm long and there is no evidence of deep contamination. In a type II injury, the wound is greater than 1 cm long and there is no extensive soft tissue injury. A type IIIA open fracture has a large, open wound, but the bone fragments remain adequately covered by soft tissues. If the wound is large and open and the bone is stripped of periosteum and exposed, the fracture is classified as type IIIB. The most serious open fracture is type IIIC, which comprises an open wound and an arterial injury that requires surgical repair.

Studies by Gustilo and associates documented a minimal risk of infection with type I open fractures if immediate surgical debridement is performed. The incidence of persistent chronic infection increases substantially with more severe wounds. In one study, only 4.4% of type IIIA wounds were infected, in contrast to 52% of type IIIB wounds. When the injuries included arterial injury, both the infection rate and the amputation rate were 42%. Thus, the severity of soft tissue injury significantly alters the prognosis for recovery of satisfactory function following a fracture and often dictates the treatment.

Fracture Sites

In the initial evaluation of any fracture, the examiner must identify the specific location of the fracture within the bone (Plate 20). The different areas of the bone heal with different mechanisms and at different rates. Fractures may occur in the shaft (diaphysis), metaphysis, joint (intraarticular fracture), growth plate (physis), or epiphysis. Fractures of the shaft and metaphysis heal in very dissimilar ways. Diaphyseal bone

usually heals by the formation of an external bridging callus, whereas metaphyseal bone heals by the apposition of a callus across the trabeculae. In addition, the cancellous metaphyseal bone heals much more rapidly than the cortical diaphyseal bone.

Intraarticular fractures involve the articular surface of the bone, and this involvement has important implications for both treatment and prognosis. The articular surface must heal with anatomic congruity to minimize the risk of posttraumatic osteoarthritis (Plate 148). Epiphyseal (growth plate) fractures are quite common in children and heal more rapidly than fractures in adults.

Types of Displacement

The initial evaluation of any fracture, in addition to assessment of the degree of soft tissue injury and the location in the bone, must determine the degree of fracture displacement. All fractures must be described as nondisplaced or displaced (Plate 21). *Nondisplaced* fractures are often difficult to diagnose because there is no associated deformity except soft tissue swelling. Indeed, many nondisplaced fractures are overlooked or mistaken for a simpler injury such as a mild or moderate sprain. All patients with a musculoskeletal injury who complain of pain and exhibit

Fractures, Dislocations, and Sprains
(Continued)

Types of Fracture

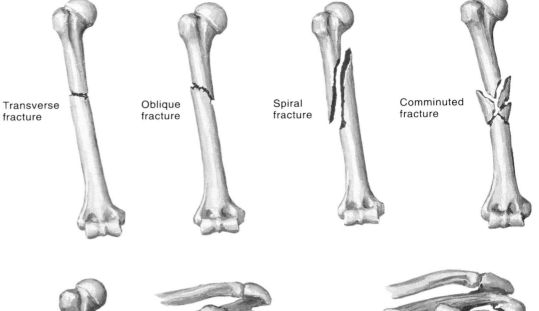

Transverse fracture

Oblique fracture

Spiral fracture

Comminuted fracture

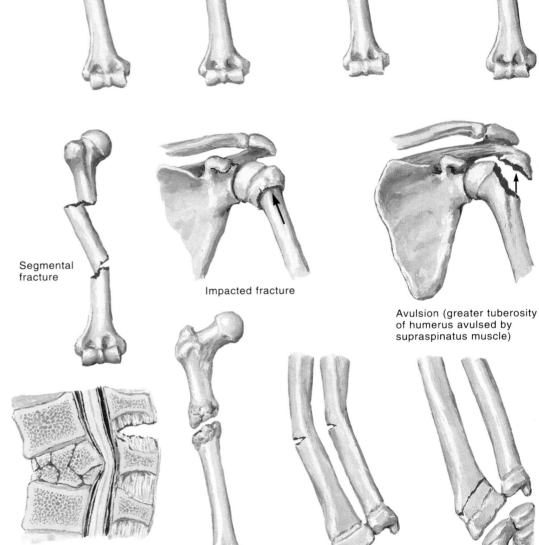

Segmental fracture

Impacted fracture

Avulsion (greater tuberosity of humerus avulsed by supraspinatus muscle)

Compression fracture

Pathologic fracture (tumor or bone disease)

Greenstick fracture

Torus (buckle) fracture

In children

swelling, ecchymosis, and point tenderness at the injury site should undergo radiographic evaluation to rule out disruption of the underlying bone architecture. If not appropriately treated, non-displaced fractures often result in serious disability.

Displaced fractures are described by the type of deformity produced by the displacement: angulation, rotation, change in limb length, or translation. Angulation at the fracture site may be in the frontal or the sagittal plane, or both. Frontal plane deformities are called varus or valgus depending on the angulation of the distal fragment at the point of fracture. When the distal fragment is angulated toward the midline, a varus deformity is produced; when the distal fragment is angulated away from the midline, a valgus deformity occurs. Sagittal plane deformities are described as either anterior or posterior angulation, depending on the direction in which the apex of the angulation points.

Fracture fragments can also be rotationally displaced. After fracture, the distal fragment is rotated along the long axis of the bone by muscle spasm or by the pull of gravity, resulting in either an internal rotation or an external rotation deformity.

A third type of displacement is a change in limb length. After a fracture, the surrounding muscles go into spasm, contracting to produce limb shortening.

Finally, translation occurs when the distal fragment shifts medially, laterally, anteriorly, or posteriorly in relation to the proximal fragment.

Frequently, the displacement is a combination of several types of the patterns described. For example, a displaced intertrochanteric fracture of the hip due to a fall typically causes both shortening and external rotation of the limb. Often, a varus angulation is present as well.

Types of Fracture

Many terms are used to describe the numerous fracture patterns (Plate 22). *Transverse*, *oblique*, and *spiral* describe the pattern of fracture seen on the radiograph. A *comminuted* fracture has more than two fracture fragments. A *segmental* fracture is a type of comminuted fracture in the shaft of a long bone in which there are three large, well-identified fragments. In an *impacted* fracture, two fracture fragments are telescoped on each other; usually, this pattern of injury is quite stable. *Avulsion* fractures frequently occur at the site of attachment of a musculotendinous unit to bone; they are caused when a sudden muscular pull tears the bony attachment loose from the rest of the bone. *Compression* fractures are common in the cancellous flat bones, particularly the vertebrae. The cancellous trabeculae are compressed, or impacted, together. A *pathologic* fracture occurs at a site in a bone that is diseased or weakened, most commonly through areas weakened by tumor or by a metabolic bone disease such as osteoporosis.

Two specific terms are used to describe fractures that are unique to children. The *greenstick* fracture occurs in the shaft of the bone, with the cortex fractured on the convex side of the deformity but intact on the concave side. This pattern is identical to the way a green stick reacts when bent. A *torus*, or *buckle*, fracture occurs in the metaphysis of the long bones in response to compressive loading. Most frequently seen in the distal radius, the torus fracture usually results from a fall on the outstretched hand. □

Healing of Fracture

Bone is unique among organs in its ability to heal a full-thickness injury by complete regeneration rather than by production of scar tissue. Although the biologic response of bone to a fracture can be modified by the method of treatment, it is useful to consider the typical biologic events that occur in the healing of a simple fracture in a nonimmobilized bone. The stages of fracture healing include impact and hematoma formation, induction, inflammation, soft callus, hard callus, and remodeling (Plate 23). The blood supply, oxygen tension, and movement at the fracture site change as normal fracture healing progresses, and these changes have profound effects on subsequent events at the fracture site.

Stages of Healing

Impact and Formation of Hematoma. At impact, bone absorbs energy and fails. The stage of impact signifies both the moment of fracture and the commencement of fracture healing. The strength of bone is proportional to the square of the mass of the bone. The strength of the bone also varies according to the mechanism (eg, bending, axial loading) and rate of force loading. At impact, periosteal and medullary blood vessels are ruptured, a hematoma forms, and inflammatory mediators accumulate at the fracture site.

Induction. The stage of induction is the most elusive stage of fracture healing; that is, very little is known about the biologic events that induce the regeneration of bone. Fracture healing is truly a process of regeneration and thus of reestablishment of an embryonic pattern that recapitulates the original formation of the skeleton. Clinical and laboratory data suggest that the inductive events occur in the first several minutes to hours following fracture. The stage of induction probably involves a complex cascade of events, including release and concentration of morphogens and growth factors, activation of pluripotential cells, and myriad changes in vascular supply, oxygen tension, pH, and other biologic processes.

In addition to its role as a mineral reserve bank, bone is also a repository for numerous growth factors that modulate its own regeneration.

Inflammation. The stage of inflammation begins at impact with early hematoma formation and persists until soft tissue callus begins to form. Recent in situ hybridization and immunohistochemical studies reveal that fibrous tissue and cartilage tissue genes and their protein products are expressed long before histologic evidence of mature fibrous or cartilage tissue is seen at the fracture site. This observation is consistent with the theory that links early inductive events to the complex temporal and spatial patterns of regeneration events that occur at the fracture site.

Formation of Soft Callus. The development of soft callus involves the early formation of external bridging callus as well as the late formation of medullary callus. Soft callus formation is characterized by vigorous mitotic and metabolic activity and may at times be mistaken for a low-grade connective tissue malignancy.

Healing of Fracture

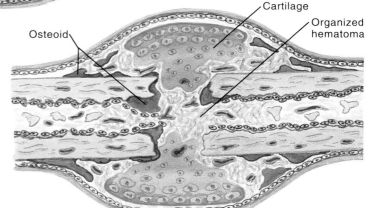

Stage of inflammation
Promptly after impact, hematoma forms as result of disruption of intraosseous, periosteal, and surrounding blood vessels. Bone at edges of fracture dies. Leukocytes, macrophages, mast cells, and fibroblasts infiltrate clot and begin to remove dead bone. Precise inductive mechanism for healing process not known

Stage of soft callus formation
Clot organized by collagen fibers and vascular elements. New vessels grow in, but P_{O_2} low, pH acidic. Osteo-progenitor cells, preosteo-cytes, and osteoblasts of cambium layer of periosteum and endosteum proliferate. Osteoblasts and chondroblasts of mesenchymal origin also appear in clot. Soft callus forms, composed of osteoid, cartilage, and collagen

Stage of hard callus formation
Osteoid and cartilage of external, periosteal, and medullary soft callus become mineralized as they are converted to fiber bone (hard callus)

Stage of bone remodeling
Osteoclastic and osteoblastic activity converts fiber bone to lamellar bone with true haversian systems. Normal bone contours restored; even angulation may be partially or completely corrected. P_{O_2} returns to normal

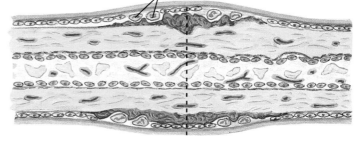

Repetitive micromovement at the fracture site is an important mechanical stimulus for the formation of soft tissue callus. The soft callus provides a mechanical scaffolding for the formation of hard bony callus, which stabilizes and eventually bridges the fracture gap. Despite the intense angiogenesis that accompanies soft callus formation, oxygen tension at the fracture site is low and pH is acidic. The intense cellularity of the soft callus far outstrips the increased oxygen supply stimulated by angiogenesis. If the vascular supply is interrupted early in fracture healing, the regenerative response is impaired, preventing normal fracture repair.

Formation of Hard Callus. The transition from soft callus to hard callus occurs 3 to 4 weeks into the fracture healing process with the appearance of calcified cartilage, and it continues until the bone ends are firmly united. The process of hard callus formation mimics similar events in the normal growth plate. Calcified cartilage provides a scaffold for osteoblasts and for the subsequent deposition and mineralization of bone matrix. Primitive fiber bone at the fracture site is eventually transformed into normal lamellar bone in both medullary and external bridging callus. Blood supply and oxygen tension at the fracture site continue to increase during this stage.

Healing of Fracture

(Continued)

Primary Union

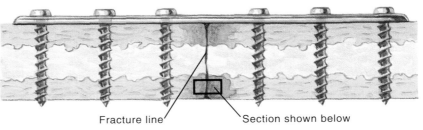

If fractured bone ends compressed securely so that no motion can take place between them, callus does not form. Dead bone at fracture site not resorbed but revitalized by ingrowth of haversian systems

Fracture line   Section shown below

Mechanism of healing by primary union

Remodeling. The final stage of fracture healing, the stage of remodeling, begins about 6 weeks after fracture and may continue for weeks or months until the process is complete. During this stage, the abundant hard callus (external bridging callus and medullary callus) is slowly remodeled from immature fiber bone into mature lamellar bone. During remodeling, the oxygen tension at the fracture site returns to normal.

Clinically, fracture healing is complete when bone strength at the fracture site has been restored to normal. This may occur as soon as 6 weeks following fracture. Radiographic evidence of healing may also be seen as early as 6 weeks following fracture. Biologically, a fracture is considered healed when all regenerative processes at the fracture site have ceased. A technetium methylene diphosphonate bone scan may show increased metabolic activity at the fracture site for months or years while remodeling continues.

Primary Union

Primary union of bone does not occur normally in nature, but it can be induced artificially with internal fixation and rigid immobilization (Plate 24). Primary cortical union is not true bone regeneration but rather the recruitment of normal remodeling processes to bridge the fracture gap. Compared with inductive callus healing, the process of primary union is extremely slow.

Complete immobilization inhibits the formation of inductive callus but promotes primary cortical union. When a rigid compression plate is affixed to a fracture, the necrotic cortical bone at the fracture site is not resorbed as in the normal process of inductive callus healing. Rather, the dead bone is recanalized by new haversian systems with mature osteons, as occurs in normal bone remodeling. New bone also arises from endosteum to bridge the fracture gap. Revascularization occurs from adjacent medullary vessels.

Unlike inductive callus formation, which includes both external bridging callus and late medullary callus, primary union of cortical bone cannot effectively bridge gaps at a fracture site. For primary union to occur, the fracture gap must be obliterated by perfect apposition and compression of the fractured bone ends. In addition, movement at the fracture site must be minimal. The bone's ability to heal by primary union depends on rigid immobilization, which enables the fragile medullary vessels to recanalize the necrotic bone and cross the fracture site. When the bone is healed, tolerance to total rigidity is excellent. The major disadvantages of primary union are its slowness compared with inductive callus formation and the need for artificial stability with rigid internal fixation to be maintained for a long period of time.

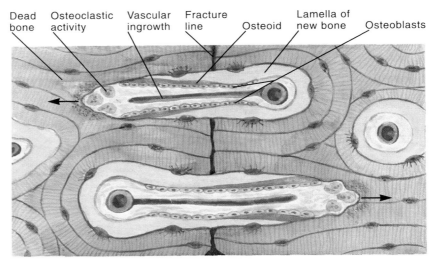

Dead bone | Osteoclastic activity | Vascular ingrowth | Fracture line | Osteoid | Lamella of new bone | Osteoblasts

Osteoclasts ream out tunnels through dead bone at fracture edges and across fracture line into opposite bone fragment. Osteoblasts line new tunnels and lay down new lamellae around them to form new osteons, restoring continuity of bone

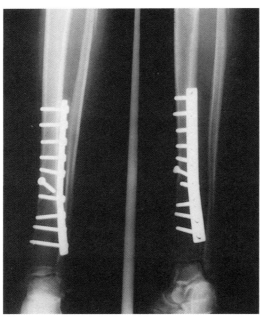

Fracture healing by primary union. Radiograph shows lack of callus formation

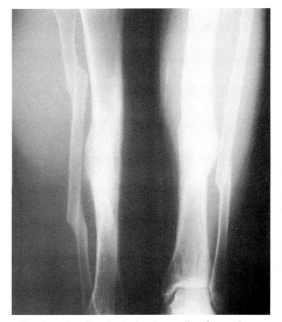

Fracture healing by inductive callus formation. Radiograph shows exuberant callus formation

Factors That Promote Bone Healing

Fracture healing is a complex regenerative process that begins at the moment of fracture and continues until all reparative events have ceased. Numerous endocrine, paracrine, autocrine, biochemical, and biophysical factors are involved in successful fracture healing, and an excess or deficiency of many of these factors impairs the regenerative response to fracture (Plate 25). While some factors play a role throughout healing, others are more critical at specific and limited times.

Peptide and steroid hormones help regulate fracture healing. Growth hormone, insulin, thyroid hormone, cortisol, and gonadal steroids all have important functions throughout the process of fracture healing; each of these hormones has cell membrane or nuclear receptors in the tissues involved in the regenerative response. Vitamin D and its active metabolites as well as parathyroid hormone are essential for normal mineralization of bone in the later stages of fracture healing. Vitamin A may also be important, but its exact role in fracture repair is not yet defined. Retinoic acid, a vitamin A analog, is believed to function as a morphogen in the formation of the skeleton and possibly also in fracture healing. Much research is focused on the role of substances such as bone

Healing of Fracture
(Continued)

morphogenetic protein (BMP) and retinoic acid in the regenerative events following fracture. Recombinant bone morphogenetic protein can stimulate endochondral ossification in an ectopic site and is a likely candidate for use in inducing the formation of external bridging callus. The roles of other growth factors, such as transforming growth factor β (TGF-β) and platelet-derived growth factor, have been studied in experimental models of fracture healing.

Vitamin C is vital in fracture healing and in posttranslational modification of collagen, the most abundant matrix component in both soft and hard callus. An adequate supply of amino acids, carbohydrates, fats, and trace elements is also critical for normal fracture healing.

Patients in a coma resulting from head injury are at risk for heterotopic ossification; in these patients, fractures often heal with excessive amounts of callus. Metabolic and humoral factors related to head injury and coma are being investigated for their roles in the promotion of fracture healing.

Physical factors such as micromovement and weight bearing are essential in the production of a normal inductive callus and are therefore essential in the promotion of bone healing. Demineralized bone matrix, bone marrow grafts, and electric stimulation are now commonly used to promote bone healing.

Factors That Delay Bone Healing

Although no factor has yet been identified that accelerates normal bone healing, numerous factors are known to retard or inhibit bone repair. Glucocorticoid excess, for example, can lead to severe osteopenia, imperiling fracture healing; juvenile diabetes has the same potential effect. A deficiency of gonadal steroids in either men or women can also result in profound osteopenia, which slows the regenerative response following a fracture. Severe anemia can alter oxygen tensions at the fracture site. Deficiencies of vitamin D or its metabolites cause abnormal mineralization of the fracture callus, delaying fracture healing or causing nonunion.

The regenerative response is interrupted by large bone gaps due to the interposition of soft tissue or by devitalization of bone by irradiation, vascular injury, loss of soft tissue, or denervation. Infections and neoplasms can retard fracture healing by some unknown mechanisms. The regenerative response can also be interrupted by components in the synovial fluid bathing the fragments of an intraarticular fracture, resulting in delayed union or nonunion. Severe osteoporosis from any cause, as well as metabolic diseases such as hyperparathyroidism, osteomalacia, Paget disease of bone, or fibrous dysplasia, can retard the regenerative response to a fracture.

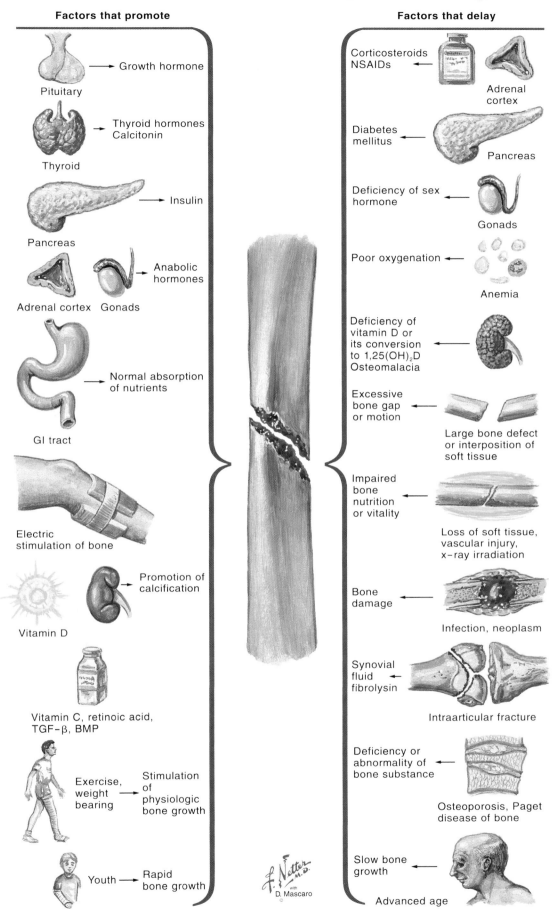

Factors That Promote or Delay Bone Healing

Fractures heal more slowly in older persons than in children and young adults. Poor general nutrition and lack of vitamin C can have a direct inhibitory effect on the production of extracellular matrix, which can disrupt the formation of both soft and hard callus. Although movement can stimulate fracture healing, too little or too much movement disrupts endochondral callus formation, which may have important clinical implications for fracture healing. □

General Principles of Prehospital Care

Prehospital Care of Musculoskeletal Injury

General Principles

Effective prehospital care of fractures, dislocations, and sprains improves the patient's chances of rapid recovery and early return to normal activity. Emergency medical technicians and paramedics are trained to recognize the common mechanisms of musculoskeletal injury and to stabilize fractures and dislocations before transporting the patient to the hospital. The emergency team always performs a *primary* survey of the injured patient in the field to ensure the adequacy of vital functions (airway, breathing, and circulation). The subsequent *secondary* survey of the patient includes a head-to-toe examination to identify specific areas of injury. When a specific limb injury is identified, the emergency personnel immediately evaluate the distal neurovascular function for limb-threatening ischemia.

The most important aspect of prehospital care of musculoskeletal injuries is effective splinting. Unless the patient's life is in immediate danger, all musculoskeletal injuries should be splinted in the field before the patient is moved. Effective splinting decreases pain, reduces bleeding at the injury site, and decreases the chance of further damage to the surrounding soft tissues, particularly the skin, muscles, nerves, and blood vessels.

The following principles govern splinting techniques (Plate 26). First, a dry, sterile compression dressing is applied to all open wounds. This controls bleeding from the open wound and prevents further contamination of the injured tissues, thus minimizing the risk of subsequent infection.

Next, the splint should be applied before the patient is moved at all, unless there is an immediate environmental threat to the life of the patient or the emergency personnel. The patient should be moved as little as possible until the injury is completely splinted, and the injured limb must always be adequately supported.

The injured limb should be splinted in the position in which it is found. The splint should incorporate the joint above and the joint below the fractured bone. If a joint is dislocated, the splint must extend along the entire length of the bones above and below the dislocated joint.

Occasionally, the fracture or dislocation creates a significant limb deformity that prevents effective splinting of the limb in the position in which it is found, making safe transportation difficult. Trained personnel may then apply *gentle* longitudinal traction to realign the limb. The goal of traction is to place the limb in a more normal and anatomic position to facilitate splinting and transportation. Traction should *not* be used routinely in the field to reduce all dislocations or fractures. Once traction is applied, it must be maintained manually until the limb is fully and effectively splinted.

After splinting, there must be frequent monitoring of neurovascular function of the injured

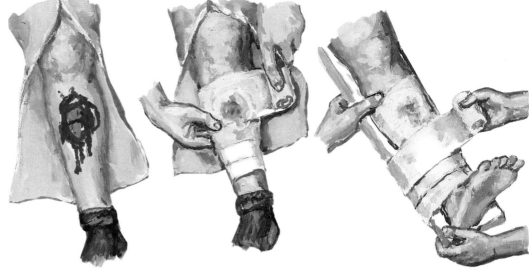

First, dry, sterile compression dressing applied to open wound to prevent further contamination and control bleeding

Next, padded board or other type of splint applied, incorporating joints proximal and distal to fracture site

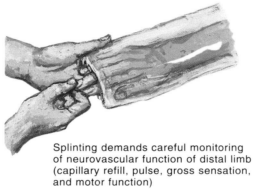

Splinting demands careful monitoring of neurovascular function of distal limb (capillary refill, pulse, gross sensation, and motor function)

Splinting must be completed before moving patient. Inflatable air splint being applied in back seat of car

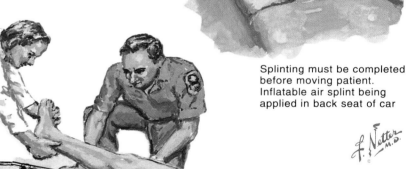

If fracture causes significant deformity of long bone, limb may be realigned with gentle traction. Traction maintained during splinting before transportation

limb by assessment of the pulse, capillary refill, gross sensation, and motor function distal to the injury. The splinted limb is elevated to minimize swelling. The upper limb can be supported on a pillow or on the supine patient's chest. In all lower limb injuries, a pillow should be used to elevate the foot slightly higher than the heart.

Proper splinting substantially lessens the pain unless there is vascular impairment distal to the injury site. If circulation to the limb is impaired or absent, immediate surgical intervention is needed. Splints are placed on the pulseless limb to minimize the risk of further damage; then the patient is rapidly transported to a medical center.

However, with most types of injury, rapid transport to the hospital is not necessary. Emergency medical teams are taught to improvise with materials on hand when standard splints are not available, as may occur in a disaster or multiple casualty situation.

After the patient is brought to the hospital, the injury should remain splinted until radiographs are taken and the treating physician is available to remove the splint. Premature removal of the splint only causes more discomfort to the patient, necessitating resplinting to reduce the pain and minimize the risk of further injury to the adjacent soft tissues.

Prehospital Care of Injury to Shoulder, Arm, and Elbow

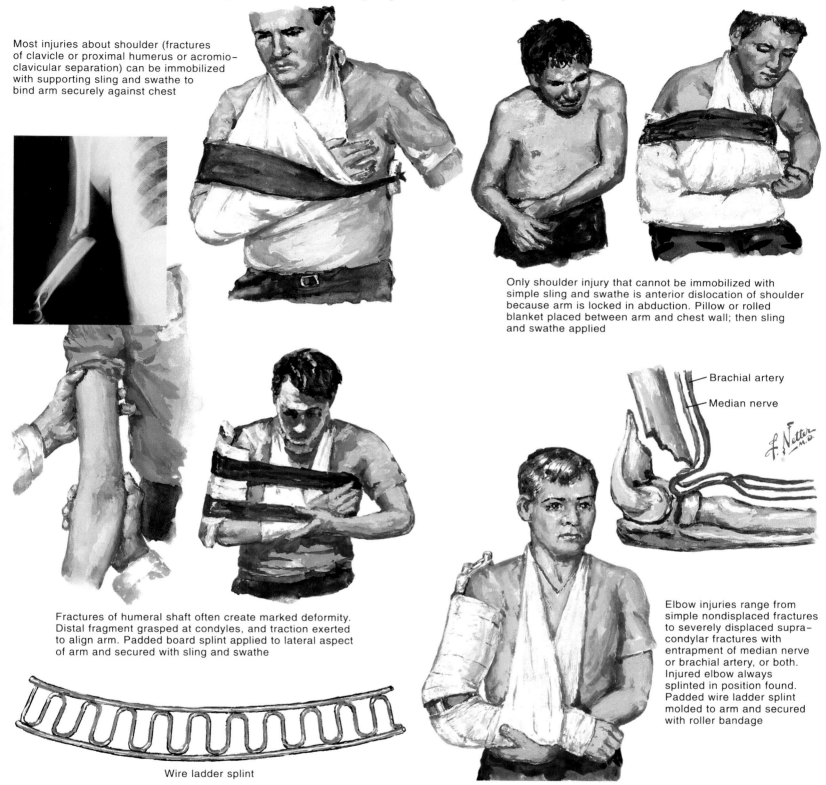

Most injuries about shoulder (fractures of clavicle or proximal humerus or acromio-clavicular separation) can be immobilized with supporting sling and swathe to bind arm securely against chest

Only shoulder injury that cannot be immobilized with simple sling and swathe is anterior dislocation of shoulder because arm is locked in abduction. Pillow or rolled blanket placed between arm and chest wall; then sling and swathe applied

Brachial artery

Median nerve

Fractures of humeral shaft often create marked deformity. Distal fragment grasped at condyles, and traction exerted to align arm. Padded board splint applied to lateral aspect of arm and secured with sling and swathe

Elbow injuries range from simple nondisplaced fractures to severely displaced supra-condylar fractures with entrapment of median nerve or brachial artery, or both. Injured elbow always splinted in position found. Padded wire ladder splint molded to arm and secured with roller bandage

Wire ladder splint

Prehospital Care of Musculoskeletal Injury

(Continued)

Types of Splints

The three general types of splints used in the prehospital setting are rigid, soft, and traction splints.

Rigid Splints. These splints are made from firm materials such as padded wooden boards, molded plastic or metal, cardboard, and malleable metal frames. Usually applied to two or three sides of the injured limb, rigid splints are secured in place with Velcro straps or roller bandages.

Soft Splints. Inflatable clear-plastic air splints come in a variety of sizes and shapes for use on both upper and lower limbs. The air splint is applied to the limb and is inflated by mouth; as it inflates, it conforms to the shape of the limb and stiffens, immobilizing the injured part without causing excessive pressure on the underlying tissues. The pressure inside the splint must be

monitored frequently, because it is affected by environmental temperature changes. The sling and swathe and the pillow splint are other soft splints that, when properly applied, effectively immobilize injured limbs.

Traction Splints. Strong muscle forces frequently cause significant deformity in the thigh after a fracture of the femur. Traction splints maintain limb alignment and effectively immobilize these fractures. The emergency medical team first restores limb alignment by applying firm longitudinal traction to the limb, maintaining the alignment manually while applying the traction splint. The splint supports the injured limb firmly,

Prehospital Care of Musculoskeletal Injury

(Continued)

and a ratchet, or windlass, mechanism exerts continuous traction on the ankle and foot. The splint also applies countertraction against the area of the ischial tuberosity.

Injury to Shoulder, Arm, and Elbow

Injury to Shoulder. Most injuries about the shoulder region, including acromioclavicular separations and fractures of the proximal humerus, scapula, and clavicle, can be stabilized with a sling and swathe (Plate 27). The sling, made of a standard triangular bandage, supports the weight of the upper limb. The knot is tied securely to one side of the neck so that, when the patient is erect, the weight of the arm is carried across the back of the neck. One or two swathes are applied over the arm in the sling to bind it firmly, but not too tightly, to the chest wall. This prevents the limb from swinging freely. The hand is left free to facilitate monitoring of the distal neurovascular function.

The only shoulder injury that cannot be effectively immobilized in a simple sling and swathe is the common anterior dislocation of the shoulder joint. Following this injury, the arm is locked in moderate abduction and cannot be brought comfortably against the chest wall. The anteriorly dislocated shoulder and the arm must be splinted in the abducted position in which they are found. A pillow or rolled blanket is used to fill the space between the arm and the chest wall. Then the elbow is flexed to a right angle and a sling applied to support the arm. The pillow and sling are secured as a unit to the chest with one or two swathes.

Injury to Humerus. Following a fracture of the humeral shaft, muscle spasm frequently produces significant deformity. When gross angulation occurs, emergency care personnel should restore overall alignment of the arm by applying longitudinal traction to the distal fragment. This is best accomplished by grabbing the condyles of the humerus with one hand, supporting the fracture site with the other hand, and gently but firmly pulling the arm distally until it is aligned against the chest wall. One person must maintain this alignment manually while a padded board splint is applied to provide additional stability on the lateral aspect of the arm. The entire injured limb and the splint are incorporated into a sling and swathe.

Injury to Elbow. Injuries of the elbow range from nondisplaced fractures to complete dislocations and severe limb-threatening injuries such as the displaced supracondylar fracture, which may impale the brachial artery or median nerve. The injured elbow is always splinted in the position in which it is found. Manipulation or the application of traction to injuries in this region may cause or aggravate an accompanying injury to a nerve or blood vessel. A malleable wire ladder splint can be molded to conform to the shape of

Prehospital Care of Fracture of Forearm Bones

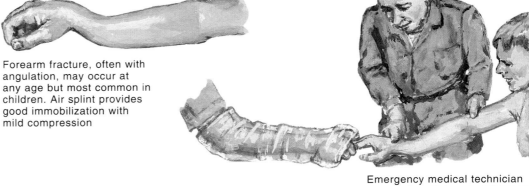

Forearm fracture, often with angulation, may occur at any age but most common in children. Air splint provides good immobilization with mild compression

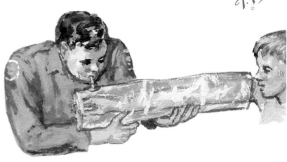

Emergency medical technician places air splint on own forearm and grasps patient's fingers, applying mild traction as assistant supports injured limb

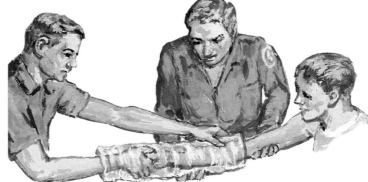

Air splint slid into place over patient's hand, forearm, and arm. Fingers left protruding from splint

Air splint inflated by mouth

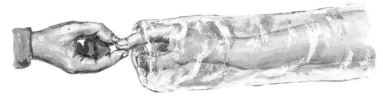

Neurovascular function tested and regularly monitored by capillary refill method

Prehospital Care of Fracture of Wrist and Hand

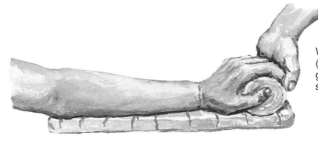

Wrist and hand splinted in functional (mild cock up) position. Hand holding gauze roll placed on padded board splint extending to elbow

Injured limb and gauze roll secured to splint with roller bandage

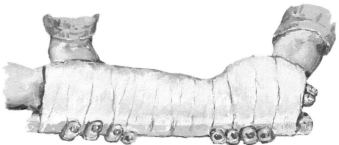

Prehospital Care of Suspected Spine Injury

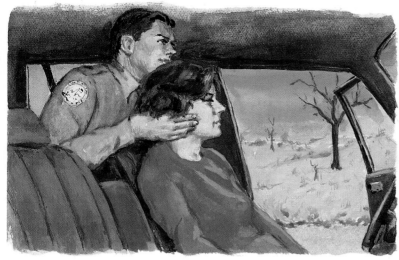

1. For all suspected spine injuries, immobilization begins with emergency medical technician providing manual support so head does not move in relation to trunk

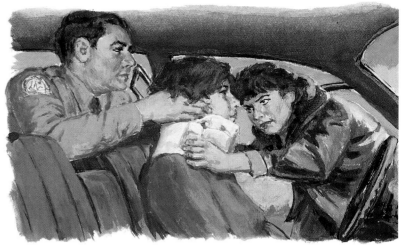

2. Firm extrication collar applied to provide partial immobilization of cervical spine

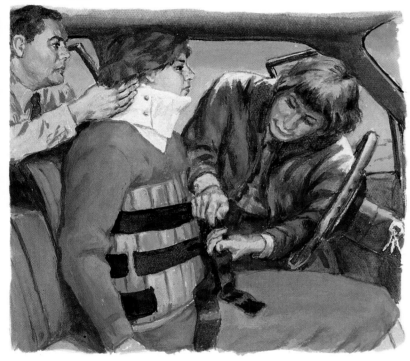

3. Spine immobilization extrication device applied to trunk and secured with straps

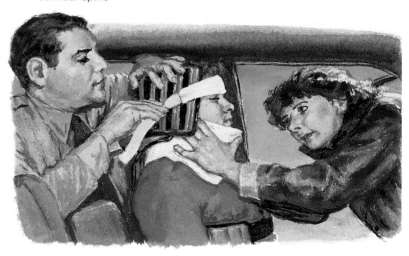

4. Patient's head secured to head extension of extrication device

5. Patient rotated as unit and laid on long spine board, fastened with straps for transportation to hospital. Prehospital immobilization of all patients with suspected spine injuries has greatly reduced incidence of paraplegia and quadriplegia

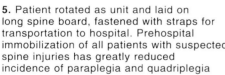

SECTION I PLATE 29   Slide 4805

Prehospital Care of Musculoskeletal Injury

(Continued)

the deformed elbow. The limb is secured to the splint *in the deformed position* with a roller bandage, and the splinted limb is then supported with a sling or with pillows while the patient is transported to the hospital.

Injury to Forearm, Wrist, and Hand

Injury to Forearm. Fractures of the forearm are particularly common in children, although they occur in persons of all ages. While significant angulation often occurs, most of these fractures can be immobilized very effectively with an air splint without manipulation or traction (Plate 28). An air splint, inflated by mouth, conforms to the deformity of the injured limb, providing gentle compression to the injury site and effectively immobilizing the fracture fragments. Two technicians are needed to apply an air splint properly. One person supports the injured limb at all times;

the other applies the splint by first sliding it onto his or her own arm, then gradually sliding it onto the patient's injured limb. The splint is inflated when it is in place. Wire ladder and padded board splints are also used in forearm fractures.

Injury to Wrist and Hand. All these injuries can be immobilized with a bulky hand dressing and a volar padded board splint. The injured hand is placed in the position of function, with the wrist dorsiflexed about 30° and the fingers gently flexed slightly as if holding a softball. A roll of soft gauze is put in the palm, and a padded board splint is placed along the volar aspect of the hand, wrist, and forearm. Then the entire limb distal to

Prehospital Care of Fracture of Pelvis

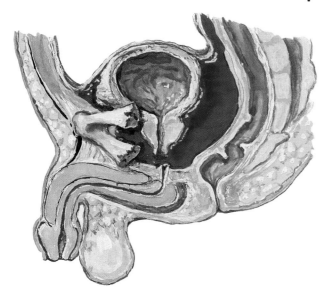

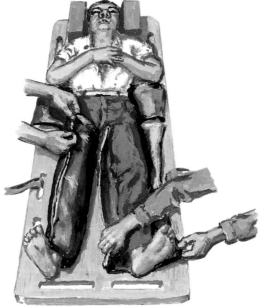

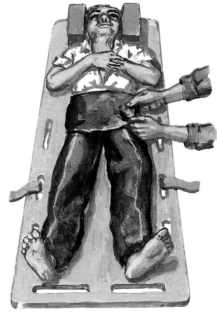

Pelvic fracture may rupture adjacent large vessels, resulting in massive retroperitoneal hemorrhage that leads to hypovolemic shock. If pelvic fracture suspected, pneumatic antishock garment needed to stabilize fracture, decrease bleeding, and shunt blood back to systemic circulation

Garment has three sections, one for each lower limb and one for lower abdomen. Patient placed on opened garment on long spine board. Lower limbs enclosed first

Abdominal section closed with Velcro fasteners, which yield if pressure excessive

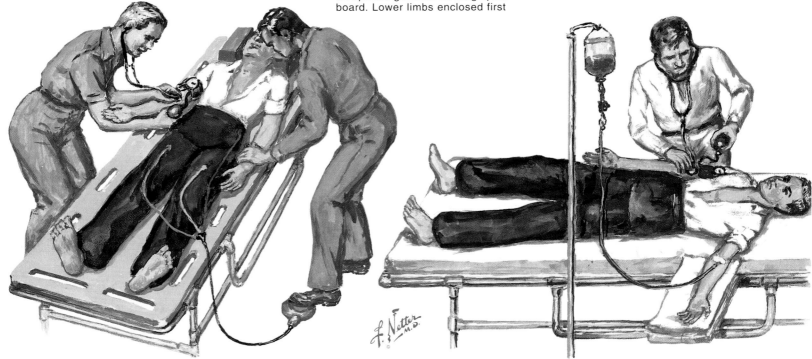

Antishock garment inflated with foot pump as blood pressure monitored. Patient transported to hospital on long spine board

Antishock garment must remain inflated until patient in hospital and blood can be transfused. Premature deflation may result in irreversible hypovolemic shock

---

Prehospital Care of Musculoskeletal Injury

(Continued)

the elbow is secured to the padded board splint with a roller bandage. To minimize swelling, the splinted hand is elevated by placing the limb in a sling or supporting it on a pillow or on the patient's chest during transportation.

Injury to Spine

Complete immobilization of the injured spine prior to hospitalization has significantly reduced the incidence of paralysis following major trauma (Plate 29). Effective splinting of the spine greatly decreases the risk of impingement on the spinal cord by unstable bony elements. Splinting is mandatory for all patients with any *suspected* spine injury (eg, patients involved in motor vehicle accidents or falls from a height or patients with head or facial injuries). Although not all patients will have a significant spine injury, this rule ensures that those few who do are protected from the

devastating complication of permanent spinal cord injury during transportation to the hospital. Emergency care personnel take great care to avoid any manipulation of the spine in the field. The only indication for realignment of the injured spine is an inadequate airway—a life-threatening problem that always takes precedence in patient care protocols.

The purpose of spine immobilization is to provide a single solid unit of head, trunk, and pelvis so that one segment does not move in relation to the other two. One emergency medical technician stands at the patient's head, holding it in his or her hands to prevent motion. Another person

Prehospital Care of Fracture of Hip

Prehospital Care of Musculoskeletal Injury

(Continued)

applies a firm extrication collar to the cervical spine to provide partial immobilization; a cervical collar alone, however, does not fully eliminate motion of the head on the trunk. After the collar is applied, a spine immobilization extrication device is secured to the patient to prevent movement between the head and trunk. The trunk and then the head are secured to the immobilization device with straps. The patient is rotated as one unit, laid on a long spine board, and secured to it with long straps. This completely and rigidly immobilizes the entire vertebral column and pelvis. After the head and spine are fully stabilized, any limb injuries are splinted as well, and the patient is transferred to the ambulance litter on the long spine board.

Fracture of Pelvis

Pelvic fractures are usually caused by high-velocity impact. Because the pelvis lies in the retroperitoneal space, close to several large blood vessels, fracture of the pelvis may result in a hemorrhage that leads to hypovolemic shock (Plate 30). Stabilizing the pelvis in the field decreases bleeding and reduces the risk of shock. The military antishock trousers (MAST), or pneumatic antishock garment, and a long spine board are most effective for immobilizing the pelvis. Inflation of the antishock garment stabilizes the pelvic fracture and decreases bleeding at the fracture sites. The three sections of the pneumatic antishock garment (one for each lower limb and one for the abdominal area) are inflated gradually while the patient's blood pressure is monitored. Because irreversible hypovolemic shock may occur when a pneumatic antishock garment is deflated, deflation should take place in the emergency department after the patient is adequately resuscitated with intravenous fluids and adequate blood is ready for immediate transfusion.

Fracture of Hip

In older persons with brittle, osteoporotic bone, falls often result in fractures of the proximal femur. Displaced hip fractures cause an obvious shortening and external rotation of the injured limb (Plate 31). Because the fracture lies so close to the hip joint, the pelvis as well as the entire lower limb must be immobilized to prevent movement at the fracture site. With pillows to support the injured limb in the position of deformity, the patient is secured to a long spine board or a scoop stretcher. To facilitate splinting and minimize pelvic movement, the scoop stretcher is disassembled at the head and foot and the two sides slid underneath the patient. The patient is secured to it with adjustable straps, and cravats are used to tie the leg and foot to the stretcher frame.

Fracture of the hip is such a common problem that all older patients should be taken to the hospital when they fall and complain of hip or knee pain. Patients with nondisplaced fractures may

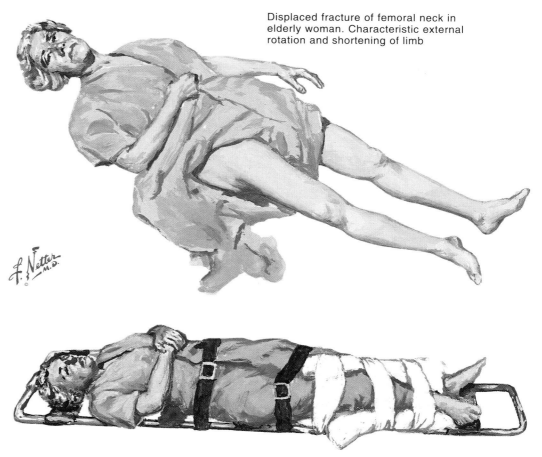

Displaced fracture of femoral neck in elderly woman. Characteristic external rotation and shortening of limb

Patient with hip fracture on scoop stretcher. Injured limb supported by pillows bound to limb and to stretcher

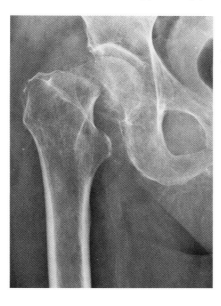
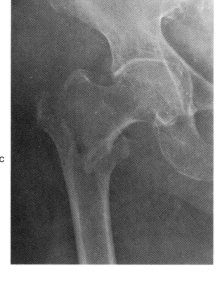

Subcapital fracture of femoral neck

Intertrochanteric fracture

have no deformity and may even be able to bear some weight on the fractured limb. Radiographic evaluation of a painful hip after a fall is essential in the diagnosis of a hip fracture.

Fracture of Lower Limb

Injury to Femur. Fracture of the femoral shaft usually occurs in young adults as the result of a high-velocity injury, particularly an automobile accident (Plate 32). Muscle spasm and the loss of stability of the underlying femur usually create a gross deformity.

Traction splints are used to immobilize fractures of the femoral shaft. First, the limb is realigned with manual traction by one emergency technician, while a second technician places the traction splint under the injured limb, fastens it with straps, and uses the windlass mechanism to maintain continuous traction on the ankle and foot during transportation. Because femoral fractures are often associated with injury of the pelvis or spine, the patient should be transported on a long spine board.

Injury to Knee. Injuries of the knee vary in severity from ligament disruptions to severe fracture dislocations. Because the risk of neurovascular injury is extremely high in this region, the injured knee must be splinted in the position

Prehospital Care of Fracture of Lower Limb

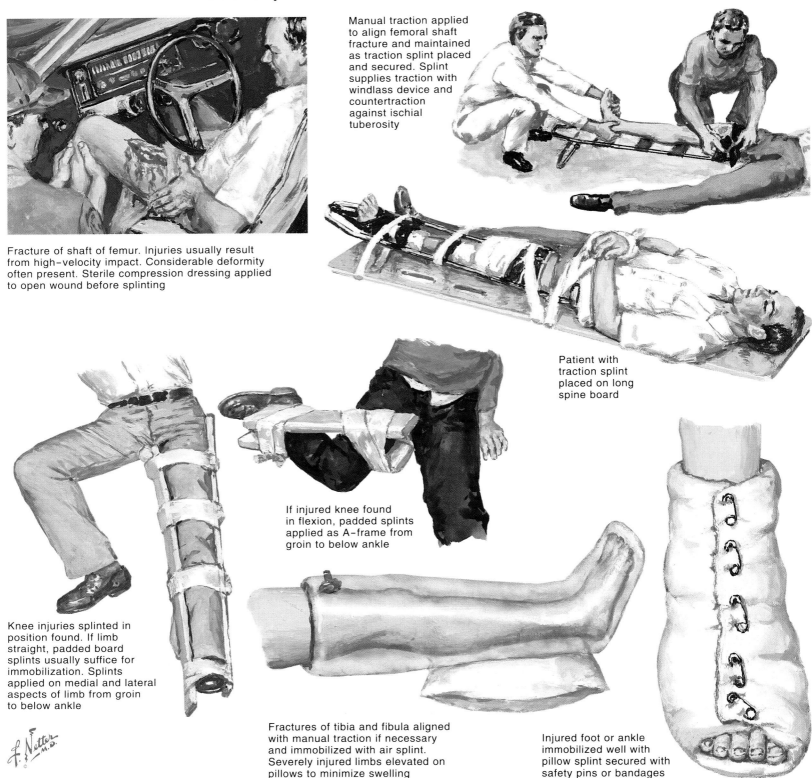

Fracture of shaft of femur. Injuries usually result from high–velocity impact. Considerable deformity often present. Sterile compression dressing applied to open wound before splinting

Manual traction applied to align femoral shaft fracture and maintained as traction splint placed and secured. Splint supplies traction with windlass device and countertraction against ischial tuberosity

Patient with traction splint placed on long spine board

Knee injuries splinted in position found. If limb straight, padded board splints usually suffice for immobilization. Splints applied on medial and lateral aspects of limb from groin to below ankle

If injured knee found in flexion, padded splints applied as A–frame from groin to below ankle

Fractures of tibia and fibula aligned with manual traction if necessary and immobilized with air splint. Severely injured limbs elevated on pillows to minimize swelling

Injured foot or ankle immobilized well with pillow splint secured with safety pins or bandages

SECTION I PLATE 32   Slide 4808

Prehospital Care of Musculoskeletal Injury

(Continued)

in which it is found. When the knee is found extended, two padded board splints are placed on the medial and lateral aspects of the limb, extending from the groin to the ankle joint and secured with several cravats. When the knee is found in the flexed position, padded board splints are applied to the medial and lateral aspects of the flexed limb in an A-frame configuration. The splints should extend from the upper end of the femur to the lower end of the tibia. After the splint is applied, distal neurovascular function must be monitored carefully during transportation to the hospital.

Injury to Tibia and Fibula. Fractures of the tibia and fibula are often associated with significant deformity. A severely displaced fracture of the tibia and fibula should be realigned with longitudinal traction and splinted with a long leg air splint or padded board splints that extend above the knee. The knee also must be completely immobilized.

Injury to Ankle and Foot. The pillow is one of many splinting devices that can be used to stabilize an injured ankle or foot. A standard pillow is wrapped around the injury and secured snugly with safety pins or a circular gauze wrap. The pillow readily conforms to the shape of the injured part, providing effective immobilization when properly secured. As with all lower limb injuries, the toes should remain exposed to allow frequent assessment of the distal neurovascular function during transportation to the hospital and in the initial evaluation in the emergency department. □

Fracture of Clavicle and Scapula

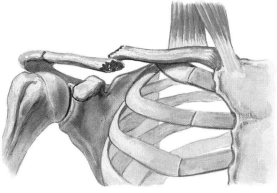

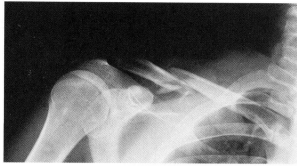

Fracture of middle third of clavicle (most common). Medial fragment displaced upward by pull of sterno-cleidomastoid muscle; lateral fragment displaced downward by weight of shoulder. Fractures occur most often in children

Anteroposterior radiograph. Fracture of middle third of clavicle

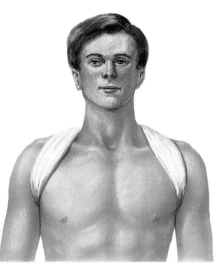

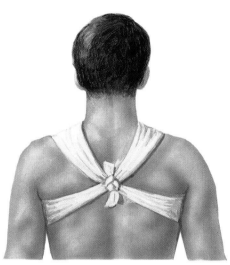

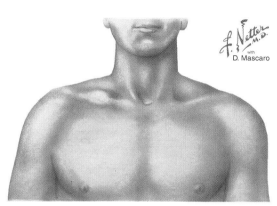

Healed fracture of clavicle. Even with proper treatment, small lump may remain

Fracture of middle third of clavicle best treated with snug figure–of–8 bandage or clavicle harness for 3 weeks or until pain subsides. Bandage or harness must be tightened occasionally because it loosens with wear

Fractures of lateral third of clavicle

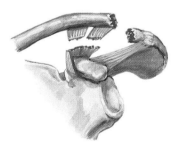

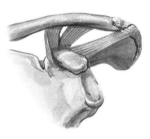

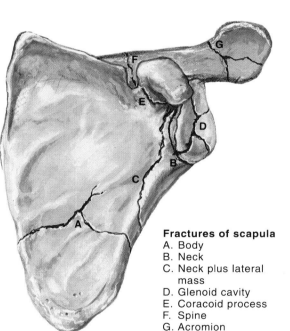

Type I. Fracture with no disruption of ligaments and therefore no displacement. Treated with simple sling for few weeks

Type II. Fracture with tear of coracoclavicular ligament and upward displacement of medial fragment. Requires open repair; if pin used, must be bent to prevent migration

Type III. Fracture through acromioclavicular joint; no displacement. Often missed and may later cause painful osteo-arthritis requiring resection arthroplasty

Fractures of scapula
A. Body
B. Neck
C. Neck plus lateral mass
D. Glenoid cavity
E. Coracoid process
F. Spine
G. Acromion

Slide 4809

Injury to Shoulder and Humerus

The shoulder region consists of three bones—the humerus, scapula, and clavicle—and three articulations—the glenohumeral, acromioclavicular, and sternoclavicular. Because full shoulder strength and motion are vital for optimal function of the upper limb, all shoulder injuries must be properly evaluated and treated.

Fracture of Clavicle and Scapula

Fracture of Clavicle. The clavicle is one of the most frequently fractured bones, and fractures are especially common in children. Most fractures are caused by indirect forces, usually a fall on the outstretched hand, although some result from a direct blow to the shoulder (Plate 33). Fractures of the medial (proximal) third of the clavicle are rare but can usually be treated with sling immobilization for 3 to 4 weeks. Fractures of the middle third usually require only support with a figure-of-8 bandage until pain subsides, generally in 10 to 14 days.

Type I fractures of the lateral (distal) clavicle are nondisplaced and are treated with a simple sling. Type II fractures are characterized by tearing of the coracoclavicular ligaments and upward displacement of the medial fragment. Because they are unstable and prone to nonunion, type II fractures often require surgical treatment, particularly if the fracture fragments are widely separated. Reducing the displaced clavicle and securing it to the coracoid process is the preferred treatment. Type III fractures of the lateral clavicle involve the acromioclavicular articulation and are treated

Dislocation of Acromioclavicular or Sternoclavicular Joint

Injury to Shoulder and Humerus
(Continued)

initially with sling immobilization for several weeks. These injuries may lead to persistent and painful osteoarthritis in the acromioclavicular joint. If conservative therapy and antiinflammatory medications do not relieve the arthritic symptoms, resection arthroplasty should be considered.

Fracture of Scapula. Most fractures of the scapula result from a direct blow to the back, and the underlying chest and lung must also be carefully examined. Fractures of the body of the scapula are treated conservatively with immobilization in a sling until pain subsides (usually 1–2 weeks). Fractures of the neck of the scapula or the glenoid rim may require open reduction and internal fixation if the fracture fragment is large or displaced enough to make the glenohumeral joint unstable.

Dislocation of Acromioclavicular or Sternoclavicular Joint

Dislocation of Acromioclavicular Joint. The most common mechanism of injury is a fall on the point of the shoulder. Plate 34 illustrates the three grades of dislocation. In a grade I injury, the acromioclavicular ligaments are sprained but joint alignment remains intact. Grade II injury refers to rupture of the acromioclavicular ligaments with disruption of the acromioclavicular joint. In a grade III injury, both the acromioclavicular and the coracoclavicular ligaments are ruptured, resulting in significant joint displacement that is apparent on clinical and radiographic examinations.

Grade I and grade II injuries can be differentiated on stress radiographs. With the patient standing or sitting, a 10-lb weight is secured to the affected upper limb. In a grade II injury, the added weight displaces the acromioclavicular articulation, increasing the distance between the clavicle and acromion. Grade I injuries remain nondisplaced.

Grade I and grade II acromioclavicular injuries are treated conservatively with sling support for 1 to 2 weeks, followed by gentle active use of the arm. Most grade III separations can be treated with sling immobilization for several weeks until the pain subsides, followed by range-of-motion and shoulder-strengthening exercises. However, some orthopedic surgeons believe that open reduction of grade III injuries is needed for optimal functional results. Surgical repair consists of fixing the clavicle to the coracoid process, plus reapproximating and repairing the coracoclavicular ligaments.

Dislocation of Sternoclavicular Joint. The sternoclavicular joint has almost no inherent stability provided by bone. Joint stability depends on the ligaments that attach the clavicle to the sternum. Despite its inherent instability, the sternoclavicular joint is rarely dislocated because its location protects it from most injury forces. A direct blow to the medial clavicle may dislocate the clavicle

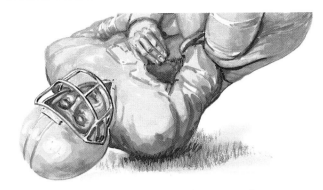

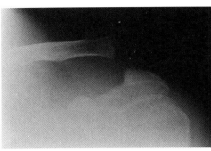

Stress radiograph. Taken with patient holding 10–lb weight, accentuating separation of acromioclavicular joint

Injury to acromioclavicular joint. Usually caused by fall on tip of shoulder, depressing acromion (shoulder separation)

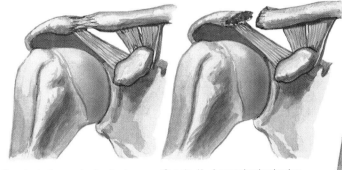

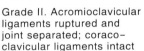

Grade I. Acromioclavicular ligaments stretched but not torn; coracoclavicular ligaments intact

Grade II. Acromioclavicular ligaments ruptured and joint separated; coraco-clavicular ligaments intact

Grade III. Coracoclavicular and acromioclavicular ligaments ruptured, with wide separation of joint

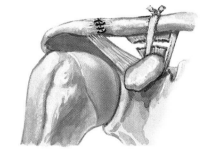

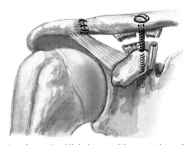

Repair of grade III injury with nonabsorbable tape (above) or screw (below)

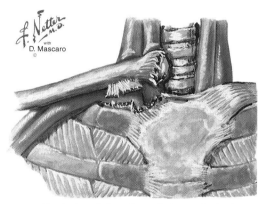

Posterior dislocation of sternoclavicular joint. Serious because of probable injury to trachea or vessels. Both posterior and anterior dislocations can usually be reduced manually or with aid of towel clip. Anesthesia needed

posteriorly, to behind the sternum. An indirect force on the lateral aspect of the shoulder may rotate the medial end of the clavicle to a point either anterior or posterior to the sternum. Displacement of the clavicle anterior to the sternum, the most common pattern of dislocation, is most easily seen on a cephalic tilt radiograph of the sternoclavicular joint. Reduction requires local or general anesthesia. The patient is placed supine on a sandbag placed between the shoulders. Traction is then applied to the upper limb in line with the clavicle and gentle manual pressure to the medial aspect of the anteriorly displaced clavicle.

Posterior dislocations are rare but are potentially much more serious than anterior dislocations because the posteriorly displaced clavicle can place direct pressure on vital structures in the neck, especially the trachea. Reduction can usually be accomplished by placing the patient on a sandbag in the same position as described above and applying longitudinal traction to the affected upper limb; general anesthesia is required. In some instances, the medial clavicle must be grasped with a percutaneously placed towel clip and pulled anteriorly to obtain reduction.

In both anterior or posterior dislocations, moderate instability often persists after reduction.

Anterior Dislocation of Glenohumeral Joint

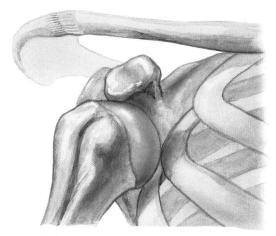

Subcoracoid dislocation (most common)

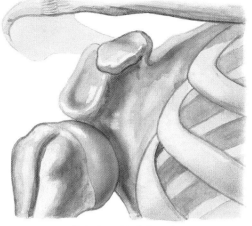

Subglenoid dislocation

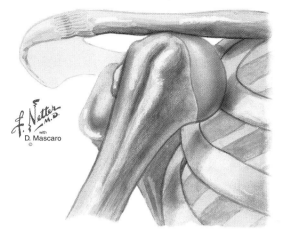

Subclavicular dislocation (uncommon). Very rarely, humeral head penetrates between ribs, producing intrathoracic dislocation

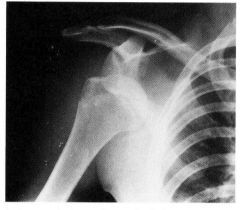

Anteroposterior radiograph. Subcoracoid dislocation

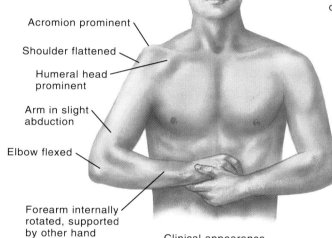

Acromion prominent

Shoulder flattened

Humeral head prominent

Arm in slight abduction

Elbow flexed

Forearm internally rotated, supported by other hand

Clinical appearance

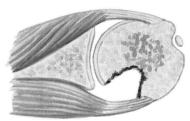

Testing sensation in areas of (1) axillary and (2) musculocutaneous nerves

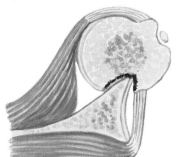

Long tendon of biceps brachii m.

Lesser tuberosity

Head of humerus

Glenoid cavity

Subscapularis m.

Infraspinatus m.

Normal indentation

Greater tuberosity

Section through normal glenohumeral joint

Stages in formation of Hill–Sachs lesion

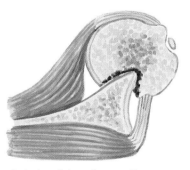

Anterior dislocation. Anterior rim of glenoid indents postero-lateral part of humeral head

Anterior dislocation continues; indentation in humeral head enlarges

After reduction. Defect persists, causing instability and predisposing to recurrent dislocation

---

SECTION I PLATE 35   Slide 4811

Injury to Shoulder and Humerus

(Continued)

Recurrent or unreduced anterior dislocations result in a visible deformity but usually remain asymptomatic. If degenerative changes persist, the medial end of the clavicle can be resected, with care to spare the costoclavicular ligament.

Anterior Dislocation of Glenohumeral Joint

About 95% of shoulder dislocations are anterior and are chiefly due to an indirect mechanism (Plate 35). Abduction, extension, and external rotation forces on the arm injure the anterior supporting structures of the shoulder, including the capsule and anterior portions of the rotator cuff.

Anterior dislocations are most commonly seen in adolescents and young adults and are often due to athletic injuries. In the older patient, a similar force is more likely to result in a fracture. The anteriorly dislocated humeral head can be

displaced to one of several positions in relation to the glenoid rim: a subcoracoid, subglenoid, or subclavicular location is possible. The clinical appearance of anterior dislocations is characteristic. Anteroposterior and lateral radiographs accurately delineate the position of the dislocated humeral head. Initial clinical evaluation includes a careful neurovascular examination of the involved limb. Before reduction is attempted, it is especially important to determine whether the axillary nerve has been injured.

Also characteristic of an anterior shoulder dislocation is a defect in the posteromedial aspect of the humeral head, called the Hill-Sachs lesion.

Reduction of Anterior Dislocation of Glenohumeral Joint

Injury to Shoulder and Humerus

(Continued)

This indentation fracture is created by impingement of the humeral head against the anterior margin of the glenoid rim. A Hill-Sachs lesion further destabilizes the glenohumeral joint, predisposing it to recurrent anterior dislocations. Special radiographic views or computed tomography is sometimes necessary to demonstrate a Hill-Sachs lesion and should be performed for recurrent anterior dislocation when surgical repair is contemplated.

Reduction of Anterior Dislocation of Glenohumeral Joint

Many methods are used to reduce anterior dislocation of the glenohumeral joint (Plate 36). Because leverage methods are more likely to cause additional injury to the shoulder, they have generally been abandoned in favor of traction methods, which involve applying a force in line with the humerus, usually combined with superior and lateral elevation of the humeral head. Simple traction is usually successful when the dislocation is only several minutes old; for dislocations treated later, both traction and countertraction are needed. Intravenous analgesics and muscle relaxants can be used, but reduction is often possible with a minimum of medication.

Hippocratic Maneuver. In the original Hippocratic maneuver, traction and countertraction are supplied by one person. The examiner must be careful not to place the heel in the axilla against the brachial plexus. Traction should be slow and gentle, with slight internal and external rotation of the arm to free the humeral head.

Stimson Maneuver. The Stimson maneuver is a gentler type of reduction but may take as long as 25 minutes. Failure of this method is usually due to insufficient muscle relaxation, which can be overcome with the use of intravenous analgesics and muscle relaxants.

Milch Maneuver. The least traumatic method of reduction, the Milch maneuver can usually be performed without intravenous analgesics. Since the patient with an anterior dislocation holds the arm in slight abduction and internal rotation, continuous traction is first applied to the arm in this position. The examiner must reassure the patient that no sudden manipulation will be performed. Patient reassurance is essential to avoid the need for heavy sedation. During 5 to 10 minutes, the direction of traction is changed gradually to bring the arm into full abduction. At the same time, the arm is brought from internal into external rotation. As the arm approaches 120° abduction and 60° external rotation, reduction usually occurs spontaneously. Sometimes, direct pressure on the humeral head is needed.

Following reduction, the shoulder is immobilized in a sling for 1 to 4 weeks, depending on the age of the patient. Patients more than 60 years

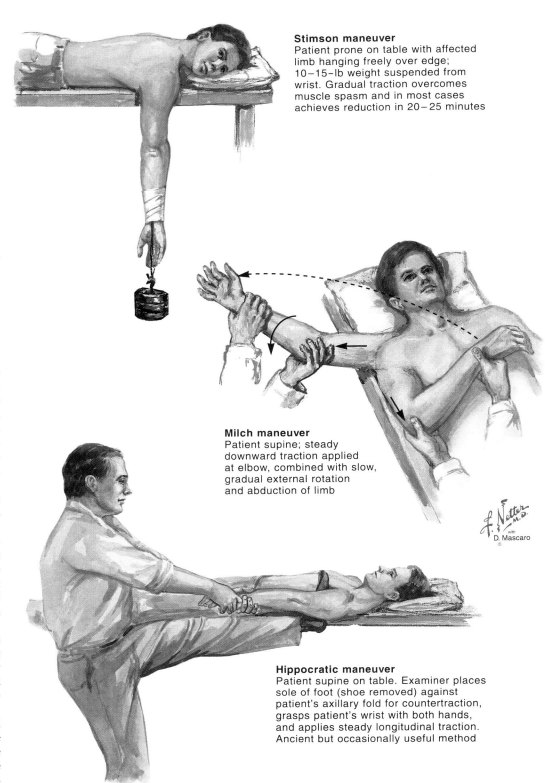

Stimson maneuver
Patient prone on table with affected limb hanging freely over edge; 10–15-lb weight suspended from wrist. Gradual traction overcomes muscle spasm and in most cases achieves reduction in 20–25 minutes

Milch maneuver
Patient supine; steady downward traction applied at elbow, combined with slow, gradual external rotation and abduction of limb

Hippocratic maneuver
Patient supine on table. Examiner places sole of foot (shoe removed) against patient's axillary fold for countertraction, grasps patient's wrist with both hands, and applies steady longitudinal traction. Ancient but occasionally useful method

of age are prone to persistent shoulder stiffness, and immobilization should be for 1 week only. Patients less than 20 years of age, who are prone to recurrent dislocation, should be immobilized for 4 weeks.

Following immobilization, gentle range-of-motion exercises are begun and gradually increased. Full activity and sports can be resumed in 4 to 6 months. Surgery is reserved for irreducible dislocations or displaced fractures of the humeral head or glenoid rim. Recurrent dislocations may require revision surgery.

The incidence of recurrent dislocations decreases with age, and recurrence is more common in men than in women. Surgical repair is needed to reconstruct the chronically stretched and insufficient structures of the anterior capsule.

Posterior Dislocation of Glenohumeral Joint

Because posterior dislocations are rare (1%) and clinical diagnosis is difficult, they often go unrecognized (Plate 37). The most common cause is a combination of indirect forces—internal rotation, adduction, and flexion—as may occur with seizures or electric shock. The humeral head is most commonly dislocated to the subacromial region. Clinical examination reveals blocked abduction and external rotation. The shoulder appears nearly

Posterior Dislocation of Glenohumeral Joint

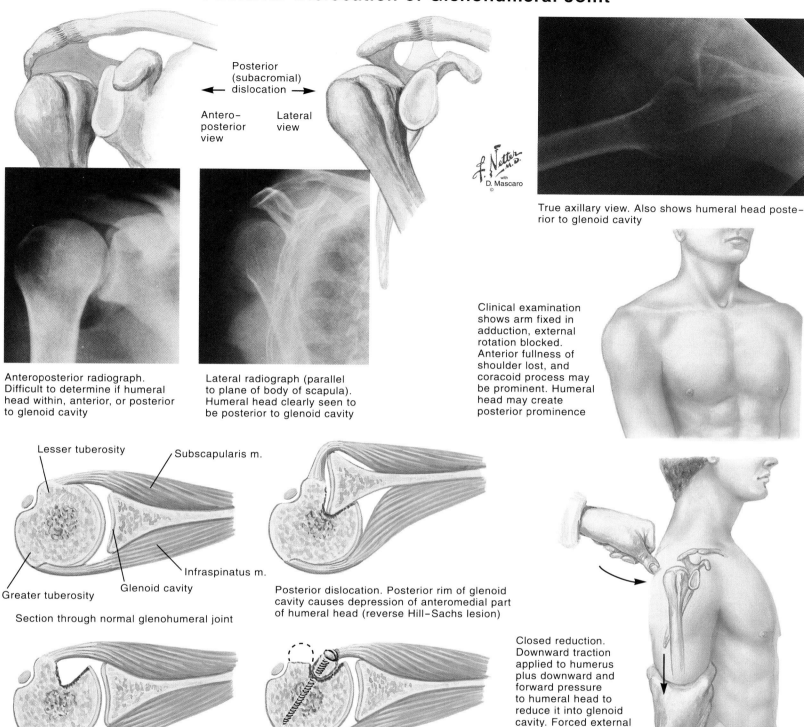

Posterior (subacromial) dislocation

← Antero-posterior view

Lateral view →

True axillary view. Also shows humeral head posterior to glenoid cavity

Anteroposterior radiograph. Difficult to determine if humeral head within, anterior, or posterior to glenoid cavity

Lateral radiograph (parallel to plane of body of scapula). Humeral head clearly seen to be posterior to glenoid cavity

Clinical examination shows arm fixed in adduction, external rotation blocked. Anterior fullness of shoulder lost, and coracoid process may be prominent. Humeral head may create posterior prominence

Lesser tuberosity   Subscapularis m.

Greater tuberosity   Glenoid cavity   Infraspinatus m.

Section through normal glenohumeral joint

Posterior dislocation. Posterior rim of glenoid cavity causes depression of anteromedial part of humeral head (reverse Hill–Sachs lesion)

Closed reduction. Downward traction applied to humerus plus downward and forward pressure to humeral head to reduce it into glenoid cavity. Forced external rotation must be avoided as fracture of head or shaft may result

Closed reduction. Persistent defect, instability, and tendency to redislocate

Open reduction. Subscapularis tendon or lesser tuberosity with tendon transplanted into defect

Injury to Shoulder and Humerus

(Continued)

normal on anteroposterior radiographs, but the injury is usually clearly visualized on the axillary lateral radiograph.

Reduction should be attempted as soon as an acute posterior dislocation is diagnosed. After the administration of intravenous analgesics and muscle relaxants, traction is applied in line with the humerus; direct manual pressure is then exerted on the humeral head to reduce it. If the shoulder is stable after reduction, a simple shoulder immobilizer is applied. Shoulder instability after reduction necessitates the use of a shoulder spica cast or orthosis to hold the limb in the reduced position, usually by securing the arm in external rotation. Exercises are begun after 4 weeks of immobilization.

Posterior dislocations frequently produce a defect in the anteromedial portion of the humeral head, the so-called reverse Hill-Sachs lesion. If the defect is large, a surgical procedure must be designed to fill the defect and prevent recurrent dislocation. If less than 20% of the joint surface is involved, the joint usually remains stable after reduction. For defects that involve 20% to 50% of the joint surface, the subscapularis tendon can be transferred into the defect (Plate 37).

A special problem is an old undiagnosed dislocation. Elderly patients with a functional range of motion and minimal discomfort require no treatment. Surgical reconstruction is indicated in younger patients and elderly patients with pain, limitation of motion, and good bone stock. Total joint replacement may be necessary.

Fracture of Proximal Humerus

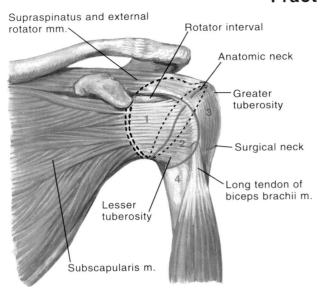

Supraspinatus and external rotator mm.

Rotator interval

Anatomic neck

Greater tuberosity

Surgical neck

Long tendon of biceps brachii m.

Lesser tuberosity

Subscapularis m.

Neer four-part classification of fractures of proximal humerus. 1. Articular fragment (humeral head). 2. Lesser tuberosity. 3. Greater tuberosity. 4. Shaft. If no fragments displaced, fracture considered stable (most common) and treated with minimal external immobilization and early range-of-motion exercise. Displacement of 1 cm or angulation of 45° of one or more fragments necessitates open reduction and internal fixation or prosthetic replacement

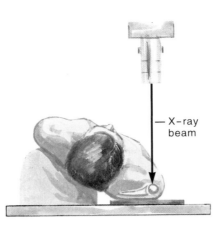

X-ray beam

Radiographic techniques for visualizing shoulder trauma

Above. Projection perpendicular to plane of body of scapula. Radiograph shows fracture of surgical neck

Below. Projection parallel to plane of body of scapula

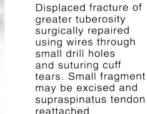

X-ray beam

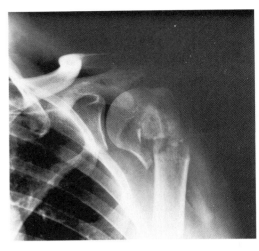

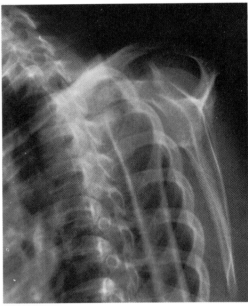

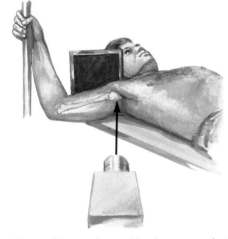

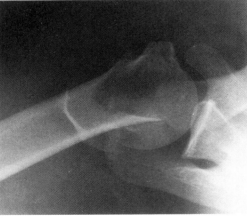

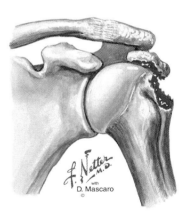

Displaced fracture of greater tuberosity surgically repaired using wires through small drill holes and suturing cuff tears. Small fragment may be excised and supraspinatus tendon reattached

True axillary radiographic view very valuable in evaluating glenohumeral fractures or dislocations, especially in determining location of humeral head fragment. Radiograph shows extracapsular fracture of shaft of proximal humerus

Injury to Shoulder and Humerus

(Continued)

Fracture of Proximal Humerus

Fractures of the proximal humerus are common, occurring most frequently in older patients from a fall on the outstretched hand (Plate 38).

The four-part classification proposed by Neer requires identification of the following four major fracture fragments and their relationships to one another on initial radiographs: (1) articular segment, (2) greater tuberosity with the attached supraspinatus muscle, (3) lesser tuberosity with the attached subscapularis muscle, and (4) humeral shaft.

The fragment is considered displaced if the displacement is greater than 1 cm or the angulation greater than 45°. On the initial axillary lateral radiograph, it is also important to determine if the articular fragment is displaced outside the joint space (ie, fracture dislocation). About 80%

of fractures are minimally displaced. Because the fragments are held in place by the intact rotator cuff and periosteum, they move together as a unit. Minimally displaced fractures are amenable to closed immobilization for approximately 4 weeks, followed by early passive motion and later active exercises. Displaced fractures are unstable and often cannot be reduced with closed means; they can also be associated with loss of circulation to the humeral head. Displaced two-part and three-part fractures require open reduction and internal fixation. Displaced four-part fractures are best treated by replacing the proximal humerus with a prosthesis.

Exercises for Fracture of Proximal Humerus

Passive stretching exercises

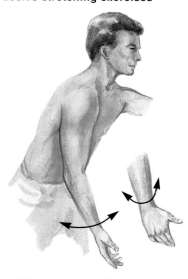

Bend forward, letting limb hang freely. Swing limb like pendulum forward and backward and side to side. Rotate hand inward and outward

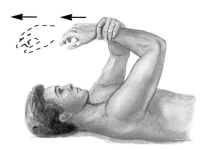

Raise hand over head, using opposite arm for power

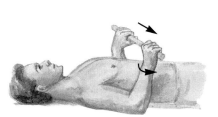

Externally rotate arm using broomstick and good arm for power

Internally rotate arm by pulling wrist backward and upward behind back with good arm

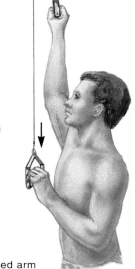

Raise affected arm with pulley placed at least 2 feet higher than reach

Active muscle–strengthening exercises

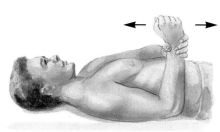

With elbow flexed, exert flexion and extension forces against resistance provided by good arm

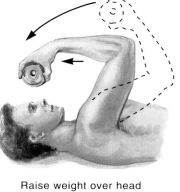

Raise weight over head with affected limb

Stretch rubber strip

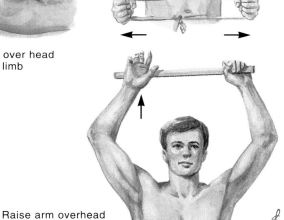

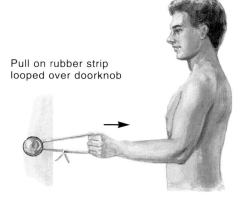

Pull on rubber strip looped over doorknob

Raise arm overhead guided by broomstick held in good hand

Push rubber strip looped over doorknob forward, away from body

f. Netter M.D. with D. Mascaro

Injury to Shoulder and Humerus

(Continued)

Exercises for Fracture of Proximal Humerus

Patients with minimally displaced fractures can begin range-of-motion exercises quite early. If the shaft fragment is not impacted, the arm must be immobilized until the shaft begins to unite with the other fragments (1–3 weeks) before exercises are started. As soon as possible, the patient begins gentle and passive exercises (Plate 39). These consist of standing pendulum swings and supine passive elevation and external rotation. After about 2 weeks, standing pulley and internal rotation exercises are added. When union has occurred and a good passive range of motion has been achieved, active exercises are added to restore strength. These begin with isometrics, with the uninjured arm assisting the recovering arm in abduction, adduction, and internal and external rotation. Supine weight lifting is then added, as well as tension exercises using rubber strips. Finally, active-assisted exercises to strengthen arm elevation are performed until the injured arm can be moved without assistance.

Fracture of Shaft of Humerus

Fractures of the humeral shaft are generally due to direct trauma. Nonsurgical treatment is generally preferred, and the choice of method is based on the type and location of the fracture, concomitant injuries, and age and condition of the patient. For closed fractures, a coaptation (sugar tong) splint or a collar and a light hanging arm cast produce good results (Plate 40). About

Fracture of Shaft of Humerus

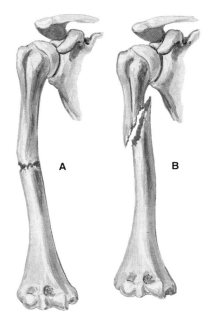

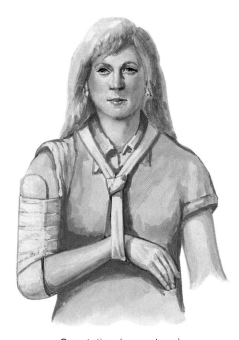

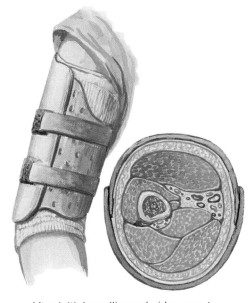

A. Transverse fracture of midshaft
B. Oblique (spiral) fracture
C. Comminuted fracture with marked angulation

Coaptation (sugar tong) splint. Effective method of closed treatment for most fractures of shaft

After initial swelling subsides, most fractures of shaft of humerus can be treated with functional brace of interlocking anterior and posterior components held together with Velcro straps

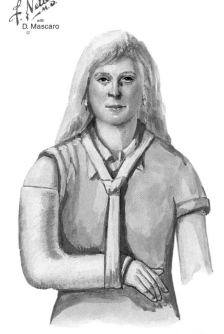

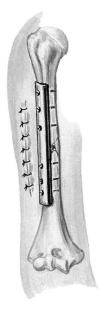

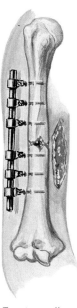

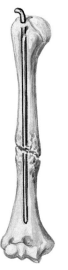

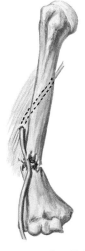

Patient with hanging arm cast and neck collar sling. Weight of cast promotes reduction, but overdistraction must be avoided because it could lead to nonunion

Open reduction and fixation with compression plate indicated under special conditions

Fracture aligned and held with external fixator. Most useful for wounds requiring frequent changes of dressing

Fixation of pathologic fracture with intramedullary Rush nail

Entrapment of radial nerve in fracture of shaft of distal humerus may occur at time of fracture; must also be avoided during reduction. Loss of nerve function after reduction requires surgical exploration

SECTION I PLATE 40   Slide 4816

Injury to Shoulder and Humerus

(Continued)

10 days after injury, when the initial swelling has subsided, the patient is fitted with a fracture brace, which allows the patient to exercise the hand, wrist, elbow, and shoulder while maintaining fracture alignment.

Fractures of the humeral shaft usually heal with no significant deformity and with excellent function. Internal fixation is indicated for (1) segmental fractures that cannot be satisfactorily aligned, (2) associated injuries of the elbow that make early motion desirable, (3) associated injuries that require several weeks of bed rest (fracture alignment may be difficult if gravity cannot be used to help control it), (4) pathologic fractures, (5) fractures associated with vascular injury, and (6) radial nerve palsy that develops after reduction. Radial nerve palsy is usually due to nerve entrapment in the fracture site during reduction. This complication necessitates surgical exploration

and decompression of the nerve. At the same time, open reduction and internal fixation are performed to avoid further injury to the nerve by moving fracture fragments.

Internal fixation usually incorporates a compression plate. Intramedullary fixation may be performed, but in most cases, intramedullary rods merely serve as internal splints to maintain alignment. External fixators have been successfully used for humerus fractures. The usual indication is a large soft tissue wound that requires frequent changes of dressing. External fixation allows access to the wound while still maintaining satisfactory fracture alignment and position. ☐

Injury to Elbow

Dislocation of Elbow Joint

Dislocations of the elbow joint are the most common dislocations after those of the shoulder and finger joints. Swelling, pain, and pseudoparalysis of the arm are acute signs and symptoms of dislocation, and elbow deformity is visible on both clinical and radiographic examinations.

Posterior elbow dislocation, the most common type, usually results from a fall on the outstretched hand (Plate 41). The elbow may also dislocate medially, laterally, or anteriorly. The rare but extensively studied anterior dislocation of the elbow is usually an open injury and may lacerate the brachial artery. Rarely, the radius and ulna dislocate in different directions, an injury called divergent dislocation.

Dislocations of the elbow are sometimes accompanied by fractures of the medial epicondyle, olecranon, radial head, or coronoid process of the ulna. Fracture dislocations of the elbow, especially displaced fractures of the olecranon and radial head, often require surgical reduction to ensure long-term stability and function of the joint. An avulsed medial epicondyle can become wedged inside the joint during reduction of the dislocation. Only occasionally can closed manipulation free the avulsed fragment from within the joint; arthrotomy is usually needed to remove the fragment and return it to its anatomic position. Generally, fractures of the coronoid process do not require anatomic fixation unless the elbow is very unstable following reduction or unless the fragment is significantly displaced.

Reduction of Dislocation of Elbow Joint

A posterior dislocation of the elbow is reduced with distal traction (Plate 42). While an assistant secures the proximal humerus, the examiner applies traction in the line of the forearm, then gently flexes the elbow joint to allow the humerus to reduce into the olecranon fossa. If the elbow is reduced immediately after dislocation, complete muscle relaxation may not be needed; if treatment is delayed, intravenous analgesics, axillary block, or general anesthesia is used to induce complete muscle relaxation. The neurovascular status of the distal limb is checked both before and after reduction. Any changes or abnormalities suggest entrapment of a nerve or vessel during reduction, which must be relieved promptly to prevent a long-term deficit.

Dislocation of Elbow Joint

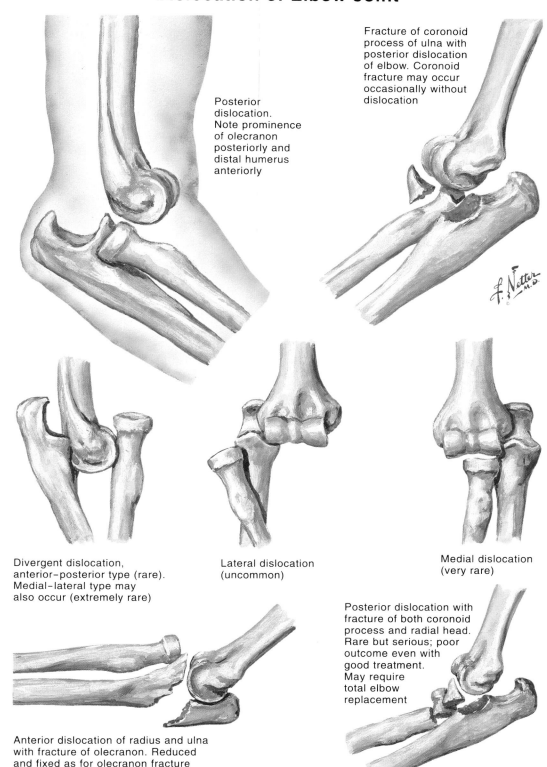

Posterior dislocation. Note prominence of olecranon posteriorly and distal humerus anteriorly

Fracture of coronoid process of ulna with posterior dislocation of elbow. Coronoid fracture may occur occasionally without dislocation

Divergent dislocation, anterior–posterior type (rare). Medial–lateral type may also occur (extremely rare)

Lateral dislocation (uncommon)

Medial dislocation (very rare)

Anterior dislocation of radius and ulna with fracture of olecranon. Reduced and fixed as for olecranon fracture without dislocation

Posterior dislocation with fracture of both coronoid process and radial head. Rare but serious; poor outcome even with good treatment. May require total elbow replacement

After the initial reduction, the examiner moves the elbow through a full range of motion to assess its stability and to check for crepitus in the joint. Crepitus strongly suggests loose fracture fragments in the joint. If the elbow remains stable through a full range of motion, it is immobilized in 90° flexion in a posterior splint. The neurovascular status of the limb is monitored frequently while the elbow is splinted to ensure that a deficit does not develop. Open reduction of elbow dislocation is reserved for (1) injuries in some high-performance athletes, (2) persistent gross instability after closed reduction, and (3) loose bone fragments within the joint.

Initially, all elbow dislocations require posterior splinting, but the splint is usually removed every day for early range-of-motion exercises. The exercises should be gentle but as active as symptoms permit. The physician's assessment of the degree of stability after reduction helps determine what range of motion to allow and when to begin the exercise program.

Elbow dislocations cause few long-term complications. By far the most common is residual joint stiffness. Although some degree of stiffness almost always persists, early active motion can minimize this problem. The older the patient, the earlier active elbow movement should be started.

Reduction of Dislocation of Elbow Joint

Injury to Elbow
(Continued)

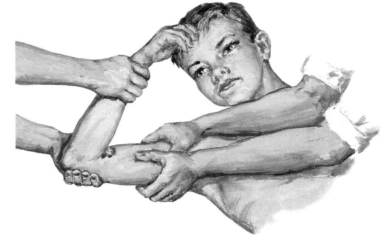

Examiner grasps patient's wrist and applies traction to forearm, keeping elbow extended as far as possible; assistant supplies countertraction. Examiner's hand at elbow applies gentle downward pressure on proximal forearm to release coronoid process from olecranon fossa and also corrects medial or lateral deviation

Myositis ossificans, another complication of elbow dislocation, results from muscle injury at the time of dislocation. Myositis ossificans is more likely to develop after severe injuries and when treatment has been delayed. Early passive motion is discouraged in patients with dislocation and muscle injury because excessive muscle stretching only precipitates the development of more myositis.

Recurrent dislocations of the elbow are uncommon and are thought to be due to damage to the posterolateral ligaments. Surgical repair of these chronically damaged ligaments may yield a reasonably good result.

Fracture of Head and Neck of Radius

Fractures of the radial head occur primarily in adults, whereas fractures of the radial neck are more common in children. The usual causes of these injuries are indirect trauma, such as a fall on the outstretched hand, and less commonly a direct blow to the elbow (Plate 43). Radial head fractures are generally classified into four groups. In type I fractures, the articular surface is nondisplaced. Type II fractures refer to fractures of the joint margin with displacement or depression of a portion of the radial head. Type III fractures are comminuted and involve the entire radial head. Type IV fractures are associated with dislocation of the elbow.

Diagnosis of a radial head fracture may be difficult. Pain, effusion in the elbow, and tenderness on palpation directly over the radial head are the typical manifestations. If the fracture is displaced, a "click" or crepitus over the radial head is detected during supination or pronation. Radiographic findings in nondisplaced fractures are minimal, and the radiograph often shows only swelling in the elbow with displacement of the anterior or the posterior fat pad. Any radiographic evidence of fat pad displacement accompanied by tenderness over the radial head strongly suggests a radial head fracture.

Initial treatment of a radial head fracture consists of a careful clinical and radiographic evaluation. If on the radiograph the fracture appears nondisplaced or minimally displaced, the elbow joint should be aspirated to remove blood and effusion. The skin over the joint is cleaned with antiseptic solution for 10 minutes. Then, a 16-gauge needle is introduced into the joint at

Elbow gently flexed as traction and countertraction maintained. Slight "click" usually heard or felt as reduction occurs. Elbow then tested through full range of motion. Reduction may be accomplished without anesthesia in some cases, but axillary block, intravenous, or even general anesthesia needed for some patients. Same procedure used for lateral, medial, or divergent dislocation with appropriate medial, lateral, or compressive pressure applied

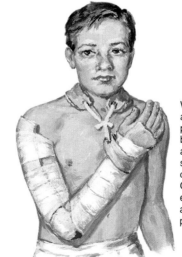

With elbow in about 110° flexion, posterior slab splint bandaged in place, and upper limb suspended with collar and cuff sling. Gentle active exercises begun as soon as pain permits

Associated fracture of coronoid process, if nondisplaced or minimally displaced, usually heals well with immobilization only. Widely separated fragment often reduced with thumb pressure; if joint remains unstable after reduction, pinning with Kirschner wires may be needed

the center of the triangle formed by the head of the radius, the lateral epicondyle of the humerus, and the tip of the olecranon. After the hematoma is aspirated from the elbow joint, 20 to 30 ml of lidocaine is injected into the joint to relieve pain and allow a thorough examination.

The examiner moves the elbow through a full range of motion to assess the degree of flexion-extension and pronation-supination and to detect any crepitus or blocked motion due to a displaced bone. If the range of motion is adequate and there is no bone block or significant crepitus, the elbow is placed in a posterior splint for 48 hours. After this period, the patient can remove the splint and

begin active range-of-motion exercises for the injured elbow. Frequent follow-up radiographs are necessary to detect any late displacement of the fracture fragment.

Controversy surrounds the treatment of displaced and comminuted fractures of the radial head or neck and fractures associated with limited range of motion due to a fracture fragment. Surgical fixation is indicated for fractures with one or two large, displaced fragments that can be effectively reduced and stabilized with screws or wires. Comminuted fractures that cannot be adequately reduced and stabilized with surgery usually require excision of the entire radial head.

Injury to Elbow
(Continued)

Fracture of Head and Neck of Radius

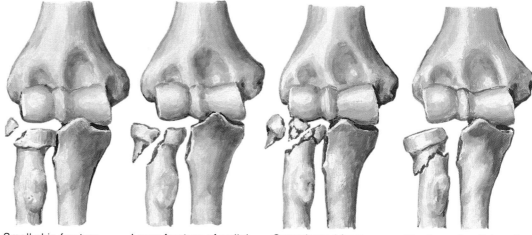

Small chip fracture of radial head

Large fracture of radial head with displacement

Comminuted fracture of radial head

Fracture of radial neck, tilted and impacted

When the radial head is removed, the annular ligament must be preserved to maintain the integrity of the ligament complex of the proximal radioulnar joint. Radial head implants made of silicone are available, but the indications for their use are limited. These implants should be used only to treat elbow instability that persists after resection of the radial head and the uncommon Essex-Lopresti fracture (fracture of the radial head plus dislocation of the distal radioulnar joint). In this type of fracture, the radius migrates proximally after the radial head is excised, which is very debilitating to the entire forearm complex. Use of the radial head implant as a spacer prevents proximal migration of the radius and minimizes long-term complications.

Dislocations of the elbow with comminuted fractures of the radial head (type IV) are serious injuries that usually involve significant soft tissue injury. Both the joint capsule and the brachialis muscle are damaged, and the joint injury often leads to stiffness, osteoarthritic changes, and myositis ossificans. If surgery is appropriate and feasible, these type IV injuries should be surgically repaired within 48 hours of injury. It is believed that prompt repair decreases the postoperative incidence of myositis ossificans.

Supracondylar Fracture of Humerus

Supracondylar fractures of the humerus are much more common in children and adolescents than in adults. In children, the fracture typically involves the thin bone between the coronoid fossa and the olecranon fossa of the distal humerus, and the fracture line angles from an anterior distal point to a posterior proximal site. In adults, supracondylar fractures are not usually confined to the extraarticular portion of the distal humerus, as in children, but extend into the elbow joint.

The most frequent cause of supracondylar fractures of the humerus is a fall on the outstretched hand (Plate 44). By far the most common fracture pattern is an extension-type injury with posterior displacement of the distal fragment; only 10% of supracondylar fractures are flexion-type injuries with anterior displacement of the distal fragment.

Supracondylar fractures are classified as (1) fractures without displacement, (2) fractures with minimal lateral displacement, (3) fractures with rotation (with or without lateral displacement), and (4) fractures with complete displacement and no contact between the fragments.

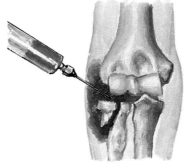

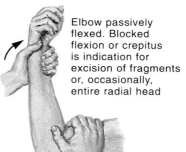

Elbow passively flexed. Blocked flexion or crepitus is indication for excision of fragments or, occasionally, entire radial head

Hematoma aspirated, and 20–30 ml of xylocaine injected to permit painless testing of joint mobility

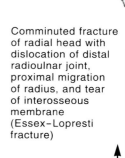

Small fractures without limitation of flexion heal well after aspiration with only sling support

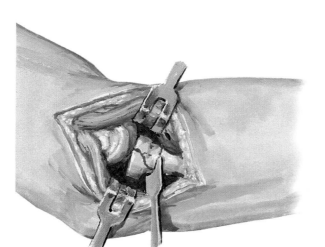

Excision of fragment or entire radial head via posterolateral incision. Radial head may be replaced with Swanson silicone implant in selected patients

Comminuted fracture of radial head with dislocation of distal radioulnar joint, proximal migration of radius, and tear of interosseous membrane (Essex–Lopresti fracture)

In the evaluation of any fracture, careful assessment of the neurovascular status is important, but this assessment is even more critical in supracondylar fractures of the elbow because of the proximity of the brachial artery to the distal spike of the proximal fragment. Vascular insult and Volkmann ischemic contracture frequently result in this type of fracture.

Before reduction, the fractured elbow should be splinted in extension so that arterial circulation is not compromised by flexion of the distal fragment. When the injury is evaluated in the emergency department, the neurovascular status of the limb should be carefully determined and

monitored. The supracondylar fracture should be reduced as soon as possible after injury, preferably with the patient under general anesthesia. Closed reduction is carried out by gentle distal traction in the line of the forearm until the humerus is restored to its full length. The medial or lateral angulation is corrected, and in extension-type injuries, the elbow is flexed greater than 90°. With the elbow in extreme flexion, the posterior periosteum and the aponeurosis of the triceps brachii muscle act as a hinge to maintain the reduction of the fragments. This position is secured with a plaster splint for 4 to 6 weeks to prevent redisplacement of the fracture fragments.

Supracondylar Fracture of Humerus

Injury to Elbow
(Continued)

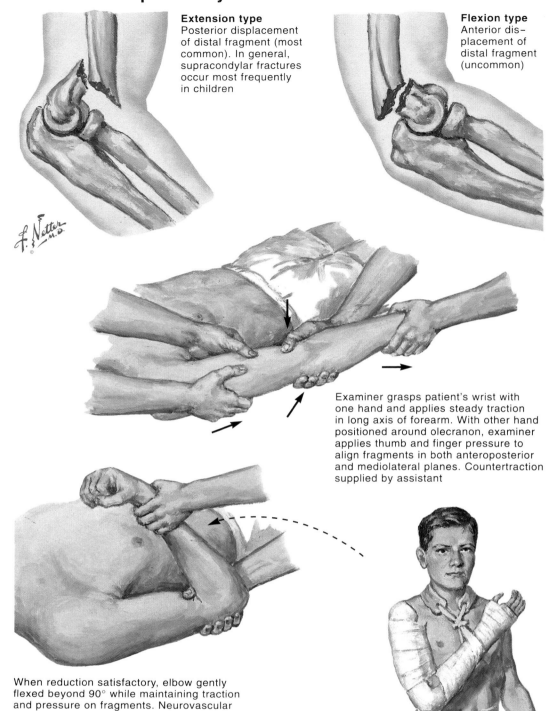

Extension type
Posterior displacement of distal fragment (most common). In general, supracondylar fractures occur most frequently in children

Flexion type
Anterior displacement of distal fragment (uncommon)

Examiner grasps patient's wrist with one hand and applies steady traction in long axis of forearm. With other hand positioned around olecranon, examiner applies thumb and finger pressure to align fragments in both anteroposterior and mediolateral planes. Countertraction supplied by assistant

When reduction satisfactory, elbow gently flexed beyond 90° while maintaining traction and pressure on fragments. Neurovascular status must be monitored carefully

With elbow in flexion, posterior slab splint bandaged in place and worn for 4–6 weeks

Note: in supracondylar fractures, entrapment of brachial artery or nerve by trauma or during reduction must be prevented to avoid Volkmann contracture

In assessing the reduction achieved, displacement in the anteroposterior plane is not nearly as important as the presence of lateral or medial angulation. If the fracture heals with the distal fragment tilted medially or laterally, a significant deformity—cubitus varus or cubitus valgus—results. Varus or valgus angulation after reduction is best diagnosed on an anteroposterior radiograph or a Jones view of the elbow, which reveals a lack of contact between the two bone fragments on one cortex.

If the adequacy of the reduction or of the vascular supply of the limb is in question, the fracture should be treated either with percutaneous pin fixation performed under image intensification or with open reduction and internal fixation. Image intensification allows closed reduction of the fracture and percutaneous insertion of two Kirschner wires. Open reduction is usually done through a lateral approach to the distal humerus. After internal fixation, the elbow can be splinted in any angle of flexion to avoid compromising the function of the brachial artery. Supracondylar fractures can also be treated with traction using a pin placed in the olecranon or with skin traction using the Dunlop method.

The major long-term complication of very severe fractures is a change in the carrying angle of the elbow, primarily cubitus varus. Neurologic injury, while not common, does occur and can involve either the median, radial, or ulnar nerve. Vascular injury is a devastating complication because it can lead to Volkmann contracture. All elbow fractures can potentially result in decreased motion.

Fracture of Distal Humerus

In adults, fractures of the distal humerus are uncommon and usually require some form of surgical fixation (Plate 45).

Fracture of Lateral Condyle. Fractures of the lateral condyle that involve the capitulum alone or extend medially to involve the lateral portion of the trochlea are usually displaced and require surgical treatment. As with any joint fracture, the method of choice is open reduction and internal fixation to reestablish the articular surface as accurately as possible and to allow early active motion. In fractures of the lateral condyles, both in adults and in children, it is important to preserve all the soft tissue attachments and thus maintain the blood supply to the fragment. With rigid internal fixation, the patient can begin active motion as soon as the soft tissues have healed.

Fracture of Medial Epicondyle. The medial epicondyle is the common origin of several flexor muscles of the hand and wrist. When the medial epicondyle is fractured, the flexor muscles pull the fragment distally. The injury is often accompanied by valgus instability of the elbow and injury to the ulnar nerve. If there is significant valgus instability of the elbow, the epicondyle must be reduced into its anatomic position and secured with a pin or a screw. During the surgical procedure, care must be taken to protect the ulnar nerve from injury.

Fracture of Capitulum. Fractures of the capitulum are also uncommon and may be difficult to diagnose if the fracture fragment is very small. Any effusion within the elbow joint together with displacement of the fat pads suggests either a capitulum fracture or a nondisplaced fracture of the radial head.

There are two types of capitulum fractures. The type I (Hahn-Steinthal) fracture involves a large part of the osseous portion of the capitulum and is treated with open reduction and fixation with one or two screws. This method makes early joint motion possible in rehabilitation. The type II (Kocher-Lorenz) fracture affects primarily the articular cartilage and very little underlying bone. Treatment includes excision of the fragment. Type II

Fracture of Condyle, Epicondyle, Capitulum, and Olecranon

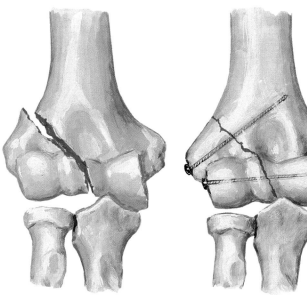

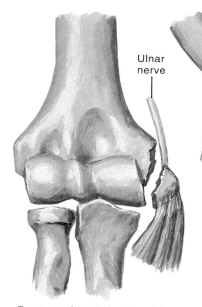

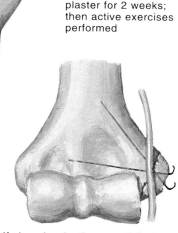

Ulnar nerve

Fragment may be reducible with thumb pressure with elbow in acute flexion. Elbow immobilized in plaster for 2 weeks; then active exercises performed

Fracture of lateral condyle of humerus. Fracture of medial condyle less common

Fractured condyle fixed with one or two compression screws

Fracture of medial epicondyle displaced by pull of flexor muscles of wrist

If closed reduction unsatisfactory, fragment fixed with pins. Ulnar nerve may be transposed anterior to epicondyle

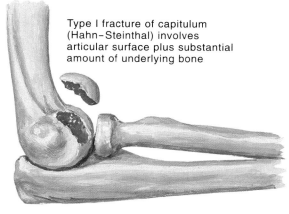

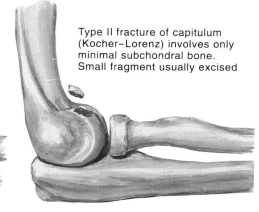

Type I fracture of capitulum (Hahn–Steinthal) involves articular surface plus substantial amount of underlying bone

Fragment reduced and held with screw, which does not penetrate articular surface. Head of radius also supplies support in flexion

Type II fracture of capitulum (Kocher–Lorenz) involves only minimal subchondral bone. Small fragment usually excised

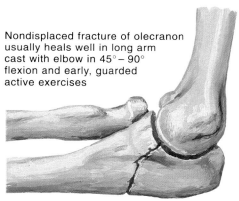

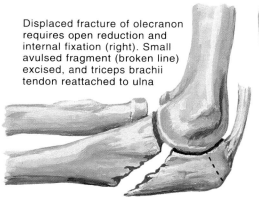

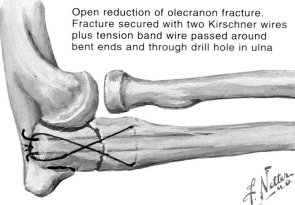

Nondisplaced fracture of olecranon usually heals well in long arm cast with elbow in 45°–90° flexion and early, guarded active exercises

Displaced fracture of olecranon requires open reduction and internal fixation (right). Small avulsed fragment (broken line) excised, and triceps brachii tendon reattached to ulna

Open reduction of olecranon fracture. Fracture secured with two Kirschner wires plus tension band wire passed around bent ends and through drill hole in ulna

Injury to Elbow
(Continued)

fractures cause few subsequent problems in the elbow joint.

Fracture of Olecranon. Nondisplaced fractures of the olecranon can be treated with posterior splinting, but displaced fractures are best stabilized with open reduction and internal fixation.

Fixation with a tension band wire using screws or Kirschner wires is common; axial screws are also used. If the fracture involves a portion of the proximal ulnar shaft, interfragmentary compression with plate fixation is the preferred method.

Excision of the olecranon is an alternative method of treating isolated, displaced fractures if the coronoid process and the anterior soft tissues remain intact. The triceps brachii tendon covers the posterior aspect of the joint capsule before it attaches to the olecranon, and a broad expanse of the aponeurosis of the triceps brachii muscle joins the deep fascia of the forearm distal to the elbow. This expanse ensures good posterior stability of

the elbow joint. Since the triceps brachii muscle is a primary extensor of the forearm, it must be accurately reattached to the distal fragment of the ulna after the olecranon is excised.

Intercondylar Fracture of Elbow Joint

Comminuted intercondylar (T or Y) fractures of the distal humerus are among the more challenging orthopedic injuries, and their reconstruction requires considerable surgical skill (Plate 46). The major complications include restricted elbow motion and early degenerative joint disease.

Surgical fixation of comminuted intercondylar fractures of the elbow is problematic: the distal

Intercondylar (T or Y) Fracture of Elbow Joint

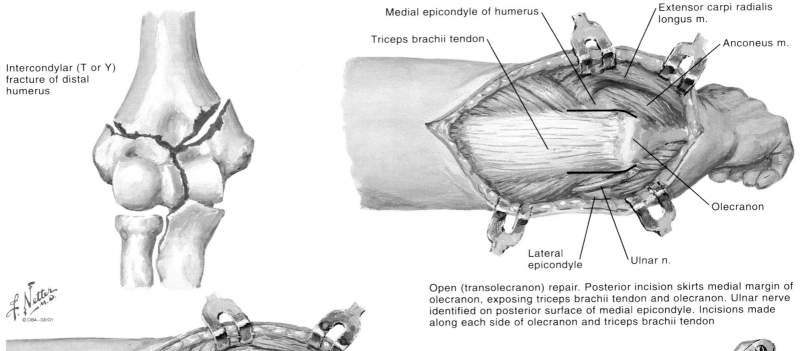

Intercondylar (T or Y) fracture of distal humerus

Medial epicondyle of humerus

Triceps brachii tendon

Extensor carpi radialis longus m.

Anconeus m.

Lateral epicondyle

Ulnar n.

Olecranon

Open (transolecranon) repair. Posterior incision skirts medial margin of olecranon, exposing triceps brachii tendon and olecranon. Ulnar nerve identified on posterior surface of medial epicondyle. Incisions made along each side of olecranon and triceps brachii tendon

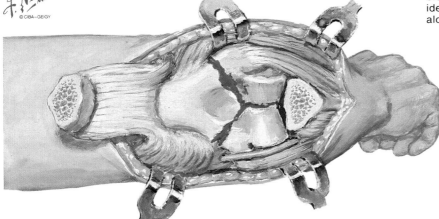

Olecranon osteotomized and reflected proximally with triceps brachii tendon

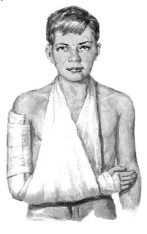

Articular surface of distal humerus reconstructed and fixed with transverse screw and buttress plates with screws. Ulnar nerve may be transposed anteriorly to prevent injury

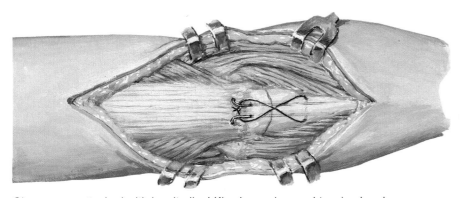

Olecranon reattached with longitudinal Kirschner wires and tension band wire wrapped around them and through hole drilled in ulna

Long posterior splint applied and worn with sling for 6–8 weeks. Guarded active range-of-motion exercises started at 5–8 days

Injury to Elbow
(Continued)

fragments are small, minimizing the number of available screw sites. The distal fragments are primarily cancellous bone, which compromises screw purchase. In addition, the surface of the fracture fragments is primarily articular cartilage, which must be protected, and the complex topography of this region makes contouring of the reconstruction plate difficult.

The structure of the distal humerus should be conceptualized as two bony columns diverging from the shaft. The medial column includes the medial pillar of the distal humerus, the medial epicondyle, and the trochlea. The lateral column includes the lateral pillar of the distal humerus plus the capitulum. To approach intraarticular fractures of the distal humerus, an intraarticular osteotomy of the olecranon is performed, and the olecranon and the aponeurosis of the triceps brachii muscle are reflected proximally, exposing the entire distal humerus. Internal fixation of the distal

humerus first involves reconstructing the articular surface and holding the fragments together with transverse Kirschner wires or lag screws. The articular surface is then reattached to the shaft with lag screws and contoured reconstruction plates to provide stability in both the anteroposterior and mediolateral planes. Attaching the contoured plates at right angles to one another enhances the stability of the repair. The olecranon is reattached with an axial screw or a tension band wire.

Protected active and active-assisted exercises are encouraged soon after the reconstruction to maintain range of motion in the elbow joint. □

Injury to Forearm

Biomechanic Considerations in Fracture of Forearm Bones

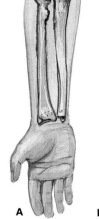
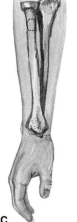
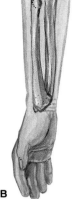
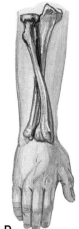

A   **B**   **C**   **D**

Tuberosity of radius useful indicator of degree of pronation or supination of radius
A. In full supination, tuberosity directed toward ulna
B. In about 40° supination, tuberosity primarily posterior
C. In neutral position, tuberosity directly posterior
D. In full pronation, tuberosity directed laterally

Biomechanic Considerations in Fracture of Forearm Bones

The forearm complex comprises two bones, the radius and the ulna, which are tethered together by an interosseous membrane. The forearm also comprises five articulations: the humeroulnar joint, humeroradial joint, proximal and distal radioulnar joints, radiocarpal joint, and many synergistic and antagonistic muscles. Any significant injury to this complex can seriously impair forearm function, particularly flexion, extension, pronation, and supination (Plate 47).

When fractures of the radius and ulna occur in the skeletally mature person, the bones must be returned to their anatomic positions. The ulna is a relatively straight, tubular bone with a very stable articulation with the humerus and runs, essentially subcutaneously, from the olecranon process to the styloid process. The radius has a more complex structure that varies in size and shape from its tuberosity at the proximal end to its wide articulation with the carpal bones. Sage described the characteristics of the radius, stressing the importance of maintaining its lateral bow when reducing fractures. The bowing of the radius is essential for maximal pronation and supination.

Major muscular forces that act to deform the fractured radius are the supinators (the biceps brachii and supinator muscles) and the pronators (the pronator teres and pronator quadratus muscles). In a fracture of the radius above the insertions of the pronator muscles, the proximal fragment is supinated by the biceps brachii muscle. When the fracture is distal to the insertion of the pronator teres muscle, the proximal fragment lies in neutral rotation, and the distal fragment is pronated.

Successful treatment of forearm fractures requires a thorough understanding of the action of the supinator and pronator muscles on the radius and ulna. These bones must be reduced to as near their anatomic positions as possible so that adequate pronation and supination of the forearm are preserved. The integrity of the interosseous membrane should also be maintained or restored; any disruption in this membrane can considerably limit pronation and supination.

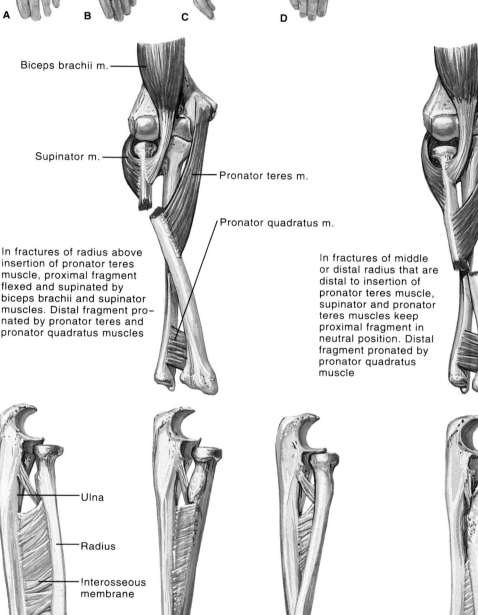

Biceps brachii m.

Supinator m.

Pronator teres m.

Pronator quadratus m.

In fractures of radius above insertion of pronator teres muscle, proximal fragment flexed and supinated by biceps brachii and supinator muscles. Distal fragment pronated by pronator teres and pronator quadratus muscles

In fractures of middle or distal radius that are distal to insertion of pronator teres muscle, supinator and pronator teres muscles keep proximal fragment in neutral position. Distal fragment pronated by pronator quadratus muscle

Ulna

Radius

Interosseous membrane

Neutral   **Pronation**   **Supination**

Normally, radius bows laterally, and interosseous space is wide enough to allow rotation of radius on ulna. Space widest when forearm is in neutral rotation, narrower in pronation and in supination. (Lateral views to better demonstrate changes in space widths)

Malunion may diminish or reverse radial bow, which impinges on ulna, impairing ability of radius to rotate over ulna

Bier Block Anesthesia

Injury to Forearm

(Continued)

Bier Block Anesthesia

In adults, significantly displaced fractures of the shaft of the forearm bones require treatment with open reduction and plate fixation. Many minimally displaced fractures, however, can be treated adequately with closed reduction and immobilization in a plaster cast. Closed reduction must be achieved in all fractures, even those definitely requiring surgery, to maintain the length of the forearm and provide comfort for the patient until the time of surgery.

Adequate muscle relaxation and anesthesia are essential for successful reduction of virtually any fracture. The usual risks of general anesthesia can be avoided with the use of regional anesthesia (Plate 48). Axillary and supraclavicular blocks are often time-consuming, and the results are not predictable, especially in patients who are in significant pain and unable to fully cooperate with the examiner.

Because of the problems encountered with axillary and supraclavicular blocks, intravenous regional, or Bier block, anesthesia is a good choice for reductions of the forearm bones. The method is safe and reliable, producing adequate muscle relaxation and pain relief to allow closed reduction of most fractures of the forearm, wrist, and hand. The Bier block is not appropriate for use in fractures about the elbow.

First, an intravenous line is established in the normal, uninjured forearm to provide immediate access for the administration of sedative medications. In the injured limb, a butterfly needle is placed in a dorsal vein in the hand, distal to the fracture site. A 0.33% lidocaine solution is given in a dose of 0.5 mg/kg. (A 1% lidocaine solution is diluted threefold with normal saline to produce a 0.33% lidocaine solution.) The syringe containing the dilute anesthetic solution is then attached to the butterfly needle. The arm is exsanguinated either by elevating it for 3 to 4 minutes or by wrapping it carefully with an elastic bandage. A double pneumatic tourniquet is placed on the arm proximal to the fracture site. The more proximal of the two cuffs is inflated to 250 to 300 mmHg. Within 1 minute after the injection, the patient usually experiences significant relief of pain. Mottling of the skin is another indication that the block is effective.

If tourniquet pain develops before reduction and radiographic examination are completed, the distal cuff of the tourniquet can be inflated and the proximal cuff released; since the area under the now inflated distal cuff is anesthetized by the block, the tourniquet can remain inflated longer without causing discomfort. Most closed manipulations with radiographic examination can

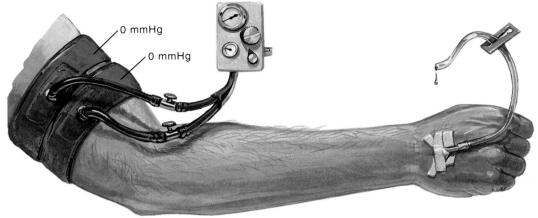

Double pneumatic tourniquet placed on arm but not yet inflated. Butterfly needle introduced into dorsal vein of hand and taped in place. Intravenous line also established in opposite limb for use if complications develop

Hand and forearm exsanguinated with Esmarch or elastic bandage up to level of distal cuff of tourniquet

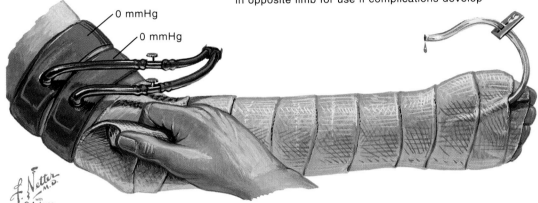

Proximal cuff inflated to about 250 mmHg and bandage removed. 0.33% lidocaine solution in dose of 2 mg/kg lidocaine instilled through needle, which is then removed

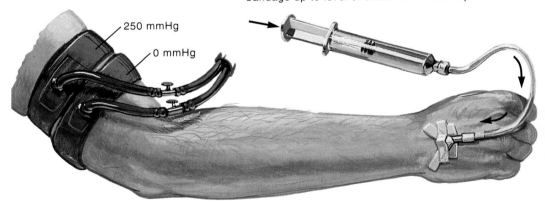

In about 10 minutes, adequate anesthesia develops from level of proximal cuff to fingertips. Distal cuff then inflated to 250 mmHg and proximal cuff deflated, transferring level of compression into anesthetized area, where it is well tolerated. Cuff remains inflated throughout surgical or manipulative procedure, after which it is slowly deflated, then inflated again, and again slowly deflated, to avoid sudden flush of anesthetic into systemic circulation. For same reason, constriction must be maintained for at least 30 minutes to allow adequate tissue binding of lidocaine. Anesthesia dissipates in about 10 minutes

Injury to Forearm
(Continued)

be accomplished in 30 minutes to 1 hour. After 30 to 45 minutes, most of the lidocaine has been bound to tissues in the forearm; therefore, removing the tourniquet at this time does not release a large dose of lidocaine into the general circulation. When the tourniquet is released, however, the patient's pulse and respirations must be monitored because cardiac arrhythmias and seizures have occurred in some patients. A recommended practice is to maintain the tourniquet for 45 minutes, then release it slowly while monitoring vital signs as shown on Plate 48.

Fracture of Both Forearm Bones

Fractures of the shafts of the radius and ulna are usually significantly displaced and are often comminuted because of the great force needed to break these strong bones (Plate 49). Anatomic reduction of the fractures, with full restoration of both the length and the bow of the radius, is essential to maintain maximal function of the forearm. Even when anatomic reduction is achieved, some long-term loss of supination and pronation can be expected.

Open reduction and internal fixation of fractures of both forearm bones are carried out through separate incisions, with a 2- to 2¾-inch (5–7-cm) skin bridge left between the two. Both fractures must be reduced and held with clamps before either is permanently fixed; this ensures that both fractures are reduced anatomically and that the reductions are maintained. After a temporary reduction is secured, the less comminuted fracture (usually the ulna) is fixed with a compression plate and screws; the more comminuted fracture is fixed subsequently using the same technique.

A number of difficulties may be encountered during the surgical procedure. Extensive comminution may make it difficult to restore the bones to their proper length. In this situation, the interosseous membrane is identified, proximally and distally, and used as a guide in restoring the bones to an adequate length. Comminution of more than 50% of the circumference of a bone indicates the need for grafting with cancellous bone taken from the iliac crest. In wound closure, the fascia is left open and only the skin is closed, because tight fascial closure combined with postoperative swelling may produce a compartment syndrome (Plate 11).

Long-term problems associated with fractures of both forearm bones include nonunion, infection, limited motion, and synostosis between the radius and the ulna. Synostosis is rare and is usually associated with comminuted fractures at the same level in the forearm that result from crushing forces. Nonunion occurs more often in fractures treated with closed reduction and plaster cast immobilization.

Fracture of Both Forearm Bones

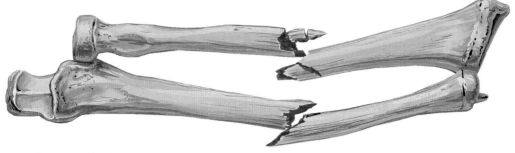

Fracture of both radius and ulna with angulation, shortening, and comminution of radius

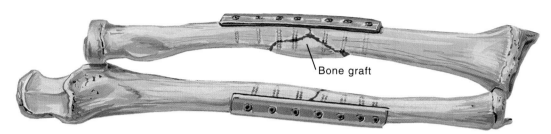

Bone graft

Open reduction and fixation with compression plates and screws through both cortices, plus bone autograft from ilium to radius. Good alignment, with restoration of radial bow and interosseous space. Postoperative immobilization in long arm cast for 6–8 weeks

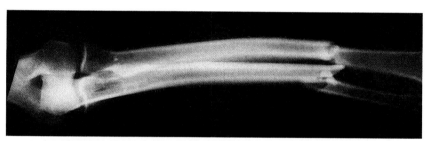

Preoperative radiograph. Fractures of shafts of both forearm bones

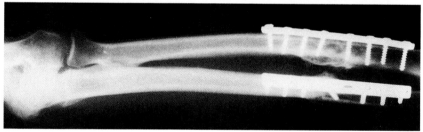

Postoperative radiograph. Compression plates applied and fragments in good alignment

Complications

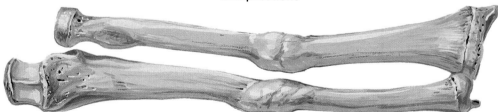

Malunion. Loss of radial bow and narrowing of interosseous space, which greatly impair pronation and supination of forearm

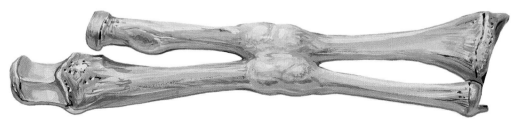

Cross union. Total loss of rotation and very difficult to correct. Separate incisions for fixation of each bone and minimal operative trauma help minimize this serious complication

Fracture of Shaft of Radius

Injury to Forearm
(Continued)

Fracture of Shaft of Radius

Single fractures of the radial shaft are often accompanied by a disruption of the distal radioulnar joint, usually at the junction of the middle and distal thirds (Plate 50). The eponyms "Galeazzi fracture" and "Piedmont fracture" are frequently used to describe this type of injury. The injury is called the fracture of (surgical) necessity because of the difficulties and generally poor results associated with closed treatment methods.

Initially, Galeazzi postulated that a direct blow to the dorsolateral wrist caused this fracture dislocation. More recent studies suggest that the usual mechanism of injury is a fall on the outstretched hand with the forearm in extreme pronation. The force across the radiocarpal joint causes fracture and shortening of the radial shaft. As further displacement occurs, the distal radioulnar joint dislocates, tearing the triangular fibrocartilage within it.

Hughston, in his classic report of 35 of 38 unsatisfactory results following closed treatment, delineated four deforming forces that lead to treatment failure: (1) the weight of the hand and the force of gravity cause subluxation of the distal radioulnar joint and dorsal angulation of the fracture; (2) the pronator quadratus muscle rotates the distal radius fragment in a volar, ulnar, and proximal direction; (3) the brachioradialis muscle rotates the distal fragment and produces shortening at the site of the radius fracture; and (4) the thumb abductors and extensors cause further shortening and displacement of the radius.

A volar surgical approach is used for open reduction and internal fixation of the fracture. Retracting the flexor carpi radialis muscle ulnarly and the radial artery and brachioradialis muscle radially exposes the fracture site, which can be fixated with a compression plate. Reduction and secure fixation of the radius fracture usually reduce the distal radioulnar dislocation as well.

After fixation of a radius fracture, the surgeon must look for any residual dislocation or subluxation of the distal radioulnar joint. Full passive supination of the forearm usually restores joint congruity. If the radioulnar joint cannot be satisfactorily aligned with closed means, the joint must be surgically reduced and secured with pins. A long arm cast is applied, with the elbow flexed 90° and the forearm in full supination. The limb is immobilized for at least 6 to 8 weeks to maintain the reduction. If a transfixation pin has been used to stabilize the distal radioulnar joint, it is left in place for 6 to 8 weeks.

If this fracture dislocation is not diagnosed and appropriately treated soon after injury, later reconstructive surgery is often needed to correct the deformity of the radius and restore the function of the distal radioulnar joint. If the distal ulna cannot be adequately reduced, ½ inch can be resected to salvage function of the distal radioulnar joint.

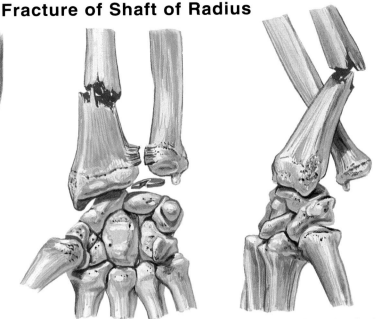

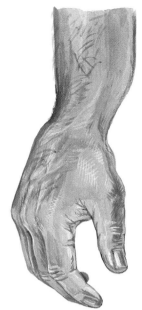

Clinical appearance of deformity due to severely displaced fracture of distal radius

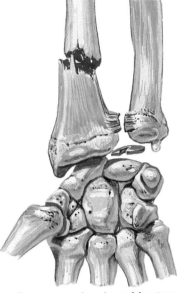

Anteroposterior view of fracture of radius plus dislocation of distal radioulnar joint (Galeazzi fracture)

Dislocation of distal radioulnar joint better demonstrated in lateral view

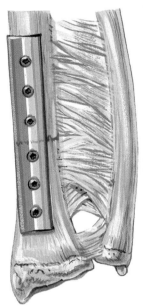

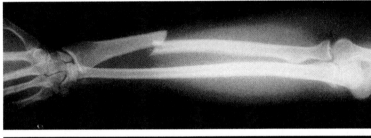

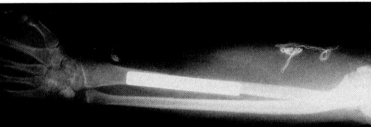

Preoperative and postoperative radiographs. Fracture of radial shaft reduced and held with compression plate

Fracture treated with open reduction and compression plate fixation using screws through both cortices. Radioulnar dislocation also reduced and normal radial bow restored

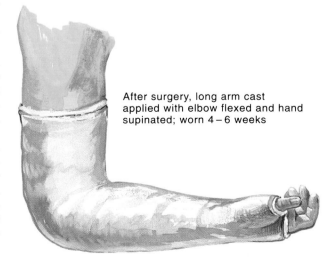

After surgery, long arm cast applied with elbow flexed and hand supinated; worn 4–6 weeks

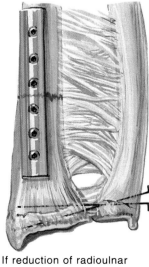

If reduction of radioulnar joint unstable, joint transfixed with crossed Kirschner wires, which are removed in 4 weeks through hole in cast

Injury to Forearm
(Continued)

Fracture of Shaft of Ulna

In 1814, Monteggia described a fracture of the ulna associated with dislocation of the proximal radioulnar joint (Plate 51). A direct blow to or forced pronation of the forearm is the usual cause of this type of fracture dislocation. Forced pronation both fractures and angulates the ulna, then causes the radial head to dislocate.

Bado classified the patterns of dislocation that occur with Monteggia fractures. Although the radial head usually dislocates anteriorly, it can also move posteriorly, medially, or laterally. The apex of the angular deformity of the ulna usually indicates the direction of the radial head dislocation. Because of the close relationship of the proximal radius to the posterior interosseous nerve, a posterior interosseous nerve palsy is not uncommon after a Monteggia fracture.

Like the Galeazzi, or Piedmont, fracture, the Monteggia fracture in adults is difficult to treat with closed methods. Achieving a stable reduction of the radial head usually requires open reduction and internal fixation of the fracture of the proximal ulna.

Treatment of the Monteggia fracture is often complicated by a variety of difficulties. Occasionally during open reduction and fixation of the ulna, the radial head does not reduce. This problem necessitates open reduction of the radial head under direct vision to ensure stability and adequate long-term function. When an open reduction is needed, the torn annular ligament should also be repaired to help stabilize the proximal radioulnar joint. When the ulna fracture is severely comminuted, it is difficult to restore the bone to its proper length, and the reduced length creates a significant problem in reducing the radial head. An extreme proximal fracture of the ulna makes plate fixation of the olecranon portion of the fracture difficult because of the configuration of the bone at the humeroulnar joint. After the fracture of the ulnar shaft is reduced, the limb is immobilized in a long arm cast for at least 6 weeks to allow healing of the ligaments of the proximal radioulnar joint.

Failure to recognize and treat Monteggia fracture soon after injury can lead to restrictions in elbow and forearm motion. Late surgical treatment includes reconstruction of the annular ligament using the triceps brachii fascia to stabilize the proximal radius. Excision of the radial head may be needed to restore supination and pronation to the forearm when the reduction of the radial head cannot be maintained or when the injury is complicated by intraarticular fractures of the radial head or the capitulum.

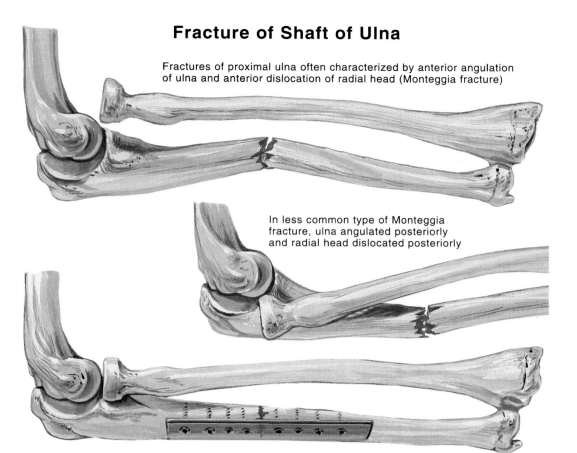

Fractures of proximal ulna often characterized by anterior angulation of ulna and anterior dislocation of radial head (Monteggia fracture)

In less common type of Monteggia fracture, ulna angulated posteriorly and radial head dislocated posteriorly

Fracture treated with open reduction and internal fixation using compression plate and screws. Dislocation of radial head reduced. If fracture is comminuted, corticocancellous bone autograft from ilium may be indicated. Postoperative immobilization in long arm cast or functional splint for 6–8 weeks. Early exercise of fingers and shoulder encouraged

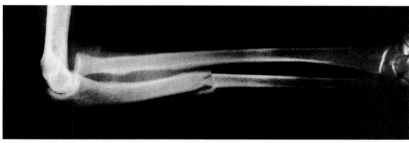

Preoperative radiograph shows anterior Monteggia fracture

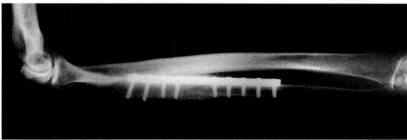

Postoperative radiograph shows compression plate in place

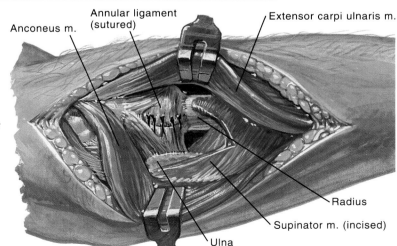

If dislocation of radial head does not reduce easily or joint remains unstable after reduction, open reduction and repair of annular ligament needed. Approach via separate incision or extension of original incision and between anconeus and extensor carpi ulnaris muscles

Anconeus m.

Annular ligament (sutured)

Extensor carpi ulnaris m.

Radius

Supinator m. (incised)

Ulna

Extension–Compression Fracture of Distal Radius (Colles Fracture)

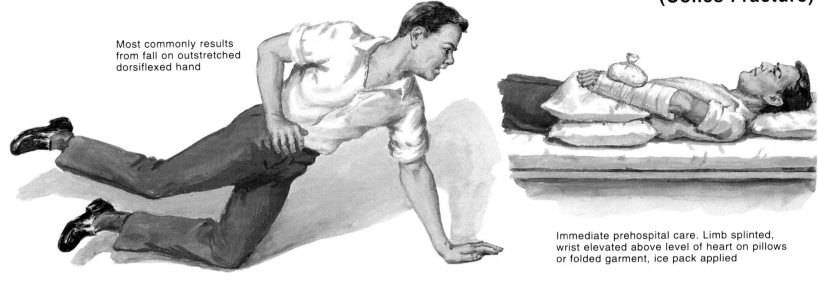

Most commonly results from fall on outstretched dorsiflexed hand

Immediate prehospital care. Limb splinted, wrist elevated above level of heart on pillows or folded garment, ice pack applied

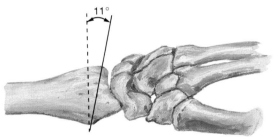

Normally, articular surface of distal radius slopes volarly, tilting about 11°

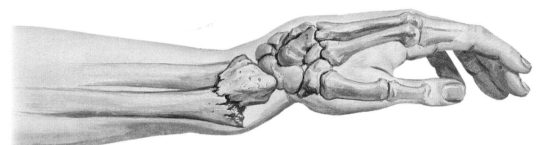

Lateral view of Colles fracture demonstrates characteristic silver fork deformity with dorsal and proximal displacement of distal fragment. Note dorsal instead of normal volar slope of articular surface of distal radius

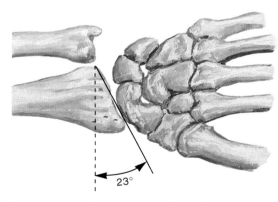

Normally, styloid process of radius extends about 1 cm beyond radioulnar joint and articular surface of distal radius slopes medially about 23°

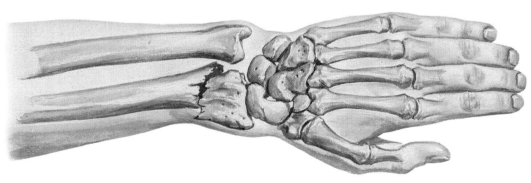

Dorsal view shows radial deviation of hand with ulnar prominence of styloid process of ulna and decrease or reverse of normal radial slope of articular surface of distal radius

Fractures of distal ends of both radius and ulna (uncommon) produce deformity identical to Colles fracture of distal radius, and treatment is same

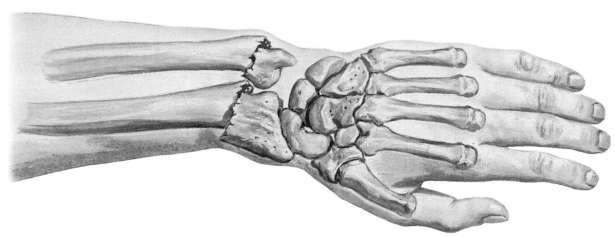

Injury to Forearm
(Continued)

Fracture of Distal Radius

Approximately 80% of fractures of the forearm involve the distal radius and the distal radioulnar joint. Fractures of the distal radius are common injuries in children, adults, and elderly persons, usually resulting from a fall on the outstretched hand. Significantly more force is required to fracture this part of the radius in adolescents and young adults than in older adults with severe osteoporosis. Fractures that involve the joint are usually caused by high impact.

Evaluation of any injury in the distal radius must include radiographs of both the wrist and the forearm. True anteroposterior, lateral, and sometimes oblique views are required to determine the extent of the injury. If intraarticular involvement is suspected, tomograms are often obtained to determine the degree of joint displacement. Fractures of the distal radius may be stable or unstable, depending on the degree of comminution. Rarely, the carpal bones are also fractured.

Extension-Compression Fracture

The precipitating injury of the extension-compression, or Colles, fracture is a fall on the outstretched hand (Plate 52). The deformity is caused by dorsal displacement of the distal radius and swelling of the distal portion of the forearm and is referred to as a "silver fork" deformity. Successful treatment involves restoration of (1) the radius to its proper length, (2) the radial and volar tilt of the distal radius, and (3) the congruity of the articular surface of the distal radioulnar and radiocarpal joints. Loss of more than 6 mm of radial length (easily measured by using the styloid process of the ulna as a reference point) may result in disability. Full restoration of the normal volar tilt is often difficult, but every attempt should be made to restore the tilt to a neutral position rather than allowing it to slope dorsally.

If more than 50% of the metaphysis of the distal radius is comminuted, the fracture is probably unstable and reduction is difficult to maintain in a plaster cast alone. This type of fracture is best visualized on the lateral radiograph. Definitive treatment is determined not only by the injury but also by the patient's age and occupation. Anatomic restoration is more important in younger, working patients, whereas some loss of radial length and tilt may be more acceptable in older patients.

Closed reduction and immobilization in a plaster cast constitute a dependable treatment for many fractures of the distal radius, but after satisfactory manipulative reduction, some Colles fractures (particularly unstable injuries in young, active adults) require fixation with an external fixator; percutaneous pin fixation with plaster cast immobilization; or open reduction and internal fixation using buttress plates, screws, and transfixing wires.

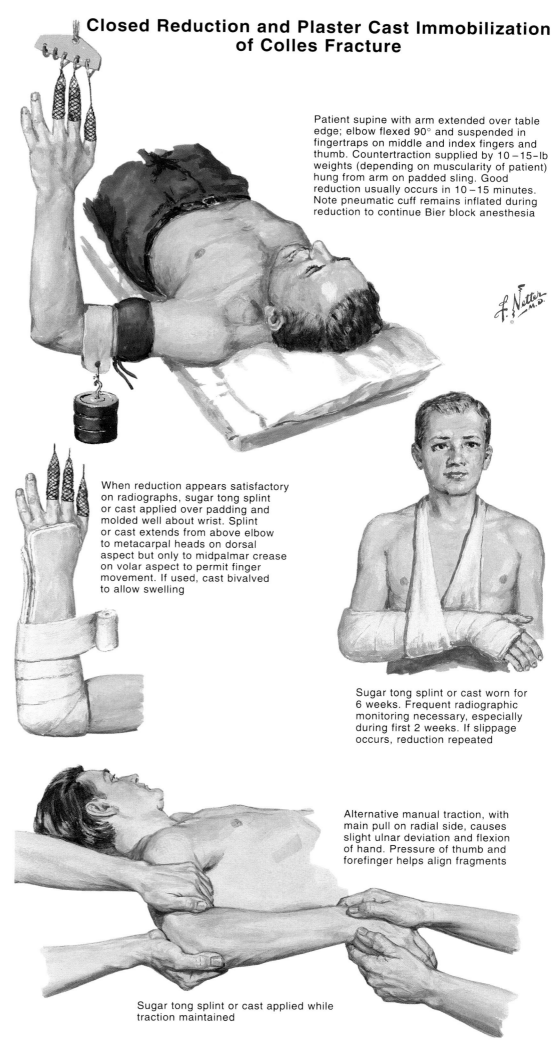

Closed Reduction and Plaster Cast Immobilization of Colles Fracture

Patient supine with arm extended over table edge; elbow flexed 90° and suspended in fingertraps on middle and index fingers and thumb. Countertraction supplied by 10–15-lb weights (depending on muscularity of patient) hung from arm on padded sling. Good reduction usually occurs in 10–15 minutes. Note pneumatic cuff remains inflated during reduction to continue Bier block anesthesia

When reduction appears satisfactory on radiographs, sugar tong splint or cast applied over padding and molded well about wrist. Splint or cast extends from above elbow to metacarpal heads on dorsal aspect but only to midpalmar crease on volar aspect to permit finger movement. If used, cast bivalved to allow swelling

Sugar tong splint or cast worn for 6 weeks. Frequent radiographic monitoring necessary, especially during first 2 weeks. If slippage occurs, reduction repeated

Alternative manual traction, with main pull on radial side, causes slight ulnar deviation and flexion of hand. Pressure of thumb and forefinger helps align fragments

Sugar tong splint or cast applied while traction maintained

Injury to Forearm
(Continued)

Treatment of Extension-Compression Fracture

The character of the fracture, whether it is stable or unstable, intraarticular or extraarticular; the life-style and age of the patient; and the experience of the treating surgeon are the best determinants of the treatment for Colles fracture.

Closed Reduction and Plaster Cast Immobilization. Colles fractures can often be reduced using manipulation or traction (Plate 53). After a sterile preparation of the forearm, local infiltration of lidocaine into the hematoma at the fracture site often provides adequate anesthesia for manipulating the fracture. Regional anesthesia, either an axillary or a Bier block, is also commonly used, but if the patient is very apprehensive or a more extensive procedure is needed, general anesthesia may be required.

Traction using fingertraps and weights is an effective method of reducing Colles fractures. The fingertraps are secured to the middle and index fingers and the thumb to suspend the arm; 10- to 15-lb weights are attached by a sling to the upper arm to provide countertraction. Gentle manual manipulation is often needed to fully reduce the fracture. Hyperextension or re-creation of the deformity should be avoided, if possible.

If the surgeon decides to manipulate the fracture without using fingertraps, an assistant is needed to hold the proximal forearm and provide countertraction. The fracture is then reduced with gentle longitudinal traction. A sugar tong splint or a long arm circular cast is applied after reduction. The sugar tong splint is easier to apply than the long arm cast and can be tightened on follow-up visits. To maintain the reduction, it is important to mold the plaster snugly to the forearm using three-point molding.

The best position for maintaining Colles fractures in plaster remains controversial. The most commonly used position comprises mild flexion, ulnar deviation, and either neutral rotation, minimal pronation, or minimal supination.

Percutaneous Pin Fixation and Plaster Cast Immobilization. In young, active adults, Colles fractures that are comminuted and unstable may require more aggressive fixation to maintain a satisfactory reduction (Plate 54). Pin fixation and a plaster cast or an external fixator may be used in these patients. Because of an increased incidence of reflex sympathetic dystrophy, pin tract infection, and other associated complications, pin fixation and plaster cast immobilization should be reserved for fractures that are very unstable and involve the joint. This method of fixation is often used in patients with bilateral injuries and in those who require elbow mobility to perform daily activities while the injury heals.

Percutaneous Pin Fixation and Plaster Cast Immobilization of Comminuted Colles Fracture

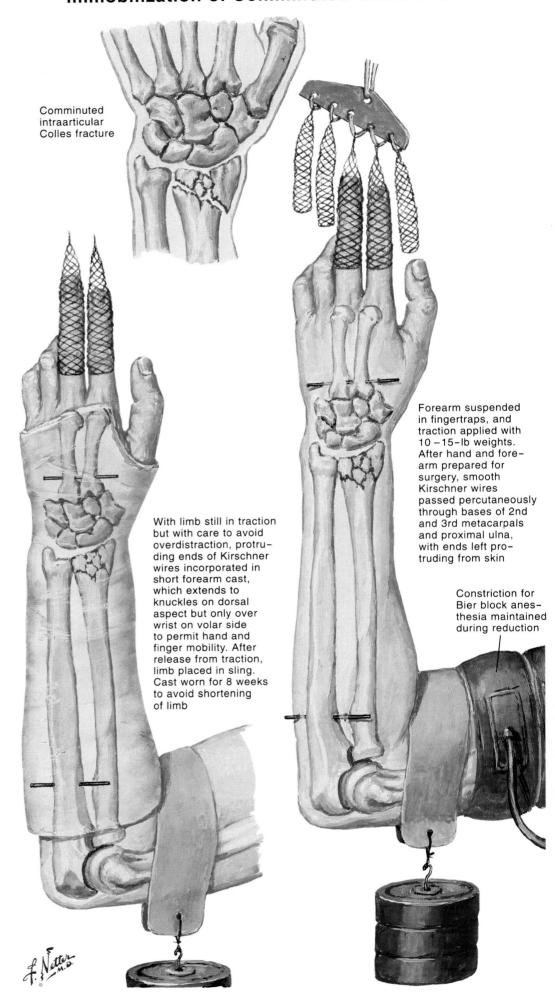

Comminuted intraarticular Colles fracture

With limb still in traction but with care to avoid overdistraction, protruding ends of Kirschner wires incorporated in short forearm cast, which extends to knuckles on dorsal aspect but only over wrist on volar side to permit hand and finger mobility. After release from traction, limb placed in sling. Cast worn for 8 weeks to avoid shortening of limb

Forearm suspended in fingertraps, and traction applied with 10–15-lb weights. After hand and forearm prepared for surgery, smooth Kirschner wires passed percutaneously through bases of 2nd and 3rd metacarpals and proximal ulna, with ends left protruding from skin

Constriction for Bier block anesthesia maintained during reduction

Injury to Forearm

(Continued)

The distal pin is inserted percutaneously into the proximal ends of the second and third metacarpals just distal to the metaphyseal flare. It is important to place the smooth pin through four cortices and within the metaphysis rather than the diaphysis of both metacarpals to ensure that loosening does not occur and to decrease the possibility of pin tract problems. After insertion, the protruding end of the pin is bent to allow the thumb to move and abduct fully without interference.

The proximal pin is placed in the ulna just distal to the olecranon process, with care not to injure the ulnar nerve. This pin should penetrate two cortices. After reduction and while traction is maintained distally, the pins are incorporated in a short arm plaster cast; securing the pin in the plaster minimizes pin movement. The fingers and the entire palm are left free. Dorsally, the plaster extends to the metacarpal heads but allows full abduction and circumduction of the thumb and full flexion of the metacarpophalangeal joints. After the pins and plaster or the external fixator device is applied, the patient must actively exercise all of the joints of the fingers and thumb to ensure the best possible outcome.

Flexion-Compression Fracture

The reversed Colles fracture, also called Smith fracture, is rare (Plate 55). In this pattern of fracture, the fragment of the distal radius is displaced volarly rather than dorsally, as in Colles fracture. Smith fractures do not produce the same disability that occurs with Colles fractures. As with Colles fractures, they can be treated with either closed immobilization or percutaneous pin fixation.

The short-term complications associated with all fractures of the distal radius are significant and demand early treatment to prevent long-term residual disability. To control edema after fracture reduction and casting, the arm is elevated on pillows or in a sling above the level of the patient's heart, and ice bags are applied over the cast. Severe swelling may necessitate splitting the cast, and the cast may need to be trimmed to prevent skin irritation. The physician should encourage frequent and full active range of motion of all the finger and thumb joints to prevent stiffness, which is common, and to reduce swelling. Any persistent pain under the cast should be investigated with the plaster removed entirely.

Acute injury of the median nerve after fractures of the distal radius is an uncommon but debilitating problem. Following injury, fracture displacement combined with swelling occasionally distorts and compresses the median nerve, causing pain or numbness. The symptoms of median nerve compression usually subside or disappear when the fracture is reduced. If symptoms

Flexion–Compression Fracture of Distal Radius
(Smith Fracture)

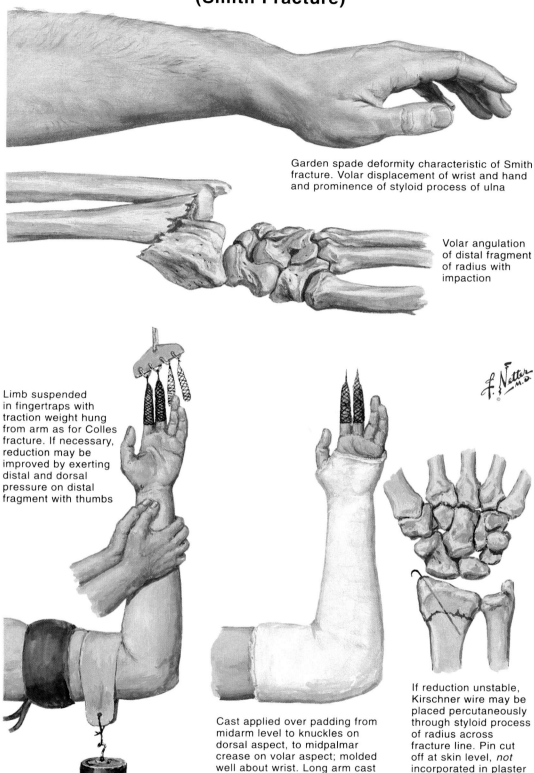

Garden spade deformity characteristic of Smith fracture. Volar displacement of wrist and hand and prominence of styloid process of ulna

Volar angulation of distal fragment of radius with impaction

Limb suspended in fingertraps with traction weight hung from arm as for Colles fracture. If necessary, reduction may be improved by exerting distal and dorsal pressure on distal fragment with thumbs

Cast applied over padding from midarm level to knuckles on dorsal aspect, to midpalmar crease on volar aspect; molded well about wrist. Long arm cast worn for 6 weeks; may be split to relieve pressure

If reduction unstable, Kirschner wire may be placed percutaneously through styloid process of radius across fracture line. Pin cut off at skin level, *not* incorporated in plaster

persist after reduction—particularly if the patient experiences burning pain in the median nerve distribution—prompt surgical decompression of the nerve in the carpal tunnel may be necessary. Mild residual numbness and tingling in the median nerve distribution usually subside with time or can be relieved following fracture healing with a carpal tunnel release. Sometimes, acute compartment syndrome of the forearm is associated with fractures of the distal radius. The characteristic symptom is excessive pain combined

with numbness and pain on passive movement of the thumb and fingers. Compartment syndromes must be recognized promptly and should be treated with fasciotomy.

Long-term complications develop in 30% to 35% of patients. Loss of the reduction is the most common problem, which can be minimized or corrected by early identification of the displacement with radiographs taken at weekly intervals in the first 3 weeks following injury. Repeat closed reduction and casting, sometimes supplemented

Fracture of Articular Margin of Distal Radius (Barton Fracture) and of Styloid Process of Radius

Injury to Forearm
(Continued)

with percutaneous pin fixation, may be needed; unstable fractures may require open reduction and internal fixation or application of an external fixator to restore and maintain alignment. After 3 weeks of healing, fractures of the distal radius have stabilized and will rarely settle with further loss of radial length. If the fracture heals with a residual deformity, usually a dorsiflexion deformity, this can be corrected with surgery. Radiocarpal and carpal instability are also associated with injuries of the distal radius. Osteoarthritis of the distal radioulnar joint may produce persistent pain. Fortunately, nonunion is rare, but if it occurs, treatment comprises open reduction, internal fixation, and bone grafting.

Rupture of an extensor tendon, most commonly of the thumb, is seen following fractures of the distal radius, as is stenosing tenosynovitis of the first dorsal compartment (de Quervain disease). Reflex sympathetic dystrophy is a very debilitating complication of any musculoskeletal injury (Plate 151). It is frequently a result of hand and wrist fractures, but it develops most often after treatment of unstable fractures with pin fixation, external fixation, or pin and plaster fixation. Early recognition and treatment of reflex sympathetic dystrophy are essential to restore good function.

Fracture of Articular Margin of Distal Radius

Fractures of the articular margin, called Barton fractures, represent a small percentage of fractures of the distal radius (Plate 56). This type of fracture is best described as a fracture dislocation of the wrist. Correct diagnosis of Barton fracture is very important because it is an inherently unstable injury and therefore difficult to manage with the traditional closed method. The injury is further defined by the direction of the dislocation. If the dorsal aspect of the articular margin, or rim, is fractured and the carpus is displaced dorsally, the injury is termed a dorsal Barton fracture; conversely, the more common volar Barton fracture refers to a fracture in which the dislocation is displaced volarly. In many cases, however, the Barton fracture is nondisplaced and can be treated with immobilization in a plaster cast.

A fall on the outstretched hand is the most common cause of the Barton fracture. The impact wedges the lunate against either the dorsal or the volar margin of the articular surface of the radius. The lunate acts as a lever against the articular surface, causing it to fracture. The carpus is then dislocated along with the fragment of the articular margin of the radius.

The stability of the closed reduction depends on the integrity of the radiocarpal ligament on the side opposite the injury. For example, the stability of the reduction of a dorsal Barton fracture is best preserved by positioning the wrist in

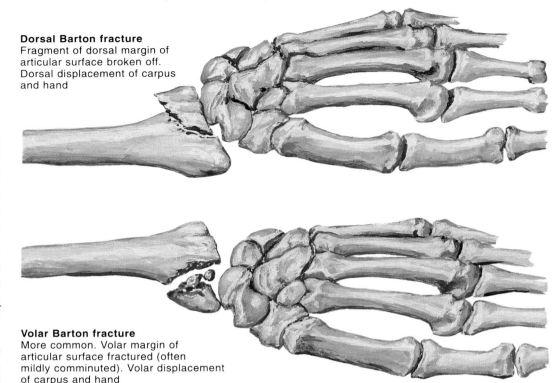

Dorsal Barton fracture
Fragment of dorsal margin of articular surface broken off. Dorsal displacement of carpus and hand

Volar Barton fracture
More common. Volar margin of articular surface fractured (often mildly comminuted). Volar displacement of carpus and hand

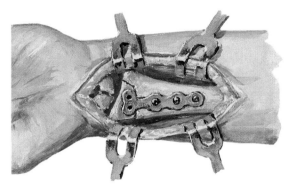

Many Barton fractures are nondisplaced and can be managed with immobilization in forearm–wrist cast and active finger exercises for about 6 weeks. For volar fractures, wrist immobilized in flexion; for dorsal fractures, in mild extension. Displaced fractures can often be reduced with traction, using fingertraps and weights hung from arm, with or without manipulation. Comminuted fractures require pin fixation and plaster casting. For unstable fractures, some surgeons prefer internal fixation using buttress plate. To avoid further comminution, plate screws not inserted into bone fragment

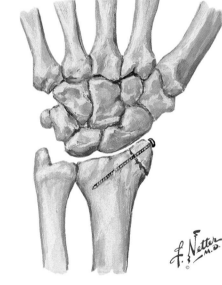

Fracture of styloid process of radius
May occur alone or with Barton fracture. Shown here fixed with screw. Nondisplaced fractures can usually be treated with immobilization in short arm cast for at least 6 weeks

extension to take advantage of the intact volar carpal ligament.

Reduction of a Barton fracture is difficult to maintain with an external fixator or with pins and plaster; therefore, treatment with open reduction and internal fixation is usually indicated for fracture dislocations that have large fragments. Barton fractures that involve a significant portion of the articular surface are usually unstable and must be treated with open reduction and internal fixation, using a small buttress plate to maintain the reduction. Buttressing the distal fragment maintains joint congruity. It is not absolutely necessary to insert screws into the distal fragment

(which may be significantly comminuted) to maintain the reduction.

Fracture of Styloid Process of Radius

Most nondisplaced fractures of the styloid process of the radius can be treated with immobilization in a plaster cast. Displaced fractures must be anatomically reduced and held with either a pin or a screw. Often, treatment with closed reduction and percutaneous pin fixation is sufficient. Fractures of the styloid process are frequently accompanied by dislocations of the lunate. Thus, with any fracture of the styloid process, the carpus should be examined for other injuries. ☐

Injury to Wrist

Dislocation of Carpus

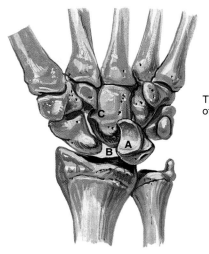
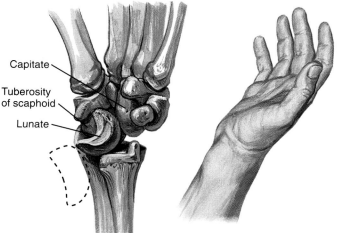

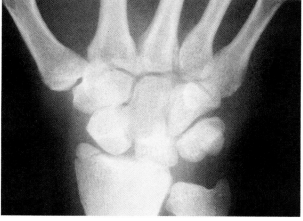

Capitate
Tuberosity of scaphoid
Lunate

Palmar view shows (A) lunate rotated and displaced volarly, (B) scapho-lunate space widened, (C) capitate displaced proximally and dorsally

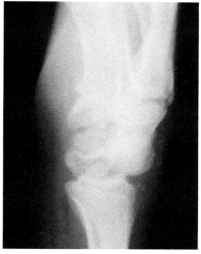

Lateral view shows lunate displaced volarly and rotated. Broken line indicates further dislocation to volar aspect of distal radius

Typical deformity. Anterior bulge of dislocated lunate

Injury to Carpus

Like fractures of the distal radius, most carpus injuries result from forces applied to the wrist when it is in varying degrees of extension or dorsiflexion. The injuries range from simple ligament sprains and tears to complex fracture dislocations.

Ligament injuries, fractures, and dislocations of the carpus must be diagnosed quickly and correctly to preserve function of the hand and wrist. The initial radiographic diagnosis of injuries to the bones and ligaments of the carpus is difficult because there are so many bones of different shapes and because the bones overlap to various degrees. Fractures and dislocations of the carpal bones are often missed because many primary care physicians are not familiar with the radiographic anatomy of the area. Detecting, diagnosing, and treating carpus fractures and dislocations therefore require a high index of suspicion.

Dislocation of Carpus

The strong volar radiocarpal ligament between the lunate, radius, and distal row of the carpal bones provides strong support for the volar aspect of the carpus; ligament support is weaker on the dorsal side. In addition, the ligament attachments from the radius to the proximal carpal row are much stronger than the attachments from the proximal carpal row to the distal carpal row. This disparity in the support between the two carpal rows and the lack of a significant lunocapitate support make the carpus particularly susceptible to dislocation and chronic instability (Plate 57).

Carpal instability results from hyperextension of the wrist, as in a fall on the outstretched hand. The amount and direction of the force determine the degree of resulting instability around the lunate. The first stage—and most minor degree—of perilunate instability is the tearing of the ligament between the scaphoid and the lunate, followed by disruption of the radioscaphoid ligament. These injuries produce a scapholunate diastasis. In the second stage, with further dorsiflexion, the radiocapitate ligament ruptures, leading to dislocation of the lunate. In the third stage of injury, the radiotriquetral ligament ruptures, resulting in perilunate dislocation associated with lunotriquetral instability. In the final stage, the hand and distal row of the carpus supinate on the triquetrum, tearing the dorsal radiotriquetral ligament and causing the capitate to push the unstable lunate volarly; these events result in a volar dislocation. The signs and symptoms of a volar dislocation of the lunate include pain and swelling in the wrist. Paresthesia and dysesthesia of the median nerve are quite common associated problems.

Anteroposterior radiograph shows rotation and volar dislocation of lunate

Lateral radiograph shows rotated lunate in front of capitate

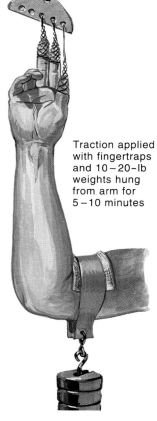
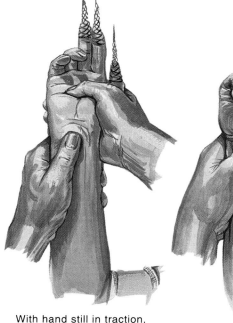
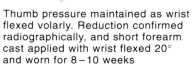

Traction applied with fingertraps and 10–20-lb weights hung from arm for 5–10 minutes

With hand still in traction, wrist dorsiflexed as firm thumb pressure applied over prominence of lunate. Reduction may be felt as distinct snap

Thumb pressure maintained as wrist flexed volarly. Reduction confirmed radiographically, and short forearm cast applied with wrist flexed 20° and worn for 8–10 weeks

Injury to Wrist
(Continued)

With lunate and perilunate dislocations, the anteroposterior radiograph often shows the lunate as wedged, or pie shaped, rather than four sided. On the lateral radiograph, the lunate appears rotated out of its articulation with the head of the capitate and pointing volarly; sometimes, the lunate is completely dislocated volarly.

Initial treatment of lunate and perilunate dislocations includes a thorough neurovascular examination followed by closed reduction of the dislocation. The reduction can be performed using regional or general anesthesia. Traction is applied by placing the fingers in fingertraps and hanging a 10- to 20-lb counterweight from the upper arm. An anteroposterior radiograph should be taken of the wrist in traction to determine the degree of ligament damage and to identify any associated osteochondral fractures.

After allowing the wrist to remain distracted for 10 to 15 minutes, the examiner places his or her thumb on the volar aspect of the wrist over the dislocated lunate. The injured wrist is gradually flexed volarly and pronated while thumb pressure is applied over the lunate to reduce it. If adequate closed reduction is obtained and post-reduction radiographs show significant lunate instability, a long arm thumb spica cast is applied with the hand in slight radial deviation and the wrist in slight flexion.

Posttraumatic carpal instability is now recognized as a common complication of these injuries, and many orthopedic surgeons prefer open reduction of lunate and perilunate dislocations and stabilization of carpus injuries with wires or screws (Plate 58). Open reduction plus internal fixation of a lunate dislocation has several advantages. The procedure achieves and maintains anatomic reduction of the fragments and allows repair of the torn ligaments at the same time. Also, the wrist joint is debrided of any loose osteochondral fragments.

Carpus dislocations may also involve fractures of the scaphoid (Plates 59–60), triquetrum, and capitate, as well as the styloid process of the radius (Plate 58). In these injuries, the dislocations cause fractures rather than ligament ruptures. The best way to ensure adequate alignment and reduce the risk of late wrist instability is anatomic reduction and rigid internal fixation.

Prompt recognition and treatment of carpus instability can restore satisfactory hand and wrist function. However, decreased range of motion and early degenerative arthritis are still common complications, particularly after severe injuries.

Fracture of Hamulus of Hamate

Fractures of the carpus usually involve the scaphoid, the dorsal tip of the lunate and triquetrum, and, less frequently, the body of the capitate. Fractures of the hamulus (hook) of the hamate are not common and are often missed on the initial examination (Plate 58). The usual

Dislocation of Carpus (continued)

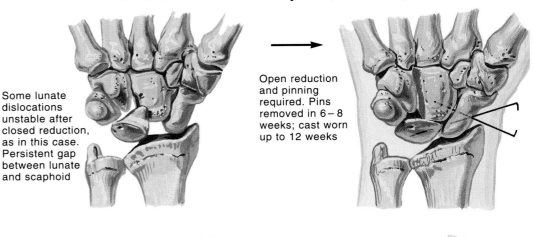

Some lunate dislocations unstable after closed reduction, as in this case. Persistent gap between lunate and scaphoid

Open reduction and pinning required. Pins removed in 6–8 weeks; cast worn up to 12 weeks

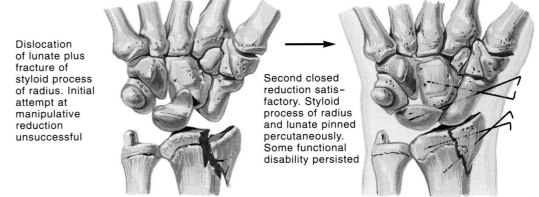

Dislocation of lunate plus fracture of styloid process of radius. Initial attempt at manipulative reduction unsuccessful

Second closed reduction satisfactory. Styloid process of radius and lunate pinned percutaneously. Some functional disability persisted

Note: if lunate badly comminuted or necrotic, as in Kienböck disease, total replacement with Swanson silicone prosthesis may be indicated

Fracture of Hamulus (Hook) of Hamate

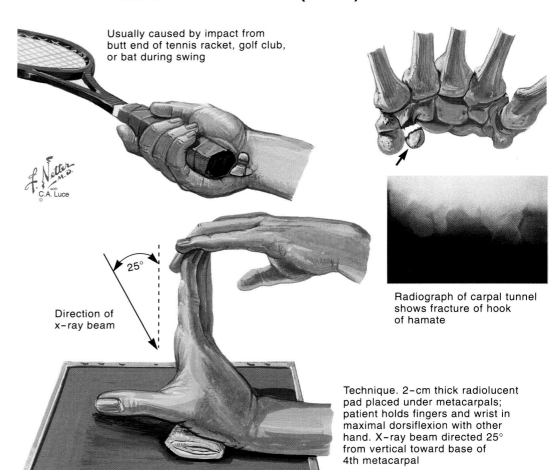

Usually caused by impact from butt end of tennis racket, golf club, or bat during swing

Direction of x-ray beam

25°

Radiograph of carpal tunnel shows fracture of hook of hamate

Technique. 2-cm thick radiolucent pad placed under metacarpals; patient holds fingers and wrist in maximal dorsiflexion with other hand. X-ray beam directed 25° from vertical toward base of 4th metacarpal

Injury to Wrist
(Continued)

cause of a hamate fracture is a fall on the outstretched hand, but this injury is also commonly seen in golfers and baseball players. For example, as a golfer hits the ground forcibly with a club, the impact may fracture the hamate.

Although the injury causes acute pain and swelling, routine anteroposterior and lateral radiographs often fail to demonstrate the fracture. The initial physical findings include a dull ache over the hypothenar eminence, tenderness over the hamate, decreased grip strength, and, occasionally, signs and symptoms of ulnar nerve impingement. The Allen test may be positive, suggesting compression of the ulnar artery. If these signs and symptoms are present but routine radiographs show no evidence of fracture, a carpal tunnel view is indicated. Tomography and computed tomography of the carpus are helpful additional diagnostic techniques.

The rate of union following these fractures is not clearly documented, but many probably fail to heal. As primary treatment, most authorities advocate surgical excision of the fracture fragment of the hamate. Most patients regain adequate or good function, although significant discomfort may persist at the surgical scar.

Fracture of Scaphoid

The scaphoid acts as a link between the proximal and distal rows of the carpus and thus is quite susceptible to injury. Most fractures of the scaphoid waist result from an extension force applied to the distal pole, with the proximal pole stabilized by the strong radiocapitate and radioscaphoid ligaments. This mechanism of injury, for example, a fall on the outstretched hand, produces the most common fracture pattern: a break through the waist of the scaphoid (Plate 59). Other patterns include fractures of the distal tuberosity and proximal pole and vertical shear fractures of the body.

The blood supply to the bone plays an important role in the healing process, and sometimes osteonecrosis is a complication of scaphoid fractures. The major blood supply enters the distal pole on the dorsal aspect, leaving the proximal pole with a relatively poor vascular supply. Fractures through the waist of the scaphoid disrupt most of the blood supply to the proximal pole, often leading to osteonecrosis.

Fractures of the scaphoid are the most commonly missed fractures of the upper limb; yet, early diagnosis is essential for successful treatment. The initial signs are tenderness and pain over the anatomic snuffbox, with some swelling and loss of the normal concavity of the dorsoradial region of the wrist. Also present is significant discomfort when the thumb is moved or the metacarpal of the thumb is compressed against the proximal carpal row.

Fracture of Scaphoid

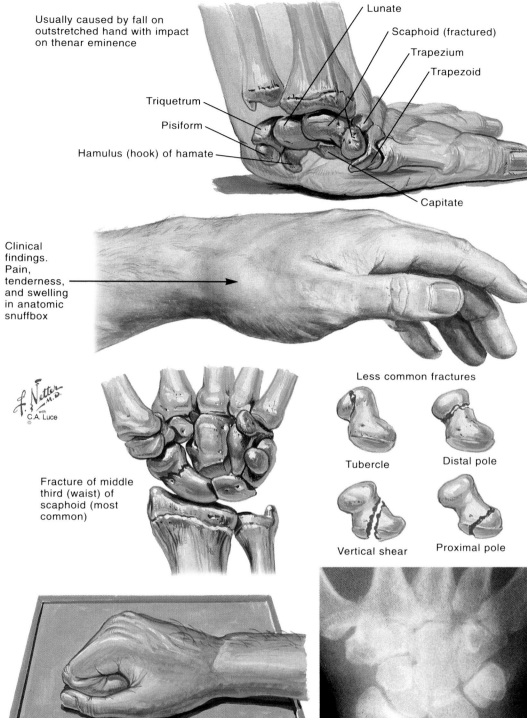

Usually caused by fall on outstretched hand with impact on thenar eminence

Lunate
Scaphoid (fractured)
Trapezium
Trapezoid
Triquetrum
Pisiform
Hamulus (hook) of hamate
Capitate

Clinical findings. Pain, tenderness, and swelling in anatomic snuffbox

Fracture of middle third (waist) of scaphoid (most common)

Less common fractures

Tubercle   Distal pole

Vertical shear   Proximal pole

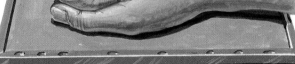

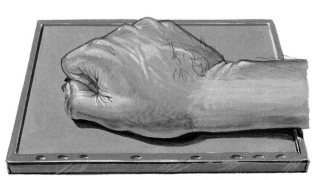

Direct posteroanterior radiograph taken with fingers clenched into fist and resting on cassette

Radiograph also taken with clenched fist in ulnar deviation

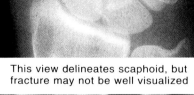

This view delineates scaphoid, but fracture may not be well visualized

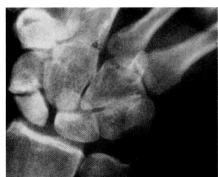

This position tends to open fracture, better visualizing it

Injury to Wrist
(Continued)

Initial radiographs may not accurately demonstrate a fracture of the scaphoid waist. Special views are needed of the hand forming a fist and of the fist in ulnar deviation, positions that bring the scaphoid into extension. An occult fracture of the scaphoid can often be visualized by aiming the x-ray beam parallel to the suspected fracture line rather than at an acute angle to it. However, even with these special views of the wrist, some acute scaphoid fractures are not clearly seen.

If symptoms are present, even if radiographs are normal, the wrist should be immobilized in a thumb spica cast for 2 to 3 weeks (Plate 60). Follow-up radiographs after the plaster cast is removed often reveal a previously occult fracture. If pain persists, the cast is reapplied.

Most nondisplaced fractures of the scaphoid can be successfully treated by placing the limb in a thumb spica cast with the hand and wrist rigidly immobilized and the thumb in abduction. Some physicians recommend the use of an above-elbow cast, at least for the first 6 weeks of treatment, on the premise that above-elbow casting of scaphoid fractures may enhance union. Prompt recognition, secure immobilization, and careful follow-up remain the essentials of closed treatment. The rate of union in fractures that are immobilized initially is close to 95%. In fractures that are not immobilized initially, the nonunion rate is significantly higher.

Any degree of displacement of a scaphoid fracture may be an indication of wrist instability. Displaced scaphoid fractures are often associated with ligament injuries that ultimately result in persistent wrist instability after the fracture heals. Displaced fractures that cannot be anatomically reduced with closed means should be treated with open reduction and internal fixation. Nonunion is much more common following displaced fractures. Therefore, a scaphoid fracture with a displacement greater than 1 mm requires open reduction and internal fixation to ensure union and wrist function.

The Herbert screw, with threads of different pitches at either end, is a very effective device for stabilizing and compressing a scaphoid fracture. In the Russe bone-grafting technique, a volar approach to the scaphoid is used to preserve the dorsal blood supply. A trough is prepared in both fragments, and most of the cancellous bone in both distal and proximal poles is curetted, creating significant cavities in both fragments. A corticocancellous bridge graft is inserted into the cavities to stabilize the fragments. Additional cancellous bone is impacted around the corticocancellous graft to enhance healing. If any instability persists, the fracture fragments are stabilized with Kirschner wires or screws. The use of bone grafts requires a long period of immobilization unless the fracture has been stabilized with metal devices. Failure to achieve union usually leads to osteoarthritis of the wrist. □

Fracture of Scaphoid (continued)

Most fractures heal well when treated with snug thumb spica cast over stockinette with wrist in 20° dorsiflexion and slight radial deviation. Cast extends to distal palmar crease on volar aspect and to knuckles on dorsal aspect. Nondisplaced fractures of waist and distal pole of scaphoid require 8–12 weeks' immobilization; displaced vertical fractures and fractures of proximal pole may need up to 18 weeks' immobilization

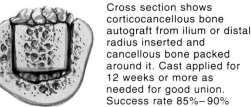

Since fractures of scaphoid often not visualized on initial radiographs, all suspected fractures with pain and tenderness in anatomic snuffbox immobilized as shown; radiographs repeated in 3 weeks with cast removed. If radiographs normal and pain or tenderness absent, cast left off; if tenderness persists, cast reapplied and radiography repeated in 3 weeks

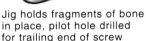

Blood supply to scaphoid enters both distal and proximal parts of bone

Radial artery

In most persons, blood supply enters only distal part of scaphoid. Fracture through waist may lead to necrosis of proximal part

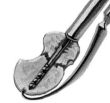

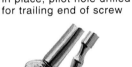

Open reduction and internal fixation

Herbert jig. Device for fixing displaced fractures or nonunion of scaphoid (after Fisher)

Jig holds fragments of bone in place, pilot hole drilled for trailing end of screw

Long drill introduced to full length of screw

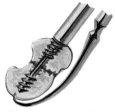

Deep end of canal tapped for leading thread of screw

Screw inserted through jig. Trailing end is self-tapping

Russe bone graft for nonunion of scaphoid

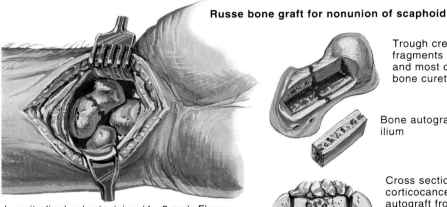

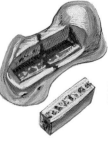

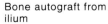

Trough created in both fragments of scaphoid, and most cancellous bone curetted

Bone autograft from ilium

Longitudinal volar incision (4–5 cm). Flexor carpi radialis tendon retracted radially, other tissues ulnarly. Joint capsule opened; radiocarpal ligaments partially incised, exposing fractured scaphoid

Cross section shows corticocancellous bone autograft from ilium or distal radius inserted and cancellous bone packed around it. Cast applied for 12 weeks or more as needed for good union. Success rate 85%–90%

Injury to Hand

Injury to Fingers

The hand has both mechanical and sensory functions. Therefore, injuries to the hand not only disrupt mechanical ability but compromise the sensory function of the upper limb. Most hand injuries cause pain, swelling, and often discoloration. Because the flexor and extensor tendons and the bones lie close to the skin, each major anatomic structure can be examined easily and its functional status determined. Radiographs of the whole hand itself are not needed if only the wrist or finger is injured, but anteroposterior, lateral, and oblique views of the specific site of injury are essential for a complete evaluation.

Fracture of Distal Phalanx. The tip of the finger is often injured by crushing forces, which cause fractures of the distal phalanx and, frequently, hematoma under the nail bed (Plate 61). Decompression of the subungual hematoma is often necessary to relieve pain. Drilling a hole in the nail bed with a heated paper clip allows the hematoma to drain. Fractures of the distal phalanx are often only minimally displaced and can be treated with splinting until pain subsides.

Mallet Finger. Hyperflexion that disrupts the extensor mechanism of the distal phalanx causes mallet finger, an injury common in baseball players. Three types of injury occur: stretching of the extensor tendon past its elastic limit, which causes multiple interstitial tears; complete disruption of the extensor tendon; and avulsion fracture of the base of the distal phalanx. The patient with mallet finger often does not appreciate the severity of the injury, and even the examining physician may not recognize the injury. The acute signs are tenderness over the dorsum of the distal interphalangeal joint and inability to actively extend the distal phalanx.

Treatment consists of splinting the distal interphalangeal joint in extension. The splint should be placed on the dorsal aspect so the volar surface of the finger can still be used in opposition; it is worn continuously for 6 to 8 weeks, then only at night for an additional 3 to 4 weeks. The patient should be warned that splinting may cause some skin loss over the dorsum of the distal phalanx and that full extension may never be regained.

Mallet finger with avulsion of a large bone fragment may be associated with volar subluxation of the distal interphalangeal joint. Surgical repair, although indicated, is difficult because the blood supply to the skin is poor, the fragment is quite small, and a good reduction with Kirschner wires is often difficult to maintain.

Avulsion of Flexor Digitorum Profundus Tendon. This tendon, which attaches to the distal phalanx on the volar side of the joint, can be disrupted by a violent traction injury. The ring finger of the dominant hand is the most common site of injury. The primary presenting sign is minor—inability to actively flex the distal phalanx—and patients often delay for weeks before seeking medical attention. Primary repair in the first 6 weeks produces acceptable functional results;

Injury to Fingers

Fractures of distal phalanx

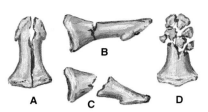

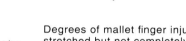

Types of fractures. A. Longitudinal B. Nondisplaced transverse C. Angulated transverse D. Comminuted

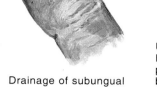

Drainage of subungual hematoma through hole made with heated paper clip relieves pain

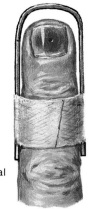

U-shaped splint held with tape protects finger but allows for swelling. Proximal interphalangeal joint left free for active motion

Mallet finger

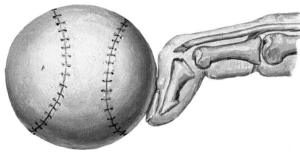

Usually caused by direct blow on extended distal phalanx, as in baseball, volleyball

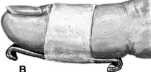

Degrees of mallet finger injury. A. Extensor tendon stretched but not completely severed; mild finger drop and weak extensor ability retained. B. Tendon torn from its insertion. C. Bone fragment avulsed with tendon. In B and C there is 40°– 45° flexion deformity and loss of active extension

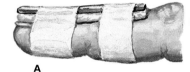

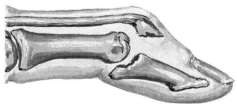

Treatment for mallet finger of tendon origin. A. Padded dorsal splint. B. Unpadded volar splint. C. Stack splint. Proximal interphalangeal joint left free for active exercise

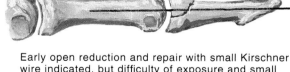

Mallet finger of bone origin. Avulsion of bone fragment and volar subluxation of distal phalanx

Early open reduction and repair with small Kirschner wire indicated, but difficulty of exposure and small size of fragment present problems. Extensor tendon may be sectioned for better exposure and subsequently repaired. One or both collateral ligaments may also have to be divided and repaired

Avulsion of flexor digitorum profundus tendon

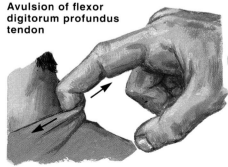

Caused by violent traction on flexed distal phalanx, as in catching on jersey of running football player

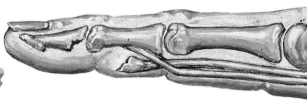

Flexor digitorum profundus tendon may be torn directly from distal phalanx or may avulse small or large bone fragment. Tendon usually retracts to about level of proximal interphalangeal joint, where it is stopped at its passage through flexor digitorum superficialis tendon; occasionally, it retracts into palm. Early open repair of tendon and its torn fibrous sheath indicated

Fracture of Proximal and Middle Phalanges

Injury to Hand
(Continued)

after 6 weeks, tendon grafting or arthrodesis of the distal interphalangeal joint is the treatment of choice.

Fracture of Proximal and Middle Phalanges

Diagnosis of fractures of the phalanges requires anteroposterior, lateral, and oblique radiographs and careful clinical examination of the soft tissues—specifically the flexor and extensor tendons—to verify the extent of the injury. Because finger injuries are often caused by crushing forces, open fractures of the fingers are common (Plate 62).

Several muscle forces contribute to deformity in fractures of the proximal or middle phalanx. The insertion of the flexor digitorum superficialis tendon along the middle phalanx affects the angulation of a fracture, depending upon the location of the break. If the fracture of the middle phalanx is distal to the insertion of the flexor digitorum superficialis tendon, the fractured bone angulates volarly. Fractures proximal to the insertion of the flexor digitorum superficialis tendon angulate dorsally. In fractures of the proximal phalanx, the insertions of the interosseous muscle at the base of the proximal phalanx tend to flex the proximal fragment, and the flexor and extensor tendons angulate the fracture volarly.

For reduction of a fracture of the phalanx, correct rotational alignment is just as essential as alignment in the anteroposterior and lateral planes. In the normal hand, the tips of all the flexed fingers point toward the tuberosity of the scaphoid. Inadequate reduction and persistent rotational malalignment adversely affect the patient's ability to grasp. Often, the rotational malalignment is not noticeable when the fingers are extended, but it is always obvious when the fingers are flexed. Although judging the reduction of any phalanx fracture in both flexion and extension may be difficult, this step is most important.

The high-energy forces that cause transverse and comminuted fractures of the phalanx often produce significant injury to the soft tissues of the finger as well. Successful treatment of phalanx fractures demands careful attention to the potential consequences of the soft tissue injuries. Even though the fracture may heal in adequate alignment, injuries to the flexor and extensor mechanisms can lead to significant long-term dysfunction.

Management of Fracture

Correction of deformity, preservation of motion, and care of the soft tissues are all important in the treatment of hand injuries (Plate 63). Adherence to the basic principles of fracture care is essential for good functional results. These principles are (1) alignment of the distal fragment with the proximal fragment, (2) adequate immobilization to allow healing, and (3) preservation of motion and soft tissue function. The primary goal in treating any hand injury is to maintain function, particularly full active motion of all joints. Persistent stiffness in the interphalangeal and metacarpophalangeal joints and adduction contracture of

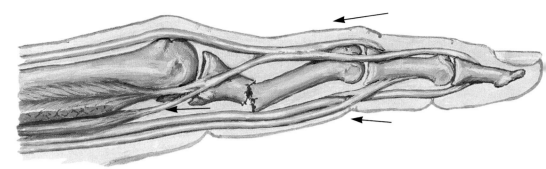

Transverse fractures of proximal phalanx tend to angulate volarly because of pull of interosseous muscles on base of proximal phalanx and collapsing action of long extensor and flexor tendons

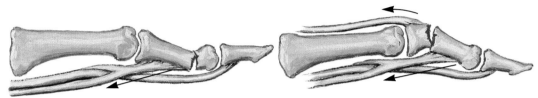

Fractures of neck of middle phalanx usually angulate volarly because of pull of flexor digitorum superficialis tendon, which inserts into proximal fragment

Fractures of base of middle phalanx often dorsally angulated by traction of central band of long extensor tendon on proximal fragment plus tension of both long flexor tendons

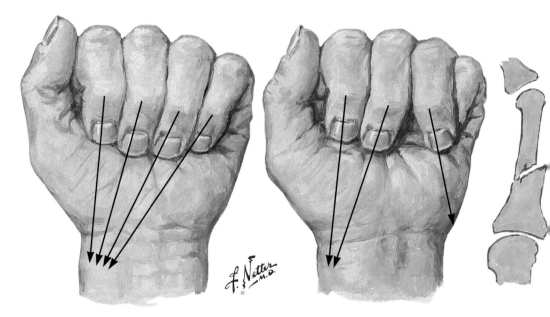

Reduction of fractures of phalanges or metacarpals requires correct rotational as well as longitudinal alignment. In normal hand, tips of flexed fingers point toward tuberosity of scaphoid, as in hand at left. Hand at right shows result of healing of ring finger in rotational malalignment. Rotational malalignment, usually discernible clinically, may also be evidenced on radiographs by discrepancy in cross-sectional diameter of fragments, as shown at extreme right. Discrepancy in diameter most apparent in true lateral radiograph but is visible to some extent in anteroposterior view

the thumb produce a functional loss that can be debilitating.

Immobilization should maintain the hand in a functional position: 45° extension of wrist, 70° flexion of the metacarpophalangeal joint, 20° flexion of the proximal interphalangeal joints, and maximal abduction of the thumb. If scarring occurs, this position will preserve as much soft tissue length and joint flexibility as possible. In any significant hand injury, only fingers requiring immobilization should be casted or splinted; the other fingers should remain free to move.

Some fractures of the phalanges are considered stable; these include most nondisplaced fractures,

long spiral fractures, and minimally displaced intraarticular fractures that do not displace with gentle early motion. Stable fractures can be treated by taping the injured finger to the normal adjacent finger (buddy taping) and initiating early active motion. Frequent and careful follow-up during the healing phase ensures that early motion does not displace the fracture fragment.

Most displaced fractures of the proximal and middle phalanges can be treated with closed reduction and cast immobilization using an ulnar or radial gutter splint. The plaster must be applied with great care to avoid excessive pressure on the soft tissues, which can cause ulceration of the skin

Injury to Hand
(Continued)

The fracture is checked at weekly intervals for 4 to 6 weeks. In fractures of the phalanges, radiographic evidence of healing appears slowly, and radiographs do not show union for many weeks. However, most uncomplicated fractures are clinically stable in 4 to 6 weeks. If examination at that time detects minimal swelling, no tenderness, and no instability, the patient can begin gentle protected motion, but the fracture should be protected for an additional few weeks with intermittent splinting or buddy taping.

Fractures that require open reduction and internal fixation or closed reduction and pin fixation include unstable fractures, fractures that cannot be adequately reduced and maintained with closed means, displaced intraarticular fractures, multiple fractures with soft tissue injuries, and fractures in patients who repeatedly remove their casts.

Oblique fractures are often unstable and tend to shorten the finger. Closed reduction under radiographic control followed by percutaneous pinning restores stability, maintains the reduction, and allows early motion. Transverse fractures of the proximal or middle phalanx are very unstable, often requiring internal fixation. Inserted through a dorsal or midaxial incision, crossed Kirschner wires stabilize the fracture with only minimal disruption of the soft tissues; the wires are removed under local anesthesia without significant soft tissue dissection. Small compression plates may be used.

When a fracture is stabilized with either closed reduction and pin fixation or open reduction and internal fixation, the finger is left undisturbed for 8 to 10 days for the initial phase of soft tissue healing; then active supervised motion is begun to preserve soft tissue function.

Massive crushing injuries with multiple fractures of the phalanges and significant destruction of soft tissue require open reduction and stabilization. Fortunately, the incidence of postoperative infection in open hand fractures is quite low.

Special Problems in Fracture of Phalanges

Management of fractures of the phalanges is complicated by numerous problems (Plate 64). Because of the intricate relationship between the flexor and extensor tendons, the joints, and the architecture of the phalanges, neglect or inadequate treatment can lead to significant disability (see CIBA COLLECTION, Volume 8/I, pages 71–73, for normal anatomy of the hand).

Treatment of Oblique Fracture. The pull of the flexor muscles tends to shorten oblique fractures of the proximal and middle phalanges. Resulting soft tissue adhesions contribute to stiffness of the proximal interphalangeal joint. In addition, a bone spike protrudes volarly, creating a mechanical block to full flexion of the proximal interphalangeal joint. Such problems can be managed in a number of ways. If the alignment of the proximal phalanx is adequate but joint motion is limited, the volar spike can be removed surgically and the tendon adhesions freed. These procedures

Management of Fracture of Proximal and Middle Phalanges

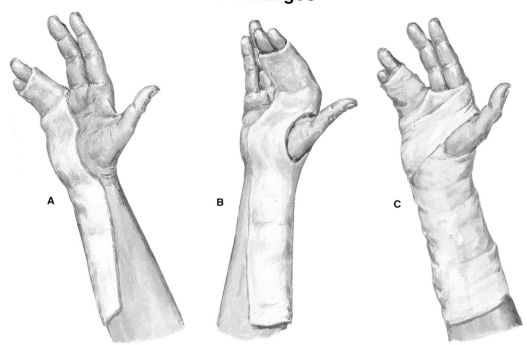

Most fractures of proximal or middle phalanx that can be treated with closed reduction and are stable can be satisfactorily immobilized in plaster gutter splint. A. Ulnar splint used for ring and little finger. B. Radial splint for index and middle fingers. C. Splints held in place with elastic bandage. Metacarpophalangeal joints flexed 70°– 90°, proximal interphalangeal joints extended

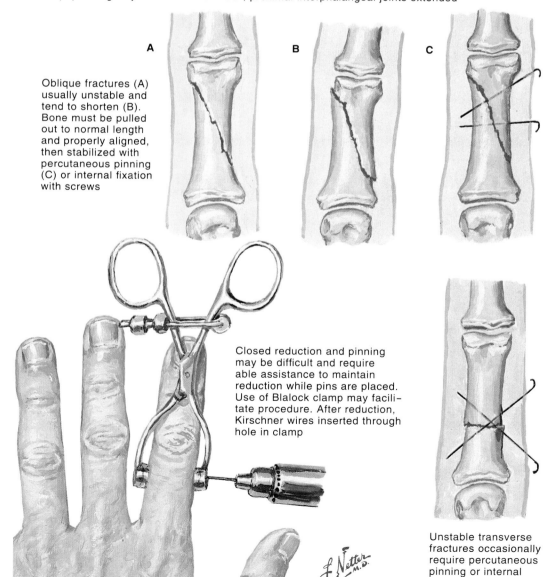

Oblique fractures (A) usually unstable and tend to shorten (B). Bone must be pulled out to normal length and properly aligned, then stabilized with percutaneous pinning (C) or internal fixation with screws

Closed reduction and pinning may be difficult and require able assistance to maintain reduction while pins are placed. Use of Blalock clamp may facilitate procedure. After reduction, Kirschner wires inserted through hole in clamp

Unstable transverse fractures occasionally require percutaneous pinning or internal fixation

Special Problems in Fracture of Middle and Proximal Phalanges

Injury to Hand
(Continued)

increase flexion and extension of the proximal interphalangeal joint. Inadequate bone alignment necessitates osteotomy of the proximal phalanx and internal fixation with Kirschner wires.

Treatment of Stable Intraarticular Fracture. Most intraarticular fractures of the metacarpophalangeal joint that have large nondisplaced fragments can be treated with buddy taping. However, close follow-up is essential to ensure that the fragment does not subsequently displace.

Treatment of Fracture of Condyles. Intraarticular fractures of the interphalangeal joints that involve the condyles of the proximal or middle phalanx are usually unstable. To avoid missing the fractured condyle and to assess the degree of displacement, radiographic examination must include anteroposterior, lateral, and oblique views. However, even following adequate open reduction, stable internal fixation, and fracture healing, stiffness usually persists in the distal or proximal interphalangeal joint.

Treatment of Boutonniere Deformity. A rare injury of the proximal interphalangeal joint, fracture of the dorsal lip of the middle phalanx results in an avulsion of the central slip of the extensor mechanism. This injury must be treated with open reduction and, if necessary, pin fixation of the fracture fragment. Failure to recognize this injury and restore the attachment of the central slip to the middle phalanx leads to a boutonniere deformity, with chronic pain and instability. If boutonniere deformity develops, arthrodesis of the proximal interphalangeal joint is often the only salvage procedure possible.

Treatment of Malunion and Nonunion. Even with proper treatment and adequate follow-up, fracture malunion may occur. In most cases, a malunion does not require any further care, but if it causes pain, limits hand function, or is cosmetically displeasing, surgical intervention should be considered. Osteotomy at the fracture site or at an adjacent area of metaphyseal bone is the usual procedure for realigning the phalanx. The osteotomy is stabilized with an internal fixation device.

Nonunion is rare in phalanx fractures and often remains asymptomatic. For symptomatic nonunion, treatment with open reduction and internal fixation combined with bone grafting usually results in healing.

Treatment of Tendon Adhesions. Because injuries to the phalanges damage soft tissue as well as bone, adhesions may develop between the flexor and extensor tendons and the fracture site. The primary clinical sign of this complication is a limitation of active flexion. The need for assistance to achieve full flexion usually indicates the presence of adhesions within the sheath of the flexor tendon. Vigorous physical therapy can help restore motion, but surgical tenolysis of the flexor sheath at the level of the healed fracture is occasionally required. Extensor tendon adhesions also limit active finger flexion and require the same treatment.

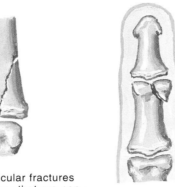
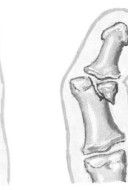
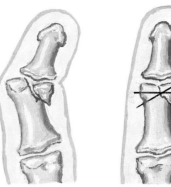

Oblique fracture of proximal phalanx with shortening. Fragment must be pulled out to avoid leaving volar spike that limits flexion of proximal interphalangeal joint

Malunion with protruding volar spike that limits joint flexion. Resection of spike may be needed later to correct disability

Intraarticular fractures of phalanx that are non-displaced and stable may be treated with buddy taping, careful observation, and early active exercise

Condylar fractures tend to angulate and require open reduction and pinning, even if fragment is small

Volar dislocation of middle phalanx with avulsion of central slip of extensor tendon, with or without bone fragment. Early repair of central slip indicated. If bone fragment present, it may be pinned. Failure to recognize and properly treat this condition results in boutonniere deformity and severely restricted function

Recurvatum (volar angulation) with compensatory flexion of proximal interphalangeal joint due to malunion of fracture of proximal phalanx. Osteotomy and realignment indicated

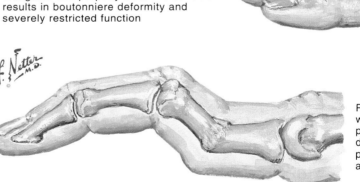

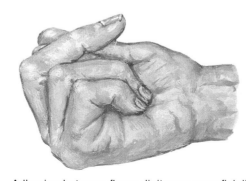

Adhesion between flexor digitorum superficialis and profundus tendons is common complication of fractures of middle or proximal phalanx. Evidenced by discrepancy between active finger flexion (left) and passive flexion (right). Illustrations depict inability to actively flex distal interphalangeal joint, which may, however, be passively flexed. Early active motion may help to avoid this disability and the need for surgical tenolysis

Injury to Hand

(Continued)

Dislocation of Proximal Interphalangeal Joint

Dorsal dislocation (most common)
Usually reducible by closed means, immobilized with palmar splint for 3 weeks, then active range–of–motion exercises begun

Palmar dislocation (uncommon)
Causes boutonniere deformity. Central slip of extensor tendon often torn, requiring open fixation, followed by dorsal splinting to allow passive and active exercises of distal interphalangeal joint

Rotational dislocation (rare)
Note middle and distal phalanges seen in true lateral radiograph, proximal phalanx in oblique view. After reduction, treated as for dorsal dislocation

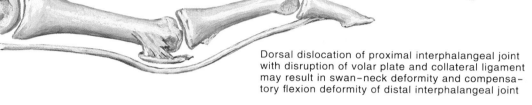

Dorsal dislocation of proximal interphalangeal joint with disruption of volar plate and collateral ligament may result in swan–neck deformity and compensatory flexion deformity of distal interphalangeal joint

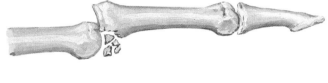

Fracture dislocation of middle phalanx with fragmented volar lip. This disabling injury often missed because of failure to take true lateral radiograph

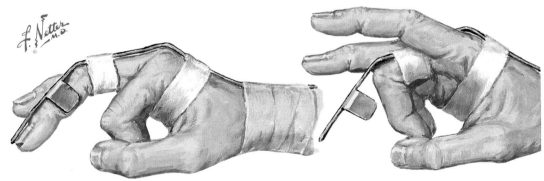

Extension block splint useful for dislocation of proximal interphalangeal joint with small or comminuted fragment from base of middle phalanx. After reduction achieved and radiographically documented, amount of flexion necessary to maintain reduction determined, and splint adjusted to permit no extension beyond that. Proximal phalanx must be secured to splint with adhesive tape. Active flexion at proximal interphalangeal joint (right) encouraged. Extension block splint gradually and progressively adjusted so that functional range of motion achieved in 3 – 4 weeks

Dislocation of Proximal Interphalangeal Joint

The proximal interphalangeal joint is basically a hinge joint supported by the architecture of the bone and by strong collateral ligaments on either side, which are in turn reinforced by a strong volar ligament, or plate. The dorsal capsule of the proximal interphalangeal joint is strengthened by the central slip of the extensor tendon and by the insertions of the lateral bands of the extensor tendon. Ligament injuries of the proximal interphalangeal joint, the most common injuries of the hand, include simple sprains of the collateral ligament or the volar plate (most common), complete dislocations, and the most severe injuries—fracture dislocations.

Any injury to the proximal interphalangeal joint can significantly affect motion and function of the finger (Plate 65). During the diagnostic evaluation, the examiner must palpate specific areas for tenderness and assess the stability of the joint both actively, as the patient flexes the finger, and passively, as the examiner moves the finger.

The most common dislocation of the proximal interphalangeal joint, the *dorsal* dislocation, is often called the coach's finger. Frequently occurring in athletic events, the dorsal dislocation is usually reduced by trainers or coaches shortly after injury. The uncommon *volar* dislocation of the proximal interphalangeal joint is a more serious injury because it disrupts the central slip of the extensor mechanism. Unless properly treated by splinting with the joint in extension, volar dislocation can result in a disabling boutonniere deformity.

Rotational dislocations are rare. A unique aspect of this type of dislocation is the appearance of the phalanges on the lateral radiograph: the proximal phalanx is seen in an oblique plane and the middle phalanx in a true lateral plane. Although closed reduction usually produces a satisfactory result, open reduction is occasionally required to restore the phalanges to their anatomic positions.

If there is evidence of instability after reduction, simple dorsal and rotational dislocations of the proximal interphalangeal joint can be treated with splinting for 3 weeks; if the joint is stable, early active motion with buddy taping is prescribed for 4 to 6 weeks. In the more severe volar dislocation, the proximal interphalangeal joint must be splinted in extension for 4 to 6 weeks to avoid creating a boutonniere deformity.

Fracture dislocations are the most severe and disabling injuries of the proximal interphalangeal joint. In addition to dislocation, a fracture disrupts the volar surface of the middle phalanx, resulting in both dorsal and volar instability. These injuries are often missed because the dislocation reduces spontaneously and the fracture of the volar lip of the middle phalanx appears quite insignificant on the radiograph.

Some fracture dislocations can be treated with closed reduction of the dislocation and use of an extension block splint. The splint allows full flexion of the finger and a range of extension that maintains the reduction and stability of the proximal interphalangeal joint. This method of treatment requires close radiographic follow-up. As healing increases the stability on the volar side, the amount of extension can be gradually increased until the joint remains stable in full extension.

Fracture of Metacarpals

Injury to Hand
(*Continued*)

Fractures of metacarpal neck commonly result from end-on blow of fist. Often called street-fighter or boxer fractures

In fractures of metacarpal neck, volar cortex often comminuted, resulting in marked instability after reduction, which often necessitates pinning

Transverse fractures of metacarpal shaft usually angulated dorsally by pull of interosseous muscles

Oblique fractures tend to shorten and rotate metacarpal, particularly in index and little fingers because metacarpals of middle and ring fingers are stabilized by deep transverse metacarpal ligaments

Most transverse fractures of metacarpals can be reduced and adequately immobilized with gutter splint, as for fractures of phalanges. Metacarpophalangeal joint should be flexed, proximal interphalangeal joint extended, and active movement encouraged to avoid flexion deformity. Frequent radiographic follow-up important

Unstable fractures, either transverse or oblique, may require fixation with smooth Kirschner wire inserted by percutaneous or open means

Fracture dislocation with a large fragment from the volar lip requires open reduction with Kirschner wire fixation. Late reconstruction of this injury involves either arthrodesis or arthroplasty of the volar plate.

In all injuries of the proximal interphalangeal joint, the patient should be informed that the joint will remain enlarged for a long time, possibly many years, and that loss of motion is quite common.

Fracture of Metacarpals

The carpal and metacarpal bones form a longitudinal arch within the osseous framework of the hand, with transverse arches formed by the metacarpals. The treatment of metacarpal fractures must restore the architecture of the hand so that the metacarpals of the mobile groups—the thumb on the radial side and the ring and little fingers on the ulnar side—maintain their important relationship with the stable central ray, which includes the metacarpals of the index and middle fingers (Plate 66).

Fracture of Metacarpal Neck. The most common metacarpal fracture occurs at the neck of the fifth metacarpal. Although often called the boxer fracture, it is more aptly named the street fighter fracture because trained boxers attempt to strike their opponent with the radial side of the hand, which is more stable than the ulnar side. Most fractures of the neck of the fifth metacarpal are significantly comminuted on the volar side, resulting in dorsal angulation at the fracture site. These fractures are usually treated with closed reduction and immobilization in an ulnar gutter splint, which holds the metacarpophalangeal joint in 70° to 90° flexion.

Most fractures heal satisfactorily. Maintaining adequate rotational alignment is important, but some residual dorsal angulation is acceptable because the flexible ulnar side of the hand can adapt to slight deformity. Some extensor lag commonly persists following fracture healing. Open reduction is indicated only if rotational alignment cannot be maintained or the fracture angulates greater than 70°. In any fracture of this type, the physician must carefully search for a laceration of the adjacent metacarpophalangeal joint caused by impact with a tooth; lacerations could lead to significant infection and marked disability if left untreated.

Fracture of Metacarpal Shaft. Most transverse fractures of the metacarpal shaft are angulated dorsally by the pull of the intrinsic muscles of the hand. The metacarpals of the middle and ring fingers, however, are stabilized by the adjacent border metacarpals and their deep transverse metacarpal ligaments; therefore, they do not generally shorten even if the fracture is comminuted. Oblique or spiral fractures of the metacarpals of the little and index fingers do tend to shorten because they are not adequately splinted by stable metacarpals on either side.

Fractures of the metacarpal shaft can be treated adequately with immobilization in a plaster cast, with the metacarpophalangeal joint flexed 70° and the proximal interphalangeal joint in full extension. This position relaxes the pull of the intrinsic muscles and allows the physician to monitor apposition, length, and rotational alignment of the metacarpals. Massive crush injuries of the hand, with multiple fractures and considerable soft tissue damage, require open reduction and internal fixation. Surgical repair allows early active motion and produces a good functional result.

Injury to Hand
(Continued)

Fracture of Base of Metacarpal of Thumb

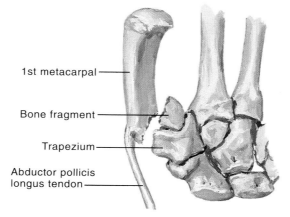

1st metacarpal ——

Bone fragment ——

Trapezium ——

Abductor pollicis
longus tendon ——

Type I (Bennett fracture). Intraarticular fracture
with proximal and radial dislocation of 1st metacarpal. Triangular bone fragment sheared off

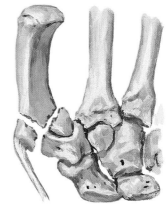

Type II (Rolando fracture).
Intraarticular fracture with
Y–shaped configuration

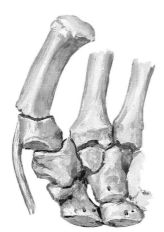

Type IIIA. Extraarticular
transverse fracture

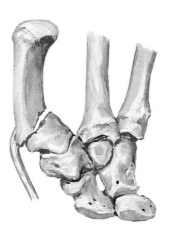

Type IIIB. Extraarticular
oblique fracture

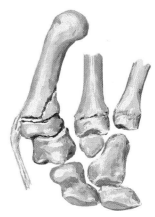

Type IV. Epiphyseal
fracture with separation
in child

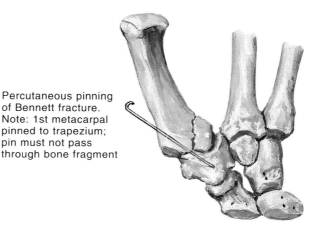

Percutaneous pinning
of Bennett fracture.
Note: 1st metacarpal
pinned to trapezium;
pin must not pass
through bone fragment

Fracture of Base of Metacarpal of Thumb

Mobility of the carpometacarpal joint of the thumb is essential for adequate hand function. Therefore, treatment of all fractures of the thumb must achieve and maintain good reduction and alignment. Two particularly troublesome fractures are intraarticular fractures of the base of the first metacarpal (Plate 67).

Type I Intraarticular Fracture (Bennett Fracture). This fracture within the joint is often associated with proximal dislocation of the metacarpal shaft. The abductor pollicis longus tendon inserts on the base of the metacarpal of the thumb and tends to abduct and pull the metacarpal shaft proximally. The very strong volar ligament, which is attached to the base of the articular facet of the metacarpal, maintains the alignment of the proximal fragment with the trapezium.

Bennett fractures usually require surgical fixation because reduction is difficult to maintain in a plaster cast. If a very small fragment of the metacarpal base remains on the ulnar side, the dislocated metacarpal can be reduced easily by applying traction and holding the thumb in abduction. The reduction is maintained with Kirschner wires inserted percutaneously. If the intraarticular fragment is very large, open reduction should be considered to restore the anatomy of the joint to as normal as possible. The reduction can be stabilized with screws, Kirschner wires, or a small buttress plate.

Often, a small displaced fragment appears innocuous on the radiograph, and the dislocation is missed. The most important aspects of the treatment of Bennett fractures are recognizing that the injury is a fracture dislocation rather than just an intraarticular fracture and achieving and maintaining an adequate reduction.

Type II Intraarticular Fracture (Rolando Fracture). This comminuted fracture involves the articular surface of the metacarpal. Unlike

the type I fracture, there is no significant proximal displacement of the metacarpal shaft. The comminution extends radially along the base of the metacarpal of the thumb and distally to the insertion of the abductor pollicis longus tendon.

In a Rolando fracture, the amount of comminution determines the method of treatment. If there are two or three large fragments that can be adequately reduced, open reduction and internal fixation can be attempted. Usually, however, good reduction is achieved only with great difficulty. Extensive comminution of the base of the metacarpal indicates the need for skeletal or skin traction to maintain the reduction.

Intraarticular fractures of the base of the thumb often lead to osteoarthritis of the carpometacarpal joint. Arthrodesis of the carpometacarpal joint of the thumb may be required later to relieve pain and instability.

Types III and IV Fractures. Type III fractures of the first metacarpal are extraarticular; that is, they do not involve the joint. Type IV (epiphyseal) fractures commonly occur in children and involve the growth plate; they should be recognized as extraarticular, not intraarticular, fractures. Extraarticular fractures are treated with closed reduction and immobilization; they rarely require surgery.

Injury to Hand
(Continued)

Thumb Injury Other Than Fracture

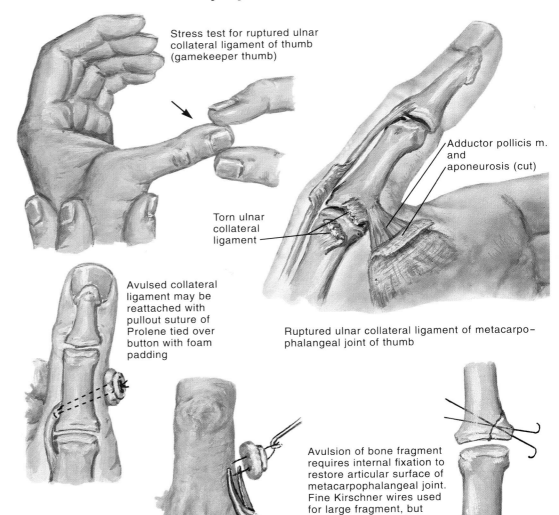

Stress test for ruptured ulnar collateral ligament of thumb (gamekeeper thumb)

Adductor pollicis m. and aponeurosis (cut)

Torn ulnar collateral ligament

Ruptured ulnar collateral ligament of metacarpophalangeal joint of thumb

Avulsed collateral ligament may be reattached with pullout suture of Prolene tied over button with foam padding

For removal, one limb of suture cut at skin level and stitch pulled out

Avulsion of bone fragment requires internal fixation to restore articular surface of metacarpophalangeal joint. Fine Kirschner wires used for large fragment, but pullout suture may be advantageous for small fragment

Pure dislocation of carpometacarpal joint of thumb without fracture is reducible but unstable. Should be pinned to trapezium, as for Bennett fracture

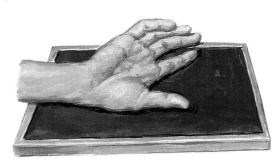

Position of hand on cassette for Robert view (true anteroposterior) radiograph. Robert view best visualizes carpometacarpal joint of thumb, and pathology may be missed if this view not taken

Thumb Injury Other Than Fracture

The thumb acts as a very mobile post that opposes the actions of the index, middle, ring, and little fingers. The stability of the thumb is therefore very important in hand function (Plate 68).

Injury to Ulnar Collateral Ligament. In the metacarpophalangeal joint of the thumb, injury to the ulnar collateral ligament destroys joint stability and impairs the ability to pinch. Known as the gamekeeper thumb, this injury is a common consequence of skiing, motor vehicle, and occupational accidents.

Any injury to the ulnar side of the metacarpophalangeal joint of the thumb must be evaluated with a stress test to determine the integrity of the ulnar collateral ligament. The stress test should be performed using digital block anesthesia. If the test shows joint instability, the ulnar collateral ligament should be repaired surgically.

Surgical examination often reveals the adductor tendon aponeurosis interposed between the torn ends of the ulnar collateral ligament; this condition, called the Stener lesion, prevents healing. A tear in the substance of the ligament itself is repaired with interrupted sutures. If the ligament is avulsed from the bone, repair with

a pull-out wire is needed. Avulsion of a bone fragment together with the ligament requires reduction of the fragment and fixation with a small screw, a pull-out wire, or Kirschner wires.

To ensure stability, a Kirschner wire is sometimes placed across the joint to relieve the tension on the repaired ligament. After ligament repair, the thumb is immobilized in a cast for at least 4 weeks. The patient can begin guarded activity at 4 weeks, after the cast and pin are removed. Early anatomic repair of gamekeeper thumb produces quite satisfactory results.

Dislocation of Carpometacarpal Joint. This thumb injury can also be quite disabling. Because

of the configuration of the carpometacarpal joint, dislocations are inherently unstable. Although reduction of the carpometacarpal dislocation is easy, maintaining the reduction in a plaster cast is very difficult. Therefore, in most carpometacarpal dislocations, the reduction must be pinned to ensure stability. The pin is placed across the joint and maintained for 4 to 6 weeks to allow the joint capsule to heal. Chronic, undiagnosed, or recurrent dislocations of the carpometacarpal joint of the thumb can be treated either with ligament reconstruction, using the flexor carpi radialis tendon, or with arthrodesis of the carpometacarpal joint. □

Common Causes of Cervical Spine Injury

Injury to Spine

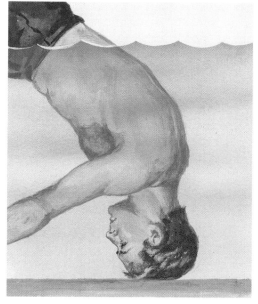

Compression injury of cervical spine may result from blow on top of head, as in diving accident

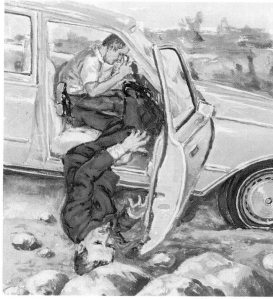

Compression–rotation injury may occur when person is thrown from car or upended in football or other sports accident

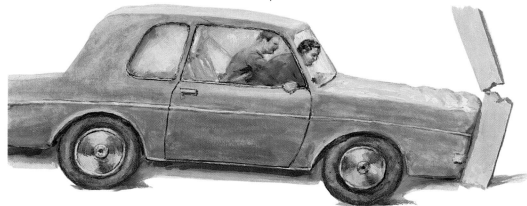

Head–on collision with stationary object or oncoming vehicle may, if seat belts not used, drive forehead against windshield. This sharply hyperextends neck, resulting in dislocation with or without fracture of cervical vertebrae

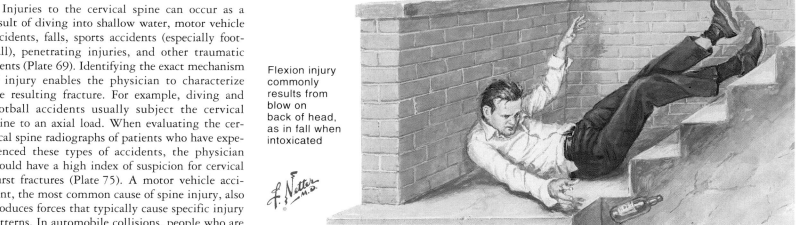

Flexion injury commonly results from blow on back of head, as in fall when intoxicated

Common Causes of Cervical Spine Injury

The cervical spine is an extremely mobile segment of the axial skeleton that provides for a wide range of flexion, extension, and rotational motion. This flexibility of movement and the relatively unprotected position of the cervical spine in the posterior aspect of the neck make it extremely vulnerable to trauma.

Injuries to the cervical spine can occur as a result of diving into shallow water, motor vehicle accidents, falls, sports accidents (especially football), penetrating injuries, and other traumatic events (Plate 69). Identifying the exact mechanism of injury enables the physician to characterize the resulting fracture. For example, diving and football accidents usually subject the cervical spine to an axial load. When evaluating the cervical spine radiographs of patients who have experienced these types of accidents, the physician should have a high index of suspicion for cervical burst fractures (Plate 75). A motor vehicle accident, the most common cause of spine injury, also produces forces that typically cause specific injury patterns. In automobile collisions, people who are not wearing seat belts usually strike the forehead against the windshield or the steering wheel. The impact sharply hyperextends the neck, often resulting in dislocation of the cervical spine with or without fracture of the cervical vertebrae. In a fall down stairs, the flexion forces applied to the cervical spine can cause a variety of cervical spine injuries, including subtle fractures of the odontoid process that might otherwise be overlooked if the mechanism of injury is not known (Plate 76). Rotational stresses often occur in combination with axial loading, flexion, or extension, thus modifying the resulting injury. Of the four types of forces, axial loading, combined with flexion or extension, is most likely to produce severe injuries of the cervical spine.

The forces that cause cervical spine injuries often cause head injuries also. Clinical manifestations include bleeding from lacerations, ecchymosis, swelling, and alteration in consciousness. These signs of head injury should not, however, distract the examining physician from searching for other injuries, especially since there is a strong association between cervical spine injuries and head injuries. Therefore, the emergency and hospital teams should presume that a patient with a head injury also has a spine injury. In all patients with head injuries, the spine should be properly immobilized and protected until radiographs and a careful neurologic evaluation have ruled out an injury of the spine.

Sensory Impairment Related to Level of Spinal Cord Injury

Injury to Spine
(Continued)

Resuscitation

All patients with suspected cervical spine trauma should first undergo the *ABCs* of resuscitation: establishment of an *A*irway with immobilization of the cervical spine, maintenance of *B*reathing and ventilation, and support of the *C*irculation with control of hemorrhage. A patent airway is initially established with the chin lift or jaw thrust maneuver and removal of any foreign objects or debris from the mouth. The cervical spine must remain immobilized with a cervical collar until lateral cervical spine radiographs have established the presence or absence of any fractures or dislocations. If a cervical injury is identified, in-line cervical traction should be applied for the remainder of the resuscitation phase until a more secure form of immobilization, such as a halo brace, can be applied.

The next phase of resuscitation involves maintenance of breathing and ventilation. If oxygenation is inadequate, supplemental oxygen is delivered via a face mask or endotracheal tube. In addition, any injuries compromising ventilation, such as a tension pneumothorax, are addressed at this time. Intravenous fluids and blood products are administered as needed to maintain circulating blood volume. Any obvious hemorrhages should be controlled with direct pressure or, in rare instances, pneumatic antishock garment. When resuscitation is complete, a thorough history is taken and a physical examination performed, including a thorough neurologic assessment with sensory, motor, and rectal examinations.

Sensory Impairment Related to Level of Spinal Cord Injury

The examiner first performs a sensory examination with a pinwheel and very light pressure, documenting the areas where sharp/dull discrimination is perceived. Areas of demonstrable changes in the patient's sharp/dull discrimination are marked with a skin marker. The demarcation between normal and abnormal areas of sensation is best identified by working backward with the pinwheel from the anesthetic areas to the sensate areas. This line marks the level of dermatomal (nerve root) sensation still present and therefore suggests the level of possible spinal cord injury (Plate 70). If the examination detects a loss of sensation, the physician must examine the patient further for any sparing of sharp/dull discrimination distal to the apparent level of injury; areas of remaining sensation may indicate an incomplete spinal cord lesion from which the patient may recover. The sacrally innervated skin is often the only area where sensation is preserved. Since this sacral sparing may be the only sign of an incomplete spinal cord lesion, assessment of

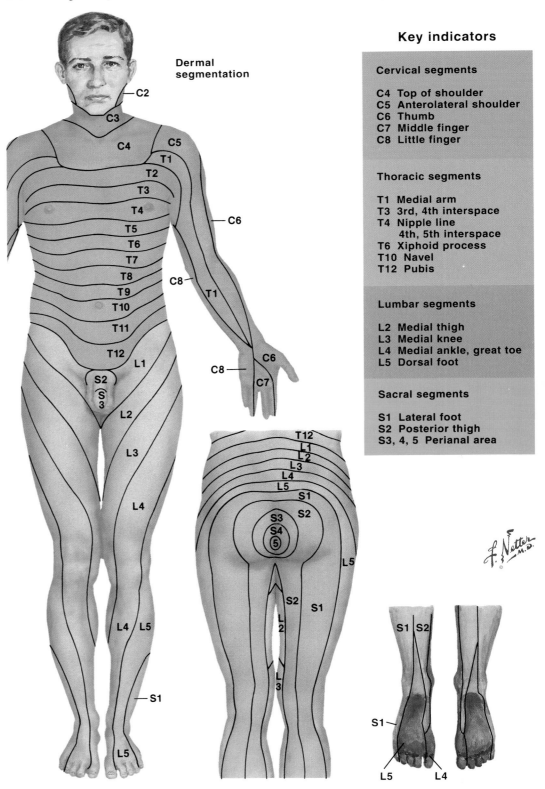

Dermal segmentation

Key indicators

Cervical segments

C4 Top of shoulder
C5 Anterolateral shoulder
C6 Thumb
C7 Middle finger
C8 Little finger

Thoracic segments

T1 Medial arm
T3 3rd, 4th interspace
T4 Nipple line
    4th, 5th interspace
T6 Xiphoid process
T10 Navel
T12 Pubis

Lumbar segments

L2 Medial thigh
L3 Medial knee
L4 Medial ankle, great toe
L5 Dorsal foot

Sacral segments

S1 Lateral foot
S2 Posterior thigh
S3, 4, 5 Perianal area

perianal sensation is mandatory in any patient with suspected spinal cord trauma.

The sensory test should also include evaluation of sensations of deep pressure, deep pain, and proprioception. Preservation of these sensations indicates an injury that has spared the posterior column of the spinal cord (Plate 75).

Although physicians do not need to memorize the complete dermatomal innervation of the body, certain areas of dermatomal innervation should be known. The C6 dermatome encompasses an area on the radial half of the forearm, the thumb, and the radial half of the index finger. The C7 dermatome includes the ulnar half of the index

finger, the entire middle finger, and the radial half of the ring finger. C8 provides sensation to the remaining ulnar border digits and the ulnar side of the forearm. Other areas of significant dermatomal innervation include the nipples (T4), umbilicus (T10), and inguinal ligament (L1). The L4 dermatome innervates the *lateral* aspect of the thigh but then rotates to innervate the *medial* aspect of the leg and foot. The L5 dermatome begins on the lateral aspect of the thigh but continues downward on the lateral aspect of the leg and then rotates slightly medially to innervate the dorsum of the foot. The S1 dermatome innervates the lateral aspect of the foot as well as the sole.

Injury to Spine
(Continued)

Motor Impairment Related to Level of Spinal Cord Injury

Immediately after the the sensory examination, the motor function of all four limbs should be assessed thoroughly (Plate 71). Each muscle tested should be graded: grade 0, no evidence of muscle contractility; grade 1, slight evidence of muscle contractility but no ability to produce joint motion; grade 2, complete range of joint motion with gravity removed; grade 3, complete range of joint motion against gravity; grade 4, complete range of joint motion against gravity with some resistance applied; grade 5, complete range of joint motion against gravity with full resistance applied.

Patients with complete spinal cord injury above the level of C4 rarely survive because sudden paralysis of all respiratory musculature usually causes death soon after the accident. The patient with an injury that spares the C5 level can actively abduct the shoulders and flex the elbows. A C6 level of motor function denotes the ability to extend the wrist and thumb, and a patient with a C7 level of function can flex the wrist and extend the finger. A C8 level of function indicates the ability to flex the fingers, and a T1 level of function indicates the use of the intrinsic muscles of the hand.

The patient with an L3 level of function can use all the musculature of the upper limbs and actively adduct the thighs. With an L4 level of function, the patient can extend the knees and usually can dorsiflex the ankle; a patient with this injury is potentially able to walk with the use of supportive devices. An L5 level of function controls active extension of the great toe, and an S1 level permits plantar flexion of the ankle.

Every patient with suspected spinal cord trauma should be evaluated with a rectal examination, which tests the lower sacral nerve roots for function and perianal sensation for sacral sparing. Intact rectal tone or sensation suggests that the spinal cord injury is only partial and that the patient has a much better chance of neurologic recovery. About 5% of patients with what appears to be a complete spinal cord injury on initial examination may actually recover a significant degree of function.

Spinal Cord Shock

Although the level of spinal cord injury can be determined with thorough sensory and motor examinations, these examinations are accurate only after the period of spinal cord shock has passed. Spinal cord shock is the absence of all spinal reflex activity below the level of the cord injury that usually persists for 24 hours after injury. The presence of spinal cord shock can be established by testing the bulbocavernosus reflex by stimulation of the trigone of the bladder. Traction on a Foley

Motor Impairment Related to Level of Spinal Cord Injury

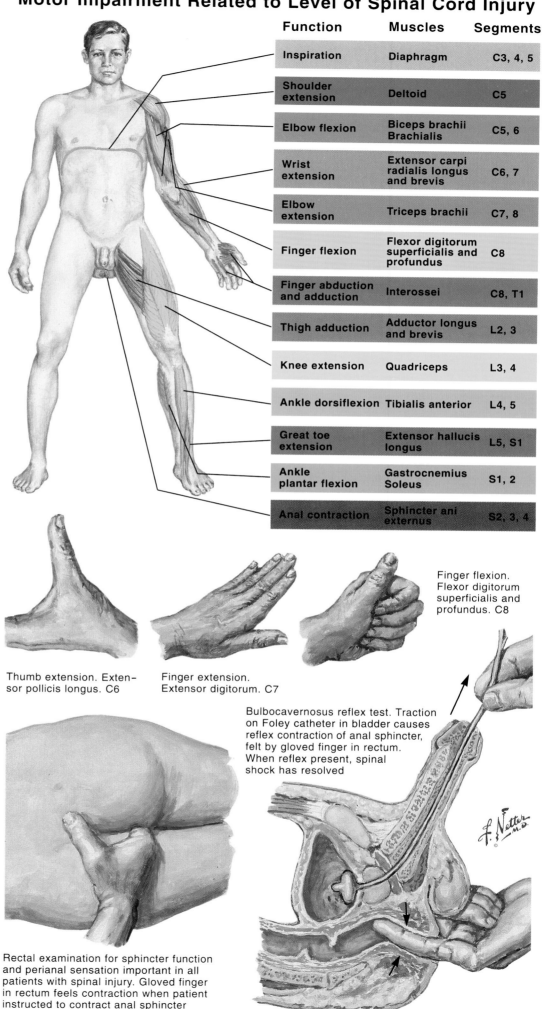

Function	Muscles	Segments
Inspiration	Diaphragm	C3, 4, 5
Shoulder extension	Deltoid	C5
Elbow flexion	Biceps brachii Brachialis	C5, 6
Wrist extension	Extensor carpi radialis longus and brevis	C6, 7
Elbow extension	Triceps brachii	C7, 8
Finger flexion	Flexor digitorum superficialis and profundus	C8
Finger abduction and adduction	Interossei	C8, T1
Thigh adduction	Adductor longus and brevis	L2, 3
Knee extension	Quadriceps	L3, 4
Ankle dorsiflexion	Tibialis anterior	L4, 5
Great toe extension	Extensor hallucis longus	L5, S1
Ankle plantar flexion	Gastrocnemius Soleus	S1, 2
Anal contraction	Sphincter ani externus	S2, 3, 4

Thumb extension. Extensor pollicis longus. C6

Finger extension. Extensor digitorum. C7

Finger flexion. Flexor digitorum superficialis and profundus. C8

Rectal examination for sphincter function and perianal sensation important in all patients with spinal injury. Gloved finger in rectum feels contraction when patient instructed to contract anal sphincter

Bulbocavernosus reflex test. Traction on Foley catheter in bladder causes reflex contraction of anal sphincter, felt by gloved finger in rectum. When reflex present, spinal shock has resolved

Radiographic Examination of Cervical Spine

Injury to Spine
(Continued)

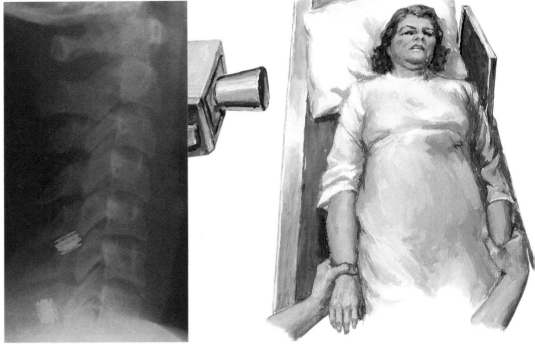

Lateral radiograph of cervical spine visualizes spine to C7–T1 articulation

Position for lateral radiograph of cervical spine. Attendant pulls down on both upper limbs

catheter normally results in a reflex contraction of the anal sphincter, which can be felt by a gloved finger in the rectum. Absence of reflex contraction indicates that the spinal cord is still in shock and that diagnosis of a complete spinal cord lesion cannot yet be made.

A patient in spinal cord shock may yet recover motor and sensory function distal to the level determined on initial neurologic evaluation. However, absence of voluntary rectal tone after spinal shock has resolved indicates a complete spinal cord injury with no chance of functional recovery distal to the cord lesion.

Imaging Techniques for Cervical Spine Injury

Radiographic Examination. Plain radiographs help define the extent of injury in the cervical spine. The initial radiographs that are needed to evaluate a cervical spine injury include lateral, anteroposterior, and oblique views, with the lateral radiograph taken first (Plate 72). It is important to remember that fracture dislocations of C6 on C7 or C7 on T1 may be missed if all seven cervical vertebrae and the first thoracic vertebra are not visualized on the lateral view. In patients whose C7–T1 level is not completely visualized, such as heavy patients with substantial shoulder mass, a special technique called a swimmer view may be required. This special lateral radiograph is obtained by abducting one arm 180° while the other arm is pulled down along the side by the application of traction. This position allows better visualization of the C7–T1 articulation on the lateral radiograph.

If the initial radiographs of the cervical spine appear normal and the neurologic examination reveals no evidence of a sensory or motor deficit, lateral views with the patient actively flexing and extending the neck may be helpful. These techniques help determine instability of the cervical spine by revealing areas of excessive motion. However, for these flexion and extension views to be obtained safely, the patient must have no neurologic loss or alterations in consciousness and must be able to perform all movements actively and without assistance.

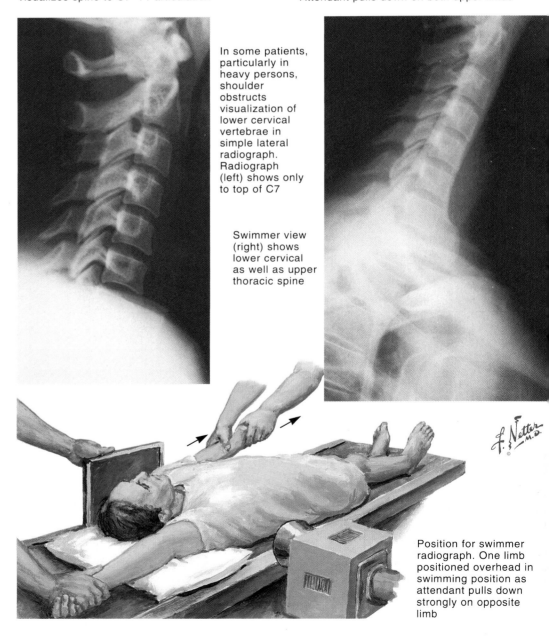

In some patients, particularly in heavy persons, shoulder obstructs visualization of lower cervical vertebrae in simple lateral radiograph. Radiograph (left) shows only to top of C7

Swimmer view (right) shows lower cervical as well as upper thoracic spine

Position for swimmer radiograph. One limb positioned overhead in swimming position as attendant pulls down strongly on opposite limb

Injury to Spine
(Continued)

Special Imaging Techniques for Cervical Spine Injury

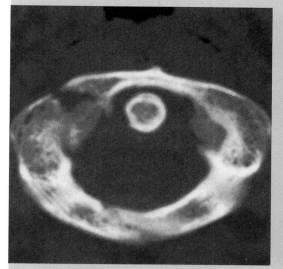

Computed tomography (CT) scan shows Jefferson fracture

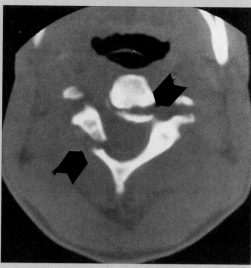

CT scan shows hangman fracture (bottom arrow)

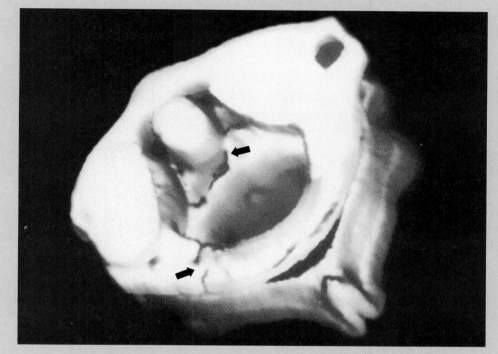

Three-dimensional CT scan of type III odontoid fracture combined with Jefferson fracture

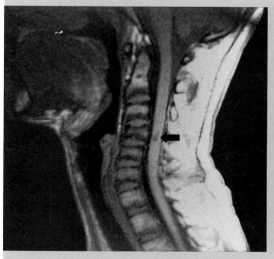

Magnetic resonance imaging (MRI) demonstrates mild spinal cord injury that resulted in some impairment of sensory and motor function below level of spinal cord damage

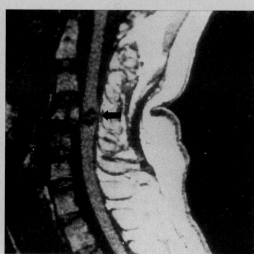

MRI reveals severe spinal cord injury. Total paralysis and sensory loss distal to spinal cord damage

Special Imaging Techniques. In addition to plain radiographs, other imaging techniques are helpful in enhancing visualization of the spine and spinal cord (Plate 73). Computed tomography (CT) is extremely useful for evaluating the bone architecture of the spine and for detecting subtle fractures that might be overlooked on plain radiographs. In addition, CT scans delineate the exact pattern and orientation of the fracture fragments better than plain radiographs.

Magnetic resonance imaging (MRI), a recent addition to orthopedic radiology, is invaluable in the diagnosis of spine or spinal cord injury because it can visualize soft tissue structures: discs, ligaments, nerves, and the spinal cord itself. High-quality MRI now allows physicians to determine the amount of permanent injury by the degree of hemorrhage, compression, and fibrosis in the spinal cord.

Magnetic resonance imaging and computed tomography provide different, useful sets of information. If both imaging techniques are available, they should be coordinated and analyzed together for a full evaluation of spinal cord trauma. Frequently, these imaging studies can be performed soon after the injury. Quick diagnosis can improve prognosis by allowing early surgical treatment of partial cord injuries when disc or bone fragments are found to be compressing the spinal cord.

Subluxation and Ligamentous Instability of Cervical Spine

Injury to Spine
(Continued)

Subluxation and Ligamentous Instability of Cervical Spine

Evaluation of the bone stability of the spine is an essential part of the diagnosis of a spine injury (Plate 74). If the fracture fragments or spine segments are likely to be displaced before healing is complete, the injury is considered *unstable*. Shifting fracture fragments in the spine can damage nerves or spinal cord at any time during the healing phase.

The concepts of acute and chronic instability of the spine are important in the selection of treatment. If a spine injury is considered *acutely stable*, it will remain stable during the entire healing process. Therefore, patients with an acutely stable injury require only treatment with analgesic medications and a soft supportive orthosis. However, a spine injury that is considered *acutely unstable* may become stable 3 months later, after bone healing has occurred and normal biomechanics are restored. Acutely unstable injuries require more aggressive management with a halo traction brace and immobilization in a rigid cast to encourage proper bone healing.

Major injury to the ligaments of the cervical spine, such as tearing of the posterior ligaments, makes the cervical spine acutely unstable. Because ligament injuries often heal poorly, this type of injury becomes *chronically unstable* if the torn ligaments do not heal adequately. Ligament injury in the cervical spine, with its high risk of chronic instability, requires stabilization with surgical procedures such as fusion (arthrodesis).

The stability of cervical spine ligaments is difficult to determine on plain radiographs, and flexion and extension views may also be needed (Plate 72). Extensive investigation has established criteria for determining cervical spine stability. According to White and Panjabi, major ligament instability of the cervical spine exists if lateral cervical spine radiographs show vertebral translation greater than 3.5 mm or angulation of adjacent vertebral segments of 11° or greater. In the lumbar spine, acute instability is defined as vertebral translation greater than 2.5 mm, vertebral tilt greater than 12°, or 25% loss of disc height.

If the evaluation detects any degree of instability, cervical fusion is necessary. A bone fusion of the area of ligament instability may restore stability by bridging the weakened area. Several procedures are used for fusing unstable cervical segments, each with specific indications and surgical techniques. Posterior fusion of the cervical spine is by far the most common procedure. The Rogers technique for posterior fusion consists of wiring adjacent spinous processes together and then placing strips of autograft bone from the ilium on top of the decorticated laminae. The procedure produces a bone fusion mass on the posterior aspect of the spine.

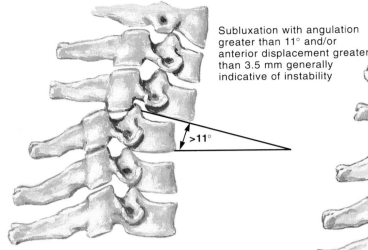

Subluxation with angulation greater than 11° and/or anterior displacement greater than 3.5 mm generally indicative of instability

Subluxation with angulation greater than 11°

Anterior displacement greater than 3.5 mm

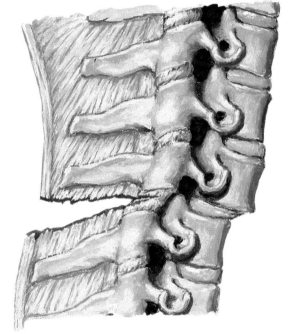

Tear of interspinal and supraspinal ligaments characteristic of anterior dislocation of spine

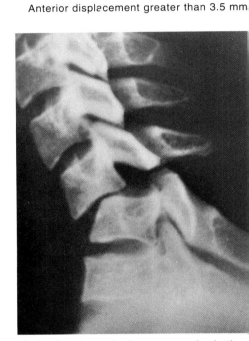

Lateral radiograph shows severe kyphotic angulation in cervical dislocation

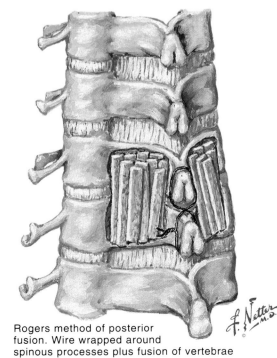

Rogers method of posterior fusion. Wire wrapped around spinous processes plus fusion of vertebrae

Postoperative radiograph shows corrected alignment and fixation wire in place

Three-Column Concept of Spinal Stability; Burst Fracture

Injury to Spine
(Continued)

Three-Column Concept of Spinal Stability

In an evaluation of the bone stability of the spine, it is helpful to think of the spine as a series of columns (Plate 75). Holdsworth described the spine in terms of two stabilizing columns—the anterior column and the posterior column. Denis added to this concept by proposing another column, called the middle column. In this concept, the anterior column is formed by the anterior longitudinal ligament, anterior annulus fibrosus, and anterior one-half of the vertebral body. The middle column consists of the posterior longitudinal ligament, posterior annulus fibrosus, and posterior one-half of the vertebral body. The posterior column comprises the posterior ligament complex of the supraspinal ligament, interspinal ligament, and ligamentum flavum, as well as the facet joints and capsules and the posterior neural arch.

The concept of three columns stabilizing the spine is particularly helpful in an analysis of bone injuries and spine stability with computed tomography. If two of the three columns are disrupted, the injury is considered unstable.

Burst Fracture

In a burst fracture, axial compression of the spine disrupts the anterior as well as the middle column (Plate 75). A burst fracture is therefore considered unstable, and fragments of bone from the vertebral body are often retropulsed into the vertebral canal, causing compression of the spinal cord itself. The number of retropulsed fragments and the degree of compression are best determined with CT scans.

Similar to a burst fracture, a compression fracture of the vertebral body is also caused by axial loading. In compression fractures, however, only the anterior part of the vertebral body is compressed, or wedged, and thus only the anterior column is involved. As a result, this injury is considered stable and requires only supportive treatment.

Immediate intervention is crucial for burst fractures with associated neurologic deficit due to compression of the anterior spinal cord by retropulsed fragments or a bulging posterior longitudinal ligament. Anterior corpectomy, as described by Bohlman, decompresses the spinal cord by removing any offending retropulsed fragments. The procedure produces long-term stability by the placement of an autograft between adjacent, unaffected vertebral bodies to maintain normal vertebral height. Thus, an unstable burst fracture is converted into a stable configuration, which minimizes the risk of late spinal deformity.

The three-column theory illustrates why posterior decompression by laminectomy is contraindicated in the treatment of many spine injuries.

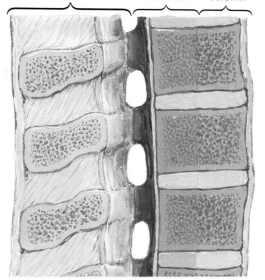

Posterior column   Middle column   Anterior column

Three-column concept. If more than one column involved in fracture, then instability of spine usually results

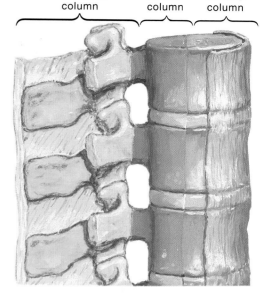

Posterior column   Middle column   Anterior column

Lateral view. Note that lateral facet (zygapophyseal) joints are in posterior column, with intervertebral foramina in middle column

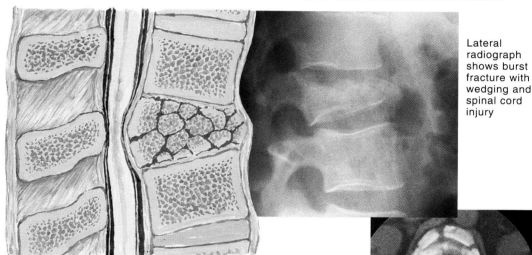

Burst fracture of vertebral body involving both anterior and middle columns resulted in instability and spinal cord compression

Lateral radiograph shows burst fracture with wedging and spinal cord injury

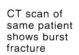

CT scan of same patient shows burst fracture

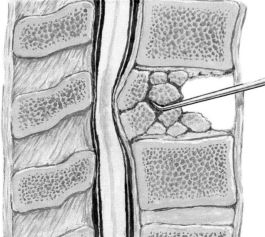
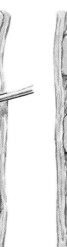

Anterior decompression of burst fracture (corpectomy) with hooked curet

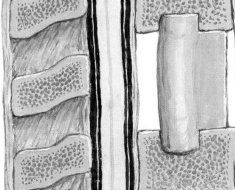

Bone graft from iliac crest restores vertebral height and stability after bone compressing spinal cord had been removed with corpectomy

Fracture and Dislocation of Cervical Vertebrae

Injury to Spine
(Continued)

Laminectomy, by removing the posterior column structures, further destabilizes the spine and compounds any instability that may already be present. In addition, laminectomy removes the posterior neural arch, which decreases the area available for the formation of a bone fusion mass; it is this mass of fused bone that eventually provides long-term stability to the spine. Finally, laminectomy does not correct the anterior compression of the spinal cord by burst fracture fragments, because during the procedure, the spinal cord cannot be retracted to allow visualization and removal of these pieces of bone.

Fracture and Dislocation of Cervical Vertebrae

Odontoid Fracture. Fractures of the second cervical vertebra (axis) usually involve the odontoid process (dens). Odontoid fractures are commonly classified as type I, type II, or type III (Plate 76).

Type I refers to an avulsion of the tip of the odontoid process. This fracture pattern is a stable injury that generally heals well when immobilized with a simple cervical orthosis.

A type II odontoid fracture occurs at the junction of the base of the dens with the body of C2. Type II fractures, which are considered unstable, are usually reduced with cervical tong traction and immobilized with a halo brace for 3 months. Unfortunately, nonunion is a serious complication with type II fractures, with some studies indicating a nonunion rate of 30% to 60% in patients treated with these conservative measures. Therefore, criteria have been established to identify patients at risk for nonunion, including persons more than 65 years of age and patients with posterior translation of the odontoid process or a greater than 5-mm displacement of the odontoid process. For such patients, the current recommended treatment is a primary posterior fusion (arthrodesis) of C1–2.

Type III odontoid fractures extend down into the body of C2. These injuries have a high rate of union and are best managed with a period of immobilization with a halo brace after reduction with cervical tong traction.

Jefferson Fracture. A burst fracture of the first cervical vertebra (atlas) is called a Jefferson fracture. The arch of C1 may be broken in one or more places. Jefferson fractures usually result from axial loading of the cervical spine, as occurs with a blow to the top of the head. In most patients with a Jefferson fracture, neurologic function is intact, and the fracture site is stable after bone healing. Generally, the recommended treatment is cervical tong traction followed by immobilization with a halo brace for 3 months.

Hangman Fracture. A fracture of the pedicles of C2 is called the hangman fracture because it is caused by sudden distraction of the cervical spine, as occurs in hanging. The majority of patients who survive the initial traumatic episode remain

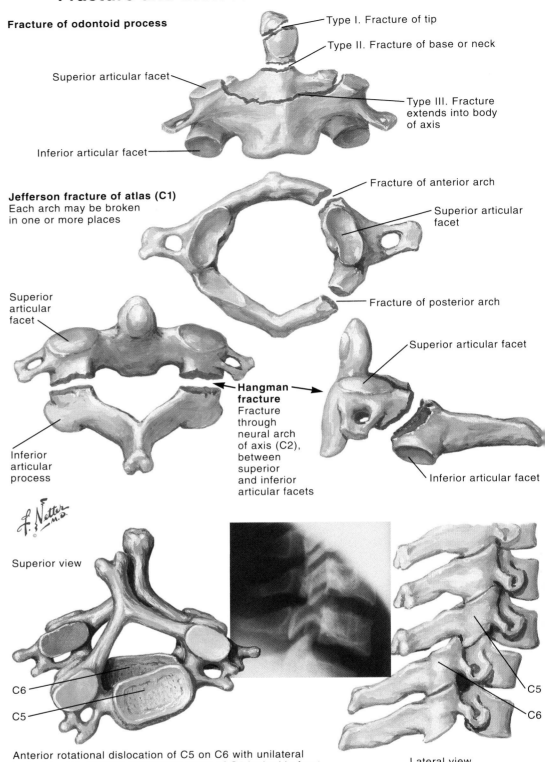

Fracture of odontoid process
Type I. Fracture of tip
Type II. Fracture of base or neck
Superior articular facet
Type III. Fracture extends into body of axis
Inferior articular facet

Jefferson fracture of atlas (C1)
Each arch may be broken in one or more places
Fracture of anterior arch
Superior articular facet
Superior articular facet
Fracture of posterior arch
Superior articular facet
Inferior articular process
Hangman fracture Fracture through neural arch of axis (C2), between superior and inferior articular facets
Inferior articular facet

Superior view
C6
C5

Anterior rotational dislocation of C5 on C6 with unilateral locked facets. Inferior articular process of C5 locked in front of superior articular process of C6

Lateral view
C5
C6

neurologically intact. Treatment of hangman fractures includes reduction with cervical tong traction and immobilization with a halo brace for 3 months. The treatment usually results in spontaneous C2–3 fusion, but if nonunion of the fractured pedicles of C2 occurs, surgical arthrodesis of C2–3 may be required.

Locked Facet Dislocation. Another injury that commonly occurs in the cervical spine is dislocation of the facet (zygapophyseal) joints of a vertebral segment. Dislocation of one of the facet joints is called unilateral locked facet. The superior facet is displaced anterior to the inferior facet and locked in position so that the edges of the

facet joints prevent spontaneous reduction. The mechanism of injury is rotation with associated flexion; continuation of the rotation-flexion will dislocate both facet joints (bilateral locked facets).

Plain lateral radiographs clearly differentiate unilateral and bilateral facet dislocations. An acute grade I spondylolisthesis between adjacent segments indicates a unilateral locked facet, whereas grade II spondylolisthesis at the injury site is evidence of bilateral locked facets. (In grade I spondylolisthesis, the vertebral body is translated 25% or less of its diameter relative to its adjacent segment; in grade II spondylolisthesis, the displacement is 25%–50% of the diameter of the vertebral body.)

Injury to Spine
(Continued)

Stable Fracture of Thoracolumbar Spine

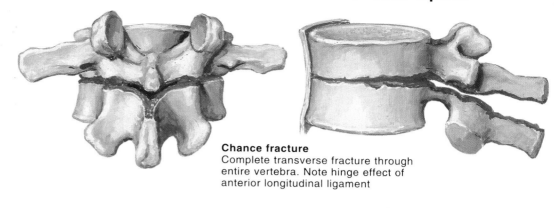

Chance fracture
Complete transverse fracture through entire vertebra. Note hinge effect of anterior longitudinal ligament

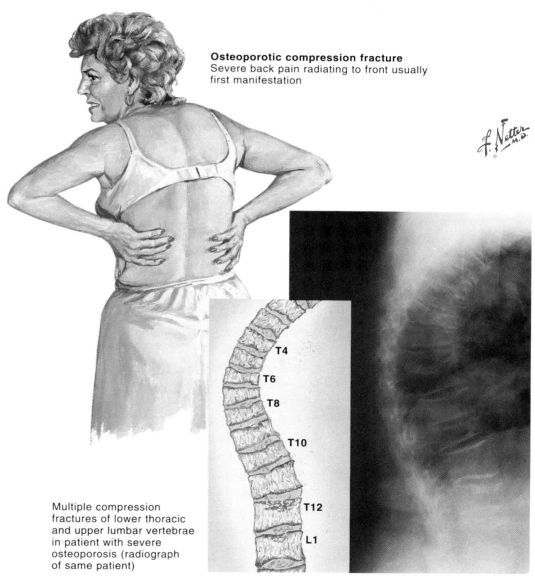

Osteoporotic compression fracture
Severe back pain radiating to front usually first manifestation

Multiple compression fractures of lower thoracic and upper lumbar vertebrae in patient with severe osteoporosis (radiograph of same patient)

Locked facet dislocations frequently involve injury to the middle column as well as to the posterior column of the spine, making these injuries unstable (Plate 75). Initial treatment of the dislocation consists of reduction with cervical tong traction. If the injury is solely a facet joint dislocation and if reduction can be maintained easily without spontaneous subluxation or dislocation, then reduction and fixation with a cervical orthosis are probably sufficient. If the dislocation is unstable after reduction or if the posterior column is disrupted because of torn posterior ligaments, then a posterior fusion at the level of injury is necessary.

Stable Fracture of Thoracolumbar Spine

Two common fractures of the thoracolumbar spine are the Chance fracture and the compression fracture (Plate 77).

A Chance fracture occurs through both the superior and inferior halves of a vertebra in the thoracolumbar spine and is best visualized on a sagittal radiograph. The Chance fracture, also called seat belt fracture, frequently results from motor vehicle accidents in which the patient wears a lap belt without a shoulder belt. With sudden deceleration, the patient's spine experiences a flexion moment, with the lap belt as the pivot point. As a result, a distraction (tension) force is applied to the spine starting at the posterior aspect of the spinous process. As the distraction moment continues, the fracture propagates anteriorly, involving all three columns of the vertebra and producing a so-called bony Chance fracture.

Frequently, the fracture reduces spontaneously after the distraction force ends, and on radiographs the injury appears to be a nondisplaced fracture. However, because all three columns of the vertebra are damaged, the Chance fracture is acutely unstable. It becomes stable only after immobilization has allowed the fracture to heal.

Occasionally, this deceleration-distraction force results in a so-called ligamentous Chance fracture.

In this variant of the injury, the transverse plane of cleavage occurs through soft tissue rather than through bone. The posterior ligament complex (supraspinal and interspinal ligaments and ligamentum flavum), facet joints and capsules, and intervertebral disc are all disrupted. Because all three spinal columns are involved, the injury results in spine instability. And because this is a ligament injury, which has little chance of healing spontaneously, surgical fusion is necessary to restore stability to the affected site.

A compression fracture most commonly occurs in older patients with osteoporosis. It is a stable fracture of the thoracolumbar spine and usually

results when a flexion force applied to the spine compresses the anterior portion of the vertebral body. As long as the anterior compression is limited to 50% of the vertebral body, a compression fracture remains stable because only the anterior column is involved. Treatment is usually symptomatic: pain medication and, occasionally, a corset for comfort. Generally, the fracture becomes stable after the bone heals. In rare instances when the height of the anterior vertebral body is reduced more than 50%, the middle column is disrupted in addition to the anterior column. A fracture of this degree is unstable and requires more intensive treatment.

Unstable Fracture of Thoracolumbar Spine

Injury to Spine
(Continued)

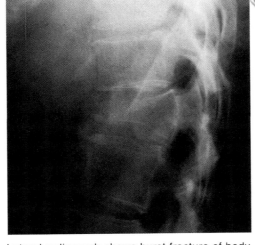

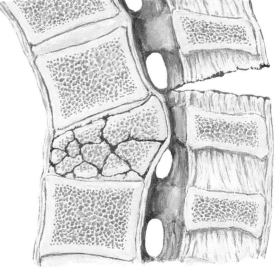

Lateral radiograph shows burst fracture of body of T12 with wedging, kyphosis, and retropulsion of fragments into spinal canal

Sagittal view of fracture shown in radiograph at left

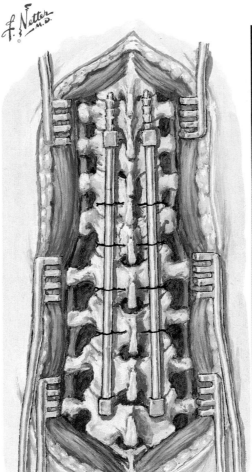

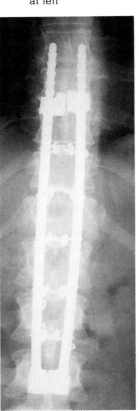

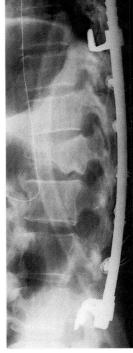

Harrington rods installed in spine reduce, realign, and stabilize vertebrae. Wisconsin wires through spinous processes secure both rods. Anteroposterior and lateral postoperative radiographs show restoration of height of crushed vertebral body

Unstable Fracture of Thoracolumbar Spine

The thoracolumbar junction is vulnerable to several different mechanisms of injury: flexion, rotation, axial loading, or any combination of these forces. Fracture dislocations are common in this region, where the rather immobile segments of the thoracic spine meet the highly mobile segments of the lumbar spine. A fracture dislocation of the thoracolumbar junction is a severe injury because the spine is inherently unstable at that point. The instability is due to the change in the orientation of the facet joints and the loss of the support provided by the ribs and their interconnecting ligaments. Any treatment of thoracolumbar fracture dislocations is directed at restoring stability to this crucial area (Plate 78).

After fracture, stability at the thoracolumbar junction is most successfully achieved with surgery.

The Harrington rod system for internal fixation is frequently used for these injuries because it reduces the fracture dislocation and stabilizes the fracture site by fixing the injured segment to the more stable uninjured segments above and below it.

Numerous developments in internal fixation systems now allow effective stabilization of the spine while reducing the number of vertebrae that must be wired. Whereas the Harrington rod system requires immobilization of four or five vertebral segments to achieve stability, in the newer systems only two or three segments are immobilized, leaving more vertebrae available for motion. Also, compared to the Harrington rod system,

the newer fixation systems are more rigid and better able to resist deforming forces after implantation. Some surgeons still prefer the Harrington rod for fixation of unstable fracture dislocations of the thoracolumbar region because it is a relatively simple and inexpensive technique of rigid immobilization. An advantage of the Harrington rod system is that it permits the use of computed tomography and magnetic resonance imaging for accurate visualization of the spinal cord and anterior vertebral structures. With fixation systems that use pedicle screws and hooks, the metal artifacts make postoperative MRI and CT scans unreadable. □

Fracture of Pelvis Without Disruption of Pelvic Ring

Avulsions

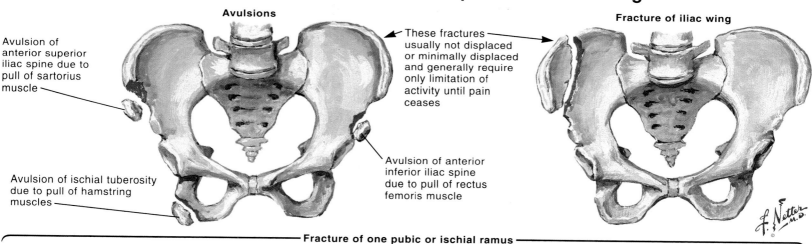

Avulsion of anterior superior iliac spine due to pull of sartorius muscle

← These fractures usually not displaced or minimally displaced and generally require only limitation of activity until pain ceases →

Avulsion of anterior inferior iliac spine due to pull of rectus femoris muscle

Avulsion of ischial tuberosity due to pull of hamstring muscles

Fracture of iliac wing

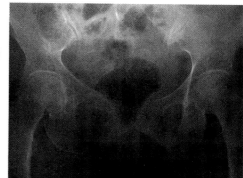

f. Netter M.D.

─── Fracture of one pubic or ischial ramus ───

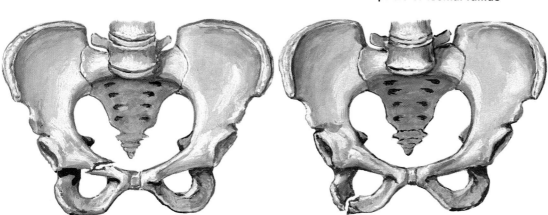

Isolated fracture of one pubic or ischial ramus requires only bed rest until pain diminishes, followed by limited activity for 4–5 weeks, provided there is no visceral or vascular injury

Radiograph shows fracture of right superior pubic ramus

─── Fractures of sacrum ───

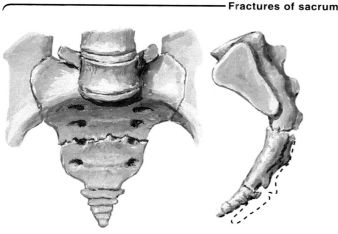

Impacted transverse fracture that is minimally displaced is most common type. Conservative treatment sufficient unless there is nerve injury

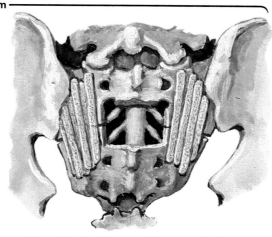

Sacral laminectomy and bone grafts from ilium used for sharply angulated fractures with nerve injury

─── Fracture of coccyx ───

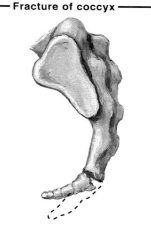

Fracture usually requires no treatment other than care in sitting; inflatable ring helpful. Pain may persist for long time

Injury to Pelvis

Fracture Without Disruption of Pelvic Ring

Injuries to the pelvis range from the most trivial to the most life threatening. In general, the severity of an injury is determined by the degree of disruption to the pelvic ring. Fortunately, many fractures about the pelvis do not affect its integrity at all (Plate 79).

Avulsion. In athletes, avulsions of bone from the pelvis due to strong muscle contractions are relatively common. These fractures occur at the anterior superior iliac spine as a result of the strong pull of the sartorius muscle, at the anterior inferior iliac spine from the pull of the rectus femoris muscle, and at the ischial tuberosity from the forceful contraction of the hamstring muscles. Most fractures can be treated with activity modification and medications until pain ceases. Patients may gradually resume athletic activities, usually attaining complete functional recovery within 3 months.

Fracture of Iliac Wing. An isolated fracture of the iliac wing, or Duverney fracture, is not uncommon, usually resulting from a direct compressive force to the lateral aspect of the pelvis. The strong muscle attachments on the fragment usually minimize its displacement, and although blood loss may be substantial, shock is not common. Radiographic examination must determine whether the acetabulum is involved or if the sacroiliac joint is disrupted. Management of the fracture involves bed rest on a firm mattress until the patient is comfortable enough to be mobilized, followed by gradual, protected weight bearing until all symptoms resolve. Occasionally, an ileus

Injury to Pelvis
(Continued)

develops that is not due to abdominal visceral injury. This complication is usually relieved with nasogastric suction and intravenous administration of fluids.

Fracture of Pubic or Ischial Ramus. An isolated fracture of a single pubic or ischial ramus is a fairly uncommon injury; it usually occurs in elderly persons as a result of a fall. In this type of fracture, the pelvis remains extremely stable because the obturator foramen is a rigid, bony circle. A fracture of a pubic or ischial ramus must be differentiated from an impacted fracture of the femoral neck because treatments differ markedly. A fracture of one pubic or ischial ramus without visceral or vascular injury requires only bed rest until symptoms abate sufficiently to allow progressive mobilization with a gradual increase in weight bearing.

Fracture of Sacrum. Transverse fractures of the sacrum are usually caused by direct impact and typically have a slightly anterior displacement. Diagnosis is based on a history of injury and evidence of pain, swelling, and tenderness over the posterior aspect of the sacrum. Neurologic dysfunction may occur, evidenced by urinary retention or decrease in rectal tone. The examiner must take extreme care during the rectal examination, especially during palpation along the anterior surface of the sacrum, to avoid converting a closed sacral fracture into an open fracture through the rectum, which increases the risk of serious contamination of the retroperitoneal space. If neurologic deficit is either absent or improving, conservative treatment is indicated. If a neurologic lesion compromises bowel or bladder function, surgical decompression should be considered.

Fracture of Coccyx. This fracture is usually caused by a direct blow to the posterior aspect of the coccyx. Symptomatic management suffices, but discomfort may persist for a long time.

Fracture of All Four Pubic Rami

When the pelvic ring is injured at more than one site, the potential for instability increases correspondingly. Fractures of all four pubic rami disrupt the structural integrity of the anterior portion of the pelvic ring (Plate 80). This injury commonly results from a fall on the front of the pelvis or from lateral compressive forces on the pelvic ring. In about one-third of patients, major trauma to the lower urinary tract occurs as well. Treatment focuses on preventing any further displacement of the fracture fragments. Bed rest, with the patient in a semisitting position to relax the abdominal musculature, is followed by mobilization as soon as symptoms allow.

Lateral Compression Injury

Double breaks in the pelvic ring are often due to lateral compressive forces (Plate 80). Most of these fractures are stable because the forces cause impaction of the posterior pelvic complex, leaving

Fracture of All Four Pubic Rami (Straddle Injury)

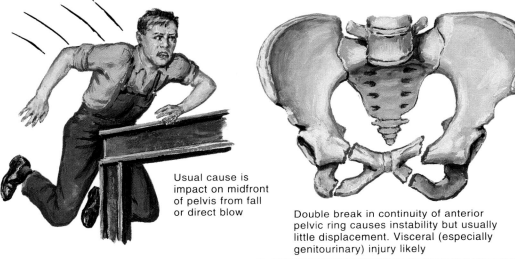

Usual cause is impact on midfront of pelvis from fall or direct blow

Double break in continuity of anterior pelvic ring causes instability but usually little displacement. Visceral (especially genitourinary) injury likely

Lateral Compression Injury (Overlapping Pelvis)

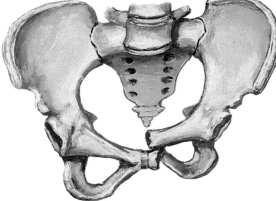

Caused by forceful blow to side of pelvis

Fracture of pubic bone or pubic rami on one side, or separation of pubic symphysis with one hemipelvis driven inward to overlap other side. Widening or subluxation of ipsilateral sacroiliac joint may occur. Displacement usually minor and may self-reduce as result of tissue recoil or with manual distraction. Conservative treatment usually adequate, but visceral or vascular injury must be considered

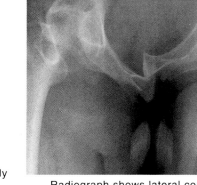

Radiograph shows lateral compression injury with overlapping pelvis

the posterior ligaments intact. If the force continues or increases, the posterior sacroiliac ligaments may tear, producing an instability in the injured hemipelvis.

This injury often includes fractures of the superior and inferior pubic rami; therefore, the anterior and posterior injuries are on the same side. When the patient is placed in the supine position, the displaced hemipelvis often reduces spontaneously. Radiographs may reveal only minimal displacement, but the examiner must remember that the degree of initial deformation of the hemipelvis is *not known*, and significant visceral injury may be present.

When a lateral compressive force is accompanied by a rotational force, the anterior fracture often occurs on the side opposite the posterior fracture; for example, an impacted fracture may occur on the left side of the sacrum, while fractures of the inferior and superior pubic rami occur on the right side. The hemipelvis then displaces superiorly and medially, causing the leg to appear internally rotated and shortened. The position of the hemipelvis generally remains stable, although the malrotation may compromise future function. Correcting this rotational deformity may create instability when the impacted posterior injury is reduced.

Injury to Pelvis
(Continued)

Anteroposterior Compression Fracture

Anteroposterior compression, or open book, fractures of the pelvis are usually caused by a forceful blow from in front of the pelvis through the anterior superior iliac spines or by force applied to externally rotated femurs (Plate 81). However, a blow from the rear against the posterior superior iliac spines may produce a similar injury that is characterized by disruption of the pubic symphysis and the anterior sacroiliac ligaments. Injuries range from an isolated rupture of the pubic symphysis to complete separation of the pubic symphysis accompanied by bilateral anterior subluxation of the sacroiliac joints. Since the sacrospinal ligaments resist external rotation of the pelvis, a separation of 2.5 cm or greater of the symphysis suggests that the sacrospinal ligaments have ruptured or have avulsed bone from the sacrum or ischial spine. Most important, the very strong posterior sacroiliac ligaments remain intact. The open book fracture is therefore relatively stable, and treatment focuses on closing the pelvic ring.

The pelvic ring can be closed with or without surgery. In nonsurgical treatment, crossover slings are used to bring the two pelvic halves together. In 3 to 4 weeks, when the soft tissues have healed sufficiently, the pelvic slings are replaced with a minispica cast and ambulatory treatment can be initiated. If surgical treatment is chosen, open reduction and internal fixation are performed, using a plate to stabilize the pubic symphysis. The planning of treatment for this injury must be clearly distinguished from the treatment for a vertical shear injury of the pelvis. Because the initial radiographs of both injuries may appear similar, differentiation requires careful physical examination and supplemental imaging, including CT scans of the posterior pelvic complex.

Vertical Shear Fracture

Vertical shear, or Malgaigne, fractures of the pelvis result from severe trauma (Plate 82). The force may cause unilateral or bilateral injuries to the posterior pelvis and severe and sometimes life-threatening injury to the soft tissue contents of the pelvic cavity. The injury to the anterior pelvis may include disruption of the pubic symphysis with or without fractures of two, three, or four pubic rami. The posterior injuries may be fractures of the sacrum, dislocations of the sacroiliac joint, fractures of the ilium, or fracture dislocations of the sacroiliac joint, including fractures of the sacrum or the ilium.

Avulsion fractures, particularly of the ischial spine or the transverse process of the fifth lumbar vertebra, also occur in major disruptions of the posterior pelvis. Complete instability of the affected hemipelvis indicates disruption of the sacrotuberal and sacrospinal ligaments. Because vertical shear fractures are caused by considerable force, many

Anteroposterior Compression Fracture of Pelvis (Open Book Fracture)

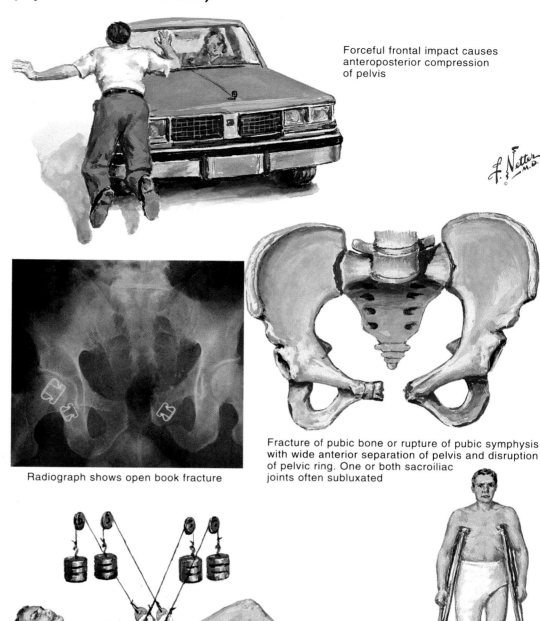

Forceful frontal impact causes anteroposterior compression of pelvis

Radiograph shows open book fracture

Fracture of pubic bone or rupture of pubic symphysis with wide anterior separation of pelvis and disruption of pelvic ring. One or both sacroiliac joints often subluxated

Application of crossover slings with enough weight to rotate halves of pelvis medially and anteriorly, thus bringing them together. Reduction maintained for 3 – 4 weeks

Minispica cast, which permits walking, then worn for 4 – 6 weeks

involve vital pelvic and abdominal tissues of the gastrointestinal, genitourinary, vascular, and nervous systems.

If the posterior hemipelvis on one side remains intact, the disrupted half can be brought to the intact side and stabilized. When both ilia are disrupted from the sacrum, stabilization is much more problematic. The aim of treatment soon after injury is to reapproximate the injured hemipelvis to the uninjured side using closed manipulation. After anesthesia or analgesia with significant muscle relaxation is obtained, the patient is positioned injured side up, with an assistant supporting the legs. The examiner pushes the displaced ilium

downward and forward. If the reduction is successful, skeletal traction is often used to maintain it until significant healing of soft tissue or bone occurs.

Because many Malgaigne fractures are grossly unstable, manipulative reduction is largely unsuccessful, and either external or internal fixation of the hemipelvis is needed. Fixation with an external fixation device provides *relative* immobilization of the hemipelvis; the stability is greater than that provided by manipulative reduction and subsequent traction. However, attempts to attain and maintain anatomic reduction with external fixators are usually unsuccessful.

Vertical Shear Fracture (Malgaigne Fracture)

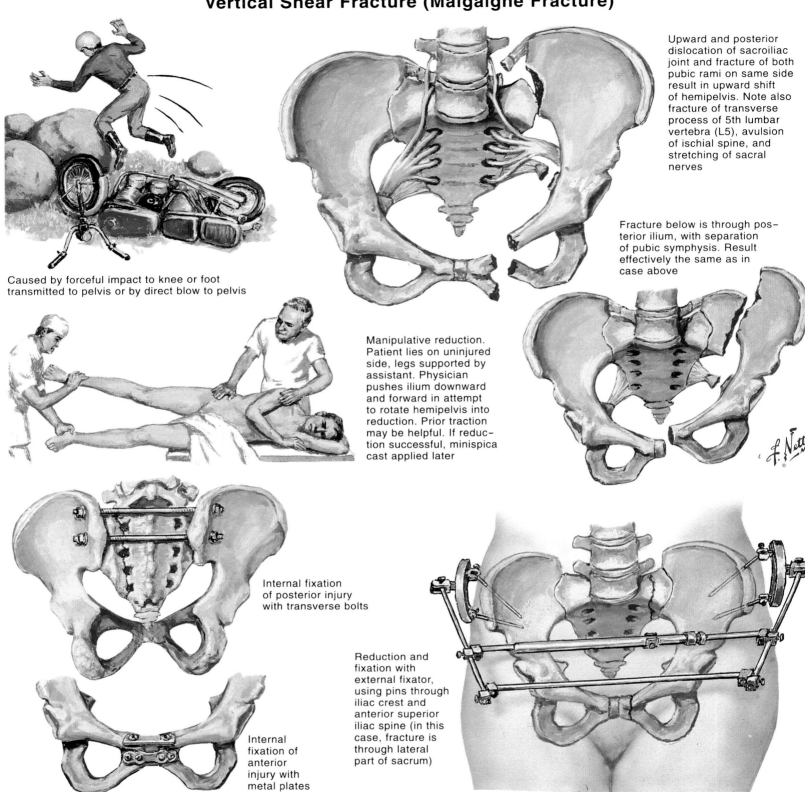

Caused by forceful impact to knee or foot transmitted to pelvis or by direct blow to pelvis

Upward and posterior dislocation of sacroiliac joint and fracture of both pubic rami on same side result in upward shift of hemipelvis. Note also fracture of transverse process of 5th lumbar vertebra (L5), avulsion of ischial spine, and stretching of sacral nerves

Fracture below is through posterior ilium, with separation of pubic symphysis. Result effectively the same as in case above

Manipulative reduction. Patient lies on uninjured side, legs supported by assistant. Physician pushes ilium downward and forward in attempt to rotate hemipelvis into reduction. Prior traction may be helpful. If reduction successful, minispica cast applied later

Internal fixation of posterior injury with transverse bolts

Internal fixation of anterior injury with metal plates

Reduction and fixation with external fixator, using pins through iliac crest and anterior superior iliac spine (in this case, fracture is through lateral part of sacrum)

Injury to Pelvis
(Continued)

Open reduction and internal fixation of both displaced components provide the best stabilization of vertical shear fractures. Two plates may be used to secure the disruptions in the pubic symphysis and two bolts inserted to stabilize a longitudinal fracture of the sacrum.

Vascular and Visceral Trauma

Vascular and visceral injuries are the chief causes of deaths associated with pelvic fractures (Plate 83). The likelihood of associated injury is directly related to the severity of the fracture.

Pelvic fractures normally cause bleeding from injured vessels of the pelvic marrow or from torn pelvic or lumbar arteries and veins and formation of a hematoma. The extent of the bleeding depends on the severity of the vascular and bone injuries, and the risk of death is directly linked to the severity of the hemorrhage. Patients with double breaks in the pelvic ring require transfusions twice as often as patients with single breaks or with fractures of the acetabulum. Persistent severe hemorrhage may warrant emergent investigation with transfemoral arteriography to identify bleeding sites and selective embolization using blood, gelatin, or other such substances. Arteriography may be used to identify injuries to large arteries. Military antishock trousers (MAST) may be used to stabilize the fracture and to help diminish blood loss.

Frequently, pelvic fractures cause injuries of the lower urinary tract. Clues to such injuries include blood at the urethral meatus or hematuria found on urinalysis. In men, rectal examination may

Vascular and Visceral Trauma in Fracture of Pelvis

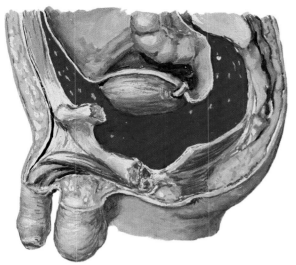

Massive retroperitoneal hemorrhage from torn arteries or veins is life–threatening complication of pelvic fractures

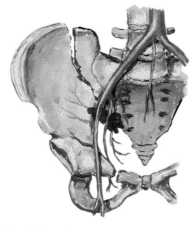

Site of bleeding may be determined with arteriography or venography and bleeding arrested with percutaneous balloon catheter embolization

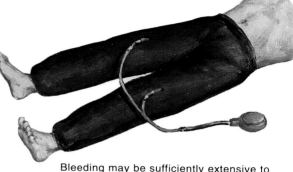

Bleeding may be sufficiently extensive to cause hypovolemic shock. Antishock garment may be applied promptly

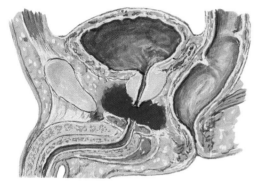

Complete supradiaphragmatic rupture of urethra due to pelvic fracture

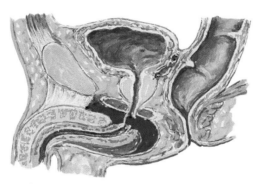

Infradiaphragmatic rupture of urethra (in this case, partial)

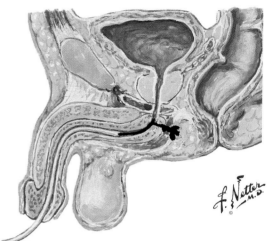

Cystourethrography used to determine site of urethral or vesical rupture. Catheter introduced short distance into urethra and dye injected. Catheter advanced farther to search for higher lesions and eventually positioned in bladder

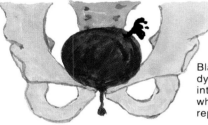

Bladder filled with dye to demonstrate intraperitoneal rupture, which must be promptly repaired

Bladder allowed to empty; residual dye evidence of extraperitoneal rupture. Repair may be delayed

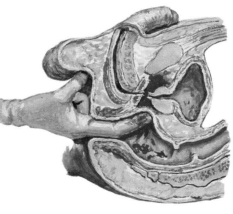

Rectal examination reveals displaced prostate. Blood on glove evidence of rectal tear

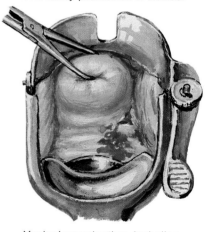

Vaginal examination, including speculum viewing, required to search for vaginal tears

Slide 4859

Injury to Pelvis
(Continued)

reveal a high-riding or free-floating prostate, which usually indicates injury to the lower urinary tract. Urethrography is performed to determine whether the anterior portion of the urethra is injured. If the urethrogram appears normal, a catheter should be passed gently through the urethra into the bladder. *The catheter must not be forced.* If this procedure is accomplished, further radiographic studies can determine whether an intraperitoneal or an extraperitoneal bladder injury is present.

Most complete transections of the urethra are treated by diverting the urine stream through a suprapubic catheter placed into the bladder and, later, with repair or reconstruction of the urethra. Intraperitoneal ruptures of the bladder are repaired with suprapubic drainage to decompress the bladder. Depending on the extent of the tear, extraperitoneal ruptures may not require surgical repair; adequate drainage of the bladder is necessary to allow the laceration to heal.

The examiner must search diligently for injuries of the lower gastrointestinal tract, especially about the rectum and the anus. Blood found on rectal examination suggests that the lower gastrointestinal tract has been lacerated by bone fragments, with possible severe contamination of the extraperitoneal pelvic space. If the rectum or anus is lacerated, standard treatment includes performing a washout of the distal rectal lumen and creating a diverting colostomy to minimize pelvic contamination. In women, a careful vaginal examination is performed to detect lacerations of the vagina, which could lead to contamination and infection of the pelvis. □

Fracture of Acetabulum

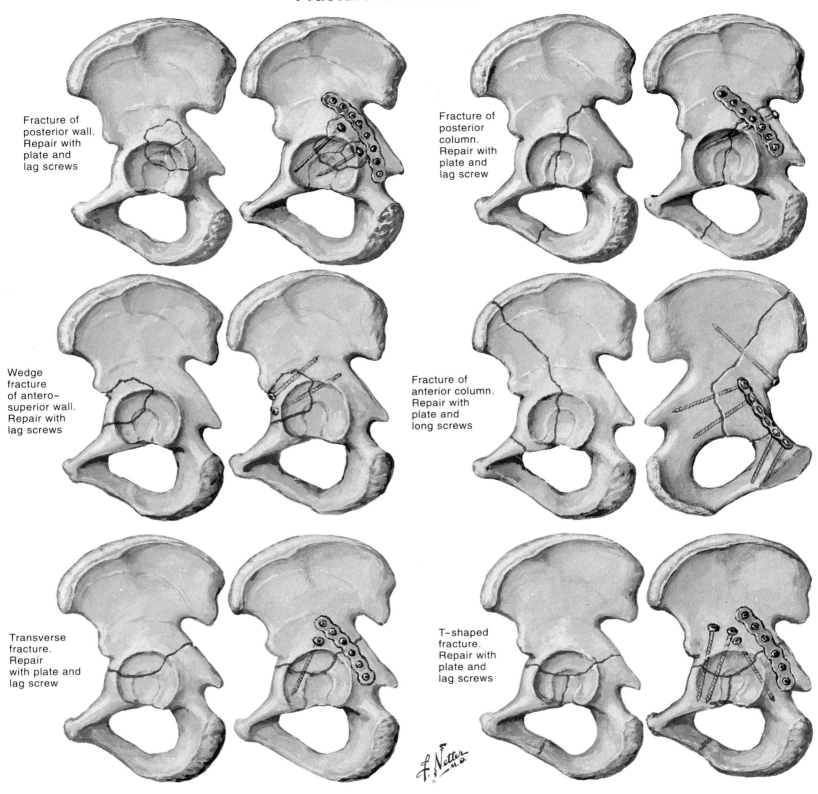

Fracture of posterior wall. Repair with plate and lag screws

Fracture of posterior column. Repair with plate and lag screw

Wedge fracture of antero-superior wall. Repair with lag screws

Fracture of anterior column. Repair with plate and long screws

Transverse fracture. Repair with plate and lag screw

T-shaped fracture. Repair with plate and lag screws

Injury to Hip

Fracture of Acetabulum

The acetabulum of the pelvis makes up the socket of the hip joint. It develops at the confluence of three epiphyseal junctions between the ilium, ischium, and pubis. The growth of the acetabulum occurs with the development of this triradiate cartilage, and its shape is influenced considerably by the shape of the femoral head with which it articulates. Acetabular injuries are not as common as other injuries to the hip joint, and most result from forces generated by the femoral head against the confines of the acetabular cup. Fractures tend to occur in younger persons and involve greater violence than the typical femoral neck or intertrochanteric fracture.

Acetabular injuries range from simple avulsions of the periphery of the acetabulum to explosions of the hip socket (Plate 84). When the acetabulum fractures, the femoral head is usually dislocated or subluxated in relation to the part of the acetabulum that remains intact. The displacement may be anterior, central, or posterior. After reduction, an incongruence often exists between the femoral head and the acetabulum. Acetabular fractures are classified as simple and associated. Simple fracture patterns are further categorized as fractures of the anterior wall, anterior column, posterior wall, and posterior column and transverse fractures. Associated fracture patterns comprise fractures of the posterior wall and posterior column, transverse fractures with posterior wall fractures, T-shaped fractures, fractures of both columns, and fractures of the anterior wall or column with an associated posterior hemitransverse fracture.

Injury to Hip
(Continued)

Patients with minimally displaced fractures of the acetabulum or those who cannot, or elect not to, undergo surgical treatment are treated with nonoperative measures. Initially, the patient is placed in traction until the acute reaction of the fracture subsides. Then the hip is moved through a range of flexion, extension, abduction, and adduction, either by a physical therapist or with the use of a continuous passive motion machine. Once these movements are achieved comfortably, the patient is mobilized using crutches, with minimal weight bearing on the injured side. Radiographs are taken frequently to assess the healing of the fracture and to check for residual displacement of the femoral head.

Central Fracture of Acetabulum

Patients with severe central fracture dislocations of the acetabulum who cannot be treated with surgery are managed with more complex traction arrangements (Plate 85). First, skeletal traction is applied with a pin through the distal femur or proximal tibia to establish a normal relationship between the superior femoral head and the dome of the acetabulum. About one-sixth of the patient's body weight is applied through the traction mechanism to restore the injured limb to its normal length. Following this maneuver, a radiograph is obtained to assess the relationship of the femoral head to the intact acetabulum. If subluxation of the femoral head persists, lateral traction, applied with a sling or with a pin placed in the femur distal to the greater trochanter, is used to extricate the femoral head from the pelvis. Traction is maintained for 6 to 8 weeks. Weight bearing on the injured lower limb is limited for at least 3 to 4 months from the time of injury. Residual subluxation may occur in the same direction as the original displacement.

Posterior Dislocation of Hip

Posterior dislocations of the hip have become more common as the occurrence of high-energy trauma has increased (Plate 86). The classic mechanism of injury is the impact of the dashboard against the flexed knee during a head-on automobile collision. The dashboard collapses, striking the knee and driving the femoral head out of the acetabular socket. Generally, the resulting posterior dislocation of the hip is not an isolated injury; multiple injuries of the lower limb often occur, including fractures of the patella and femoral shaft and injuries to the posterior cruciate ligament.

Pure dislocations of the femoral head occur with the hip adducted and flexed. In this position, the force is concentrated against the soft tissues of the hip joint capsule rather than the bone architecture of the posterior acetabulum. Indentation fractures of the femoral head occasionally occur, as do abrasions of the articular cartilage. Because of its close proximity to the posterior aspect of the hip joint, the sciatic nerve (especially the peroneal

Fracture of Acetabulum (continued)

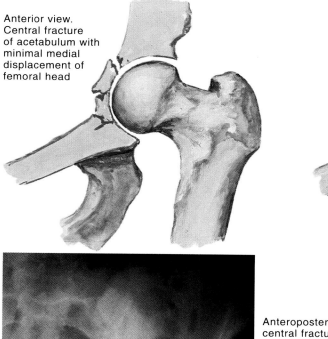

Anterior view. Central fracture of acetabulum with minimal medial displacement of femoral head

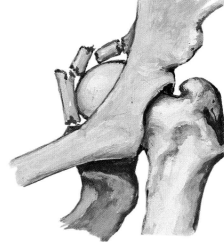

Central fracture of acetabulum with dislocation of femoral head into pelvis

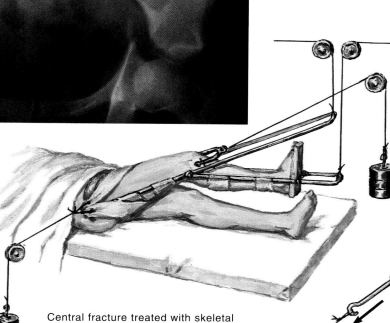

Anteroposterior radiograph of central fracture of acetabulum

Central fracture treated with skeletal traction; lateral traction also applied with sling around proximal thigh to correct medial displacement of femoral head. Initially, 20 – 25 lb of longitudinal traction and 8 – 10 lb of lateral traction used; weights modified as needed

If lateral traction with sling does not suffice, screw may be passed through greater trochanter and femoral neck for direct traction

division) is injured in 8% to 20% of patients with posterior dislocation or posterior fracture dislocation of the hip. Sciatic nerve injury is more common with fracture dislocations than with pure dislocations.

When the dislocation of the hip is posterior, the major blood supply to the femoral head is injured. Avascular necrosis of the femoral head, one of the more common complications of this injury, appears to be related to the amount of time the femoral head remains dislocated from the acetabulum.

Posterior dislocation of the hip results in a classic posture: the lower limb is flexed at the hip joint, adducted, and internally rotated. Careful

physical examination also reveals shortening of the limb. Many patients report a feeling of fullness in the buttocks. A neurologic evaluation of the limb must be performed, with emphasis on the musculature innervated by the peroneal division of the sciatic nerve.

Radiographs of the pelvis and hip reveal the absence of the femoral head from its normal articulation in the acetabulum. The displaced head usually appears smaller than the femoral head on the uninjured side and in a position proximal to the acetabulum. Radiographs are important for determining both the extent of bone injury to the hip socket and any associated fractures.

Posterior Dislocation of Hip

Injury to Hip
(Continued)

In posterior dislocation of the hip with no associated sciatic nerve injury, the hip should be reduced within 12 hours of injury. Prompt reduction helps to minimize the development of avascular necrosis of the femoral head. Dislocations with associated sciatic nerve injury are acute emergencies and must be reduced to relieve extrinsic pressure on the nerve and lessen the risk of permanent sciatic nerve palsy.

In patients with multiple injuries, the most common method of closed reduction of a posterior dislocation of the hip is the Allis maneuver. The maneuver is performed with the patient supine and allows further evaluation of associated injuries to the abdomen, chest, and airway that would be difficult to perform with the patient in a lateral or prone position. With an assistant stabilizing the pelvis, the physician applies gentle traction to the lower limb in the line of the deformity. After traction has been applied, the hip is gently flexed 90° while gentle internal and external rotation is applied until reduction is achieved. When it occurs, the reduction can be felt by both the physician and the assistant.

If the dislocation is an isolated injury, the Stimson gravity reduction maneuver can be used. The patient is placed prone and the injured hip flexed over the end of the examining table. An assistant stabilizes the pelvis by pressing down on the sacrum or by extending the uninjured limb. The physician flexes the involved hip and knee 90° and applies gentle downward pressure behind the flexed knee. As pressure is applied, gentle internal and external rotation is added. As in the Allis maneuver, both the physician and the assistant can feel the reduction when the femoral head relocates into the acetabulum.

After reduction, it is extremely important to reassess the neurologic status of the injured limb, focusing on the function of the sciatic nerve and its peroneal division. If sciatic nerve dysfunction is now apparent, surgical exploration of the nerve should be considered. Radiographs and CT scans should be examined for evidence of joint space widening or for the presence of small bone fragments within the joint that might prevent congruence between the femoral head and the acetabulum. After successful reduction, the limb is placed in light skin traction to allow the injured hip to rest. When the local reaction to the injury subsides, the patient can be mobilized and begin gentle active range-of-motion exercises, including extension, flexion, abduction, and adduction.

Guidelines for weight bearing after this injury are not well established and remain controversial. Generally, early motion of the hip is promoted but weight bearing is delayed. If evidence of avascular necrosis develops, weight bearing is postponed even longer to prevent collapse of the femoral head. Although recurrence of posterior dislocation or subluxation of the hip is rare, posttraumatic osteoarthritic changes of the hip are not uncommon. Follow-up should continue for at least 2 years to detect any arthritic or necrotic changes.

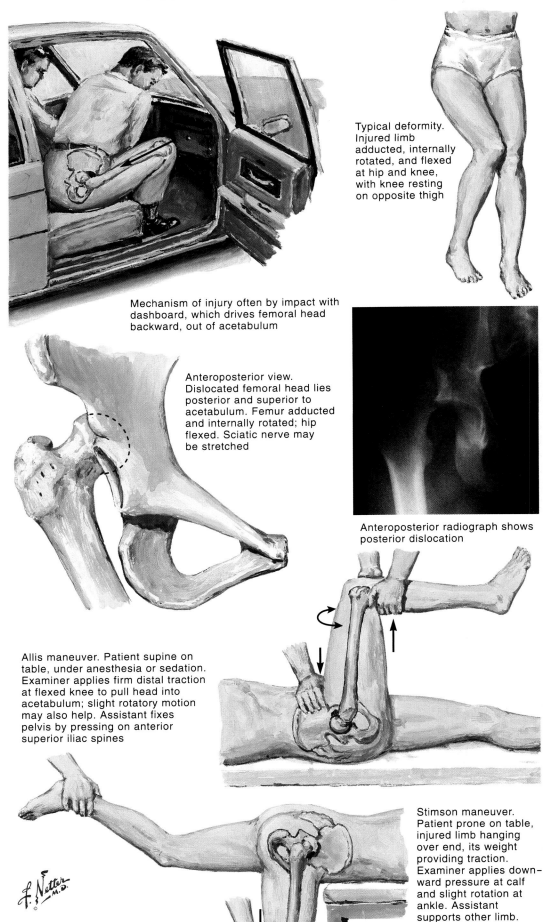

Typical deformity. Injured limb adducted, internally rotated, and flexed at hip and knee, with knee resting on opposite thigh

Mechanism of injury often by impact with dashboard, which drives femoral head backward, out of acetabulum

Anteroposterior view. Dislocated femoral head lies posterior and superior to acetabulum. Femur adducted and internally rotated; hip flexed. Sciatic nerve may be stretched

Anteroposterior radiograph shows posterior dislocation

Allis maneuver. Patient supine on table, under anesthesia or sedation. Examiner applies firm distal traction at flexed knee to pull head into acetabulum; slight rotatory motion may also help. Assistant fixes pelvis by pressing on anterior superior iliac spines

Stimson maneuver. Patient prone on table, injured limb hanging over end, its weight providing traction. Examiner applies downward pressure at calf and slight rotation at ankle. Assistant supports other limb. Anesthesia may not be necessary; sedation may suffice

Injury to Hip
(Continued)

Anterior Dislocation of Hip

About 10% to 15% of traumatic dislocations of the hip are anterior dislocations, either the superior type or the more common obturator type (Plate 87). Anterior dislocation occurs when the hip is abducted, externally rotated, and flexed and the knee strikes a fixed object. Either the neck of the femur or the greater trochanter levers the head of the femur out of the acetabulum through a disruption of the anterior hip capsule. As the femoral head leaves the anterior aspect of the acetabulum, transchondral or indentation fractures of the femoral head can occur. Since the introduction of computed tomography, the incidence of this type of fracture has been shown to be much greater than previously thought.

The characteristic clinical appearance is the limb flexed at the hip, abducted, and externally rotated. In assessing the neurovascular status after an obturator dislocation, the examiner must pay special attention to the presence of an injury to the obturator nerve resulting in paresis of the hip adductor musculature. Similarly, in the superior dislocation, the femoral nerve, artery, or vein can be damaged and must be assessed before reduction attempts are made. Radiographic evaluation of the injury should include anteroposterior and Judet views (oblique at 45°) of the pelvis to help delineate associated injuries of the acetabulum, femoral head, and femoral neck.

The Allis maneuver is generally recommended for obturator dislocations. Strong intravenous analgesics or spinal anesthetics are given to provide adequate muscle relaxation. If closed reduction is not successful, open reduction is required. An anterior iliofemoral approach allows identification and treatment of the obstruction to the dislocation.

After reduction, new radiographs are taken to determine the extent of associated injuries to the femoral neck, acetabulum, or femoral head. Polytomography or computed tomography may demonstrate a nondisplaced fracture of the femoral head or indentation fracture resulting from impingement of the femoral head against the acetabulum. Reassessment of the neurovascular status of the limb distal to the hip is also important. Posttraumatic osteoarthritis requiring later reconstructive surgery eventually develops in one-third of patients. Avascular necrosis may also be a residual complication. Recurrent dislocations are not common.

Postreduction care involves light traction with early active range-of-motion exercises, including extension, flexion, abduction-adduction, and rotation but avoidance of extremes of flexion, abduction, and external rotation. Just when weight bearing should begin is not clear, and the available guidelines are not consistent. Usually, as pain diminishes, the patient is allowed to begin weight bearing using crutches for support. Weight bearing is gradually increased until the support can be discarded. Follow-up should continue for at least 2 years to monitor for avascular necrosis or posttraumatic osteoarthritis.

Anterior Dislocation of Hip, Obturator Type

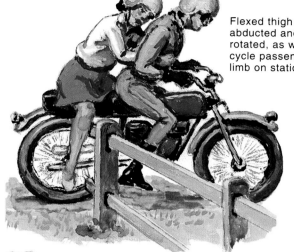

Flexed thigh sharply abducted and externally rotated, as when motorcycle passenger catches limb on stationary object

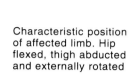

Characteristic position of affected limb. Hip flexed, thigh abducted and externally rotated

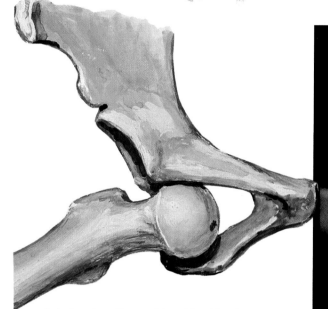

Anterior view. Femoral head in obturator foramen of pelvis; hip flexed and femur widely abducted and externally rotated

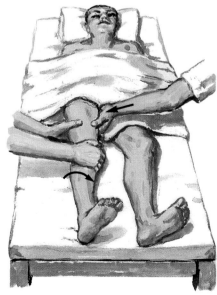

Anteroposterior radiograph shows obturator-type dislocation

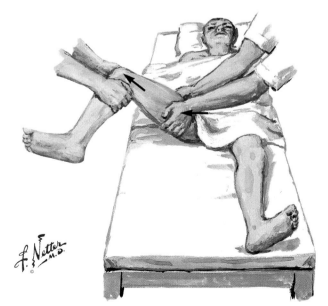

Allis maneuver. Patient supine; examiner applies manual traction in line of dislocated femoral shaft, as assistant applies lateral pressure to proximal thigh. Usually performed with patient under anesthesia or sedation

With continued traction, thigh adducted, internally rotated, and extended, thus reducing hip. No more than two attempts at reduction should be made; if they fail, open reduction indicated

Dislocation of Hip With Fracture of Femoral Head

Injury to Hip
(Continued)

Dislocation of Hip With Fracture of Femoral Head

As posterior dislocations and fracture dislocations of the hip have increased in frequency, associated femoral head fractures have also become
more common (Plate 88). These injuries are
believed to occur with the hip flexed 60° or less
and in neutral abduction. The force of the trauma
drives the femoral head against the posterosupe-
rior portion of the acetabulum, resulting in the
dislocation and shear fracture of the femoral head.

Pipkin delineated four types of fracture dislocations of the hip and assigned higher numbers
to the injuries with the worst prognoses. In
type I injuries, fracture of the femoral head occurs
inferior to the fovea of the head of the femur.
Type II injuries include a fracture that is superior
to the fovea. In type III injuries, a type I or type II
fracture may occur in association with a femoral
neck fracture, and type IV injuries involve a
type I, type II, or type III injury in association
with an acetabular fracture.

Since these injuries are associated with posterior hip dislocations, the neurovascular status of
the limb must be determined and radiographs of
the hip, including anteroposterior and Judet views,
obtained before reduction is attempted. The posterior dislocation should be reduced as soon as
possible to minimize avascular necrosis of the
femoral head. Reduction can be performed using
the maneuvers described for reduction of a
simple posterior dislocation of the hip. Careful
evaluation must be made of the reduction of the
femoral head in the acetabulum and the reduction of the fractured portion of the femoral head
to the intact head. The femoral head must be con-
centrically reduced in the acetabulum. The amount
of step-off and gap that exists at the fracture
surface must also be determined.

In type I or II injury, the fragment of the
femoral head need not be removed as long as it
does not impede hip motion and the hip is congru-
ently reduced and stable. If a congruent reduction
was not achieved, removal or internal fixation of
the fragment to the remaining surface of the
femoral head should be considered. After closed
reduction, incongruence resulting in either an offset or gap greater than 2 mm should be used as
the criterion for open reduction or excision of the
fragment. As much as one-third of the femoral
head can be removed, but many surgeons prefer
internal fixation of fragments of this size.

In type III and IV injuries, the adequacy of
the reductions of the femoral head fracture and
dislocation are assessed first; then the reduction
of the femoral neck or the acetabulum or both
must be evaluated. Displaced fractures of the
femoral neck may require internal fixation, and
severe displacement may necessitate total hip
replacement. Internal fixation of acetabular injuries
should be considered if this will optimize the
anatomic reconstruction of the hip joint. ☐

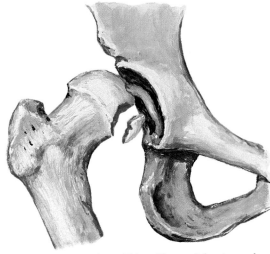

Posterior dislocation of hip with small fracture of
femoral head inferior to fovea that does not involve
weight-bearing surface of femoral head. Such small
fragments may be excised or left alone

Dislocation with fracture of large fragment
of femoral head extending proximal to fovea
that does involve weight-bearing surface.
May require open repair to restore articular
congruity and hip joint stability

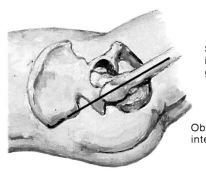

Skin and fascial incision

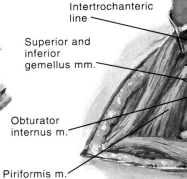

Intertrochanteric line

Superior and inferior gemellus mm.

Obturator internus m.

Piriformis m.

Sciatic n.

Gluteus maximus muscle split by separation
of fascicles, exposing piriformis and short
external rotator muscles and sciatic nerve.
Nerve must be carefully preserved

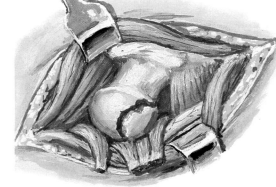

Piriformis and short external rotator
muscles divided and reflected. Hip
joint opened, exposing femoral head
and fracture fragment. If small,
fragment removed

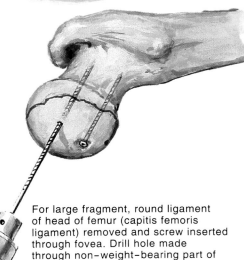

For large fragment, round ligament
of head of femur (capitis femoris
ligament) removed and screw inserted
through fovea. Drill hole made
through non-weight-bearing part of
fragment and femoral head into femoral
neck for placement of second screw

Second screw inserted. Both
screws countersunk to prevent
abrasion of acetabular cartilage

Intracapsular Fracture of Femoral Neck

Injury to Femur

Intracapsular Fracture of Femoral Neck

Femoral neck fractures are very common injuries, especially in older persons. In young persons, these injuries are usually caused by severe trauma. In older patients, especially those with osteoporosis, they are associated with falls, and it is possible that the fracture occurs before the fall.

Garden has classified femoral neck fractures into four categories (Plate 89). In type I fracture, the superior portion of the femoral neck is impacted into the femoral head. Type II is a complete fracture that remains nondisplaced. Type III is a fracture with partial displacement between the femoral head and neck. In a type IV fracture, the femoral head is completely displaced from the femoral neck. The Garden classification is useful because it correlates the incidence of fracture nonunion and avascular necrosis of the femoral head with fracture displacement. The incidence of these complications is very low in type I injury, whereas the type IV fracture has a 33% risk of nonunion and a 30% risk of symptomatic avascular necrosis.

Management of femoral neck fractures involves reducing the fracture in both the anteroposterior and lateral planes and achieving secure internal fixation of the fracture fragments. Most fractures can be reduced with closed means, using a variety of reduction techniques. In the Leadbetter maneuver, reduction occurs with the hip in 90° flexion. Other techniques involve reduction with the hip in extension or in only slight flexion. Regardless of what method is used, near-anatomic reduction must be achieved in both fracture planes; this is especially important in younger patients. After reduction, the femoral neck fracture is securely fixated to allow for impaction of the fracture fragments. Plate 89 shows fixation with multiple cannulated (Asnis) screws that, through a lag effect, compress the two fracture surfaces together.

After surgery, the patient can begin gentle active and passive range-of-motion exercises if the fixation is secure. Active straight-leg raising is best avoided for the first 3 months. Patients who are able to cooperate with a rehabilitation program are allowed gradual weight bearing as healing of soft tissue and bone progresses. Patients who are not able to cooperate are mobilized early from bed to chair, but weight bearing on the injured limb is delayed.

Periodic follow-up is important to monitor fracture healing and to check for development of avascular necrosis of the femoral head (Plate 149). Initially, this tends to occur in the anterolateral segment of the femoral head, where damage to the vasculature is greatest. If avascular necrosis is detected, intervention may be required to prevent the avascular segment from undergoing late segmental collapse, which leads to degenerative changes in the hip joint.

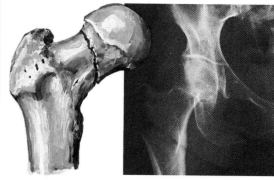

Impacted fracture

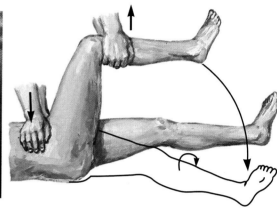

Nondisplaced fracture

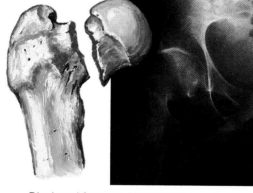

Displaced fracture. Vertical fracture line generally suggests poorer prognosis

Reduction of displaced fracture with Leadbetter maneuver. With knee flexed, slightly abducted limb slowly flexed to 90°, and upward traction applied as assistant fixes pelvis. Limb then gently extended, adducted, and internally rotated. (Near-perfect reduction essential)

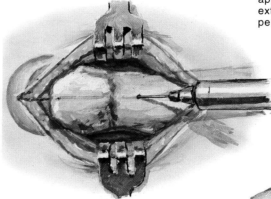

Incision 8–cm long made directly over lateral aspect of proximal femur. Guide wire drilled into femoral head at 45° to femoral shaft, starting 2.5 cm below distal margin of greater trochanter through small opening made in lateral cortex

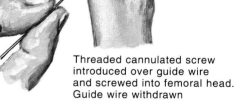

Threaded cannulated screw introduced over guide wire and screwed into femoral head. Guide wire withdrawn

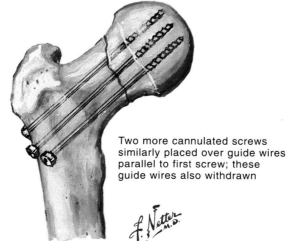

Two more cannulated screws similarly placed over guide wires parallel to first screw; these guide wires also withdrawn

Radiograph shows avascular necrosis of femoral head, which may occur despite pinning and may necessitate total hip replacement if collapse of necrotic head occurs

Intertrochanteric Fracture of Femur

Injury to Femur
(Continued)

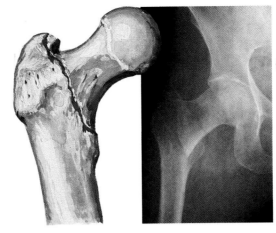

Nondisplaced fracture

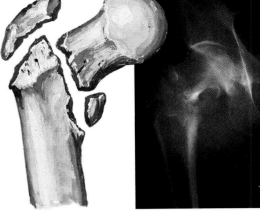

Comminuted displaced fracture

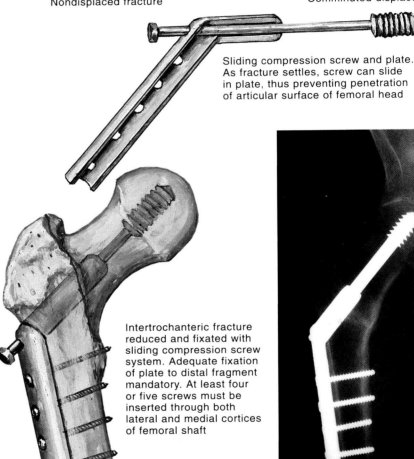

Sliding compression screw and plate. As fracture settles, screw can slide in plate, thus preventing penetration of articular surface of femoral head

Intertrochanteric fracture reduced and fixated with sliding compression screw system. Adequate fixation of plate to distal fragment mandatory. At least four or five screws must be inserted through both lateral and medial cortices of femoral shaft

Anteroposterior radiograph shows intertrochanteric fracture stabilized with compression screw and plate

Intertrochanteric Fracture of Femur

Intertrochanteric fractures of the femur typically occur in persons 10 years older than those who sustain fractures of the femoral neck (Plate 90). These fractures occur along a line that connects the greater and lesser trochanters. Fractures can result in a simple two-part displacement or in more complex, comminuted fractures. Because the fracture surfaces created in the injury are large and filled with an abundance of cancellous bone, delayed union or nonunion is rare. Although nonoperative treatment with prolonged bed rest can be employed, the fractures are most commonly treated with open reduction and internal fixation.

Of the many classifications of intertrochanteric fractures, the system developed by Evans appears to be the most useful for selecting appropriate treatment. The fractures are classified into two types, stable and unstable. The system is based on whether a stable reduction of the fracture at the medial and posteromedial aspects of the fracture surface can be achieved. If stability is attained at these two sites, the fracture is likely to heal in this position with proper fixation. Evans noted that if stability could not be achieved, patients more frequently experienced loss of fixation or loss of reduction due to collapse of the fracture into a varus and externally rotated position.

The sliding compression screw was developed to treat intertrochanteric fractures of the femur. The unstable fracture fragments telescope along the sliding portion of the device to a position of stability. The screw portion of the device is securely fixated in the femoral neck and head, and the sliding portion allows for a controlled collapse of the fracture. Recent studies have demonstrated that use of the device has reduced the incidence of complications after surgical treatment of unstable intertrochanteric fractures. However, many surgeons prefer to achieve a stable reduction of the fracture before using any device to fixate it. Stable fixation

lessens the stresses applied to the sliding compression screw, which decreases the risk of implant failure.

Postoperative management depends on the patient's ability to cooperate with a rehabilitation program, the quality of the bone in the proximal femur, and the adequacy of the reduction and fixation. Cooperative patients with good-quality bone and secure fracture fixation can be mobilized early with progressive weight bearing. Uncooperative patients or those unable to understand the postoperative treatment program are mobilized more slowly and cautiously. At first, these patients are simply moved from bed to chair. A similar

postoperative program is recommended for patients with poor-quality bone and for those with markedly comminuted fractures and fracture instability. Comminuted intertrochanteric fractures may require bone grafting at the time of fracture fixation.

Subtrochanteric Fracture of Femur

Subtrochanteric fractures of the femur occur in two separate age groups—in young adults as a result of high-energy injuries and in very elderly persons as a result of simple falls. The fractures occur just distal to the lesser trochanter (or may involve it) and with varying degrees of comminution (Plate 91).

Subtrochanteric Fracture of Femur

Injury to Femur
(Continued)

In adults, subtrochanteric fractures are usually treated with internal fixation to allow early mobilization and rehabilitation of the patient. Occasionally, closed treatment methods involving skeletal traction are used in young patients with isolated injuries.

Biomechanical analysis of the intact femur demonstrates that the highest compressive and tensile stresses on the femur are concentrated in the subtrochanteric region. Because of these very high forces, implant failure has been most commonly seen with internal fixation of this type of fracture (Plate 145). Nonunion, malunion, and implant failure occur more often with a subtrochanteric fracture than with any other type of femoral injury. Angled nail plate devices, long used to treat this injury, are more likely to fail than other implant devices; the implant often breaks opposite an area of medial comminution. For this reason, when a long nail plate is used to stabilize this fracture, bone grafting of any medial comminution or defect must always be considered to enhance bone repair and minimize the chance of implant failure due to cyclic loading.

Because of problems with the use of nail plate devices, other intramedullary devices have been developed specifically for treating subtrochanteric fractures of the femur. The Zickel nail is one of the earliest and most successful devices. The incidence of malunion and nonunion has been reduced with the use of the Zickel nail, because of its intramedullary position and firm fixation in the femoral head and neck. However, even if the Zickel nail is used, bone grafting should be considered when there is substantial comminution in the medial subtrochanteric region.

Traction may be employed in younger patients with markedly comminuted or exploded subtrochanteric fractures. The limb may be kept in traction for as long as 8 weeks; then the patient is placed in a one and one-half hip spica cast until final fracture consolidation occurs.

Postoperative management depends on the quality of fixation, the quality of bone, and the stability of fracture reduction. Patients with good bone mass, minimal comminution, and good fracture stability are mobilized early from bed to chair and then to walking using crutches for support. In patients treated with an intramedullary device, which helps distribute the load across the fracture site, weight bearing on the injured limb progresses more rapidly than in patients treated with a nail plate device. Generally, patients who are treated with a nail plate device are allowed weight bearing on the injured limb only for balance until there are signs of healing along the medial cortex of the femur. Older patients with osteoporotic bone are mobilized slowly from bed to chair. Weight bearing on the fractured limb is allowed when clinical and radiographic evaluations show adequate fracture healing.

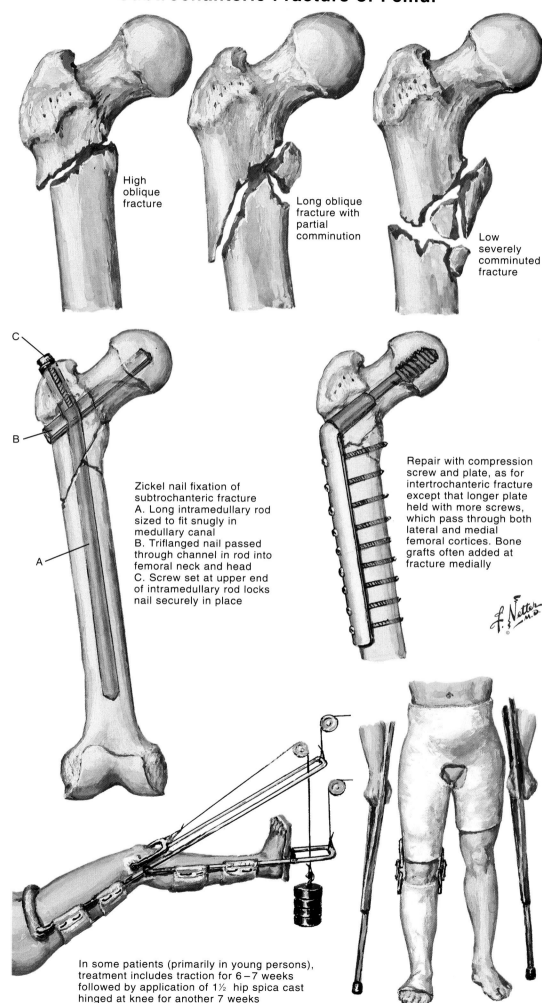

High oblique fracture

Long oblique fracture with partial comminution

Low severely comminuted fracture

Zickel nail fixation of subtrochanteric fracture
A. Long intramedullary rod sized to fit snugly in medullary canal
B. Triflanged nail passed through channel in rod into femoral neck and head
C. Screw set at upper end of intramedullary rod locks nail securely in place

Repair with compression screw and plate, as for intertrochanteric fracture except that longer plate held with more screws, which pass through both lateral and medial femoral cortices. Bone grafts often added at fracture medially

In some patients (primarily in young persons), treatment includes traction for 6–7 weeks followed by application of 1½ hip spica cast hinged at knee for another 7 weeks

Injury to Femur
(*Continued*)

Fracture of Shaft of Femur

Femoral shaft fractures occur in all age groups but are more common in younger than in elderly persons (Plate 92). Several types of fractures can result from simple trauma to high-velocity trauma. Spiral fractures are most commonly due to low-velocity torsional forces applied to the femur, whereas comminuted, segmental, and transverse fractures all result from greater forces. About 15% of femoral shaft fractures are open injuries, but associated neurovascular involvement is not common.

The traditional treatment of fractures of the femoral shaft begins with skeletal traction, which is followed by immobilization in either a hip spica cast or a fracture brace. Generally, skeletal traction is applied by placing a pin through the proximal tibia and aligning the fracture. Once fracture callus forms and the fracture site is no longer tender, traction is discontinued and a cast or brace applied.

Until recently, femoral fractures were immobilized in a one and one-half hip spica cast that did not allow knee flexion. Newer methods of immobilization, such as the fracture brace, allow early knee motion and rehabilitation of both the quadriceps and the hamstring muscles. With the fracture brace, the patient is allowed to walk using crutches and to place as much weight on the injured limb as symptoms allow.

A major advance in the treatment of femoral fractures is the use of closed intramedullary nailing guided by a C-arm image intensifier. As the complexity of femoral fractures increased, advances in the technology of intramedullary nails also occurred. Even severely comminuted femoral fractures can now be securely fixated with standard and modified intramedullary devices. However, the major impact of intramedullary nailing has been on the treatment of femoral shaft fractures in patients with multiple injuries. Early fracture stabilization allows these patients to be upright and out of bed soon after injury, which decreases the incidence of adult respiratory distress syndrome (Plate 141) and, possibly, of multiple organ system failure, which often accompanies multiple injuries.

When an isolated femoral shaft fracture is treated with intramedullary nailing, the patient is allowed out of bed very early. First mobilized using crutches, the patient increases weight bearing on the injured side based on the results of follow-up clinical and radiographic examinations.

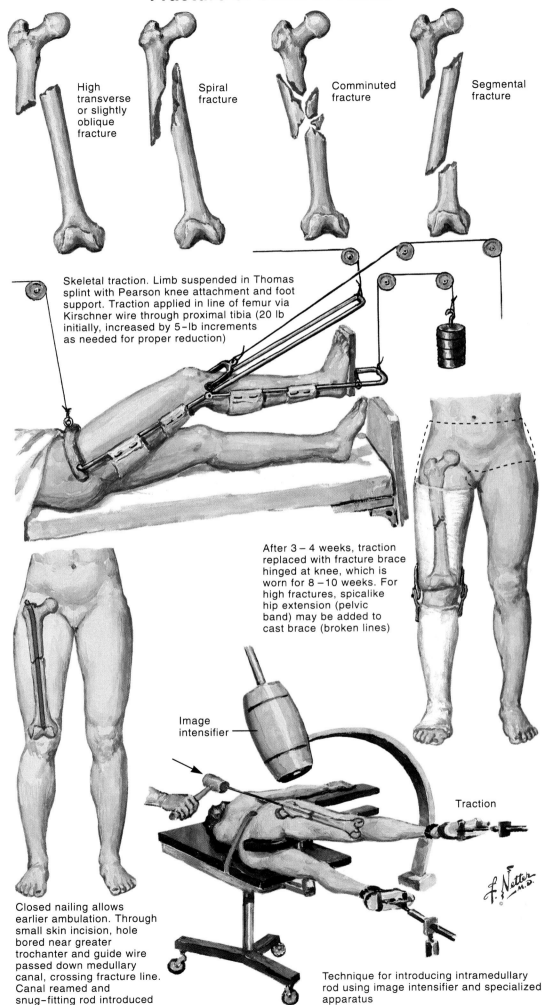

Fracture of Shaft of Femur

High transverse or slightly oblique fracture

Spiral fracture

Comminuted fracture

Segmental fracture

Skeletal traction. Limb suspended in Thomas splint with Pearson knee attachment and foot support. Traction applied in line of femur via Kirschner wire through proximal tibia (20 lb initially, increased by 5–lb increments as needed for proper reduction)

After 3 – 4 weeks, traction replaced with fracture brace hinged at knee, which is worn for 8 –10 weeks. For high fractures, spicalike hip extension (pelvic band) may be added to cast brace (broken lines)

Image intensifier

Traction

Closed nailing allows earlier ambulation. Through small skin incision, hole bored near greater trochanter and guide wire passed down medullary canal, crossing fracture line. Canal reamed and snug-fitting rod introduced

Technique for introducing intramedullary rod using image intensifier and specialized apparatus

Injury to Femur
(Continued)

Fracture of Distal Femur

Fractures of the distal femur are generally divided into two groups, those that involve the joint surface and those that do not (Plate 93). As with any intraarticular fracture, those of the distal femur can lead to significant posttraumatic osteoarthritis if reduction and fixation of the intraarticular aspect of the fracture are not satisfactory.

The many different fracture patterns that occur in the distal femur range from the fracture type that does not involve the joint surface to the type with severe comminution of both the intraarticular and extraarticular components.

Fractures with joint involvement require treatment with open reduction and internal fixation, first to achieve secure fixation of the intraarticular fragments, then to join them to the intact distal femur. Intraarticular fractures are usually treated with a blade plate or supracondylar screw plate. The success of treatment with these devices depends on a meticulous surgical technique and the availability of sufficiently strong bone for fixation.

The same problems of implant failure or fixation that occur in the treatment of subtrochanteric fractures can also complicate the treatment of the distal femur. In areas of marked metaphyseal comminution, bone grafting medially may help prevent late failure of the plate device. Patients with poor-quality bone may benefit from traction or a modified intramedullary device such as the Zickel supracondylar device.

Fractures of the distal femur that involve a single condyle may be stabilized securely with single lag screws or lag screws with a buttress plate. This technique allows early motion with minimal risk of displacement at the joint surface.

Skeletal traction is another treatment option, especially for distal femoral fractures with no intraarticular involvement. Extraarticular fractures, especially of the distal third of the femoral shaft, are very amenable to skeletal traction, with the pin placed in the proximal tibia. This form of traction allows early motion of the knee. After about 3 to 4 weeks of traction, the patient is placed in a fracture brace hinged at the knee. This appliance allows early active motion of the knee and progressive weight bearing. Generally, the cast brace is removed about 3 months after fracture.

Rehabilitation after open reduction and internal fixation is based on the security of the fixation and the quality of the bone. As clinical and radiographic examinations document healing, the patient is allowed to increase weight bearing on the injured extremity. If the quality of fixation appears tenuous or bone quality is poor, internal fixation may be supplemented with a fracture brace to protect the reduction until the fracture heals. □

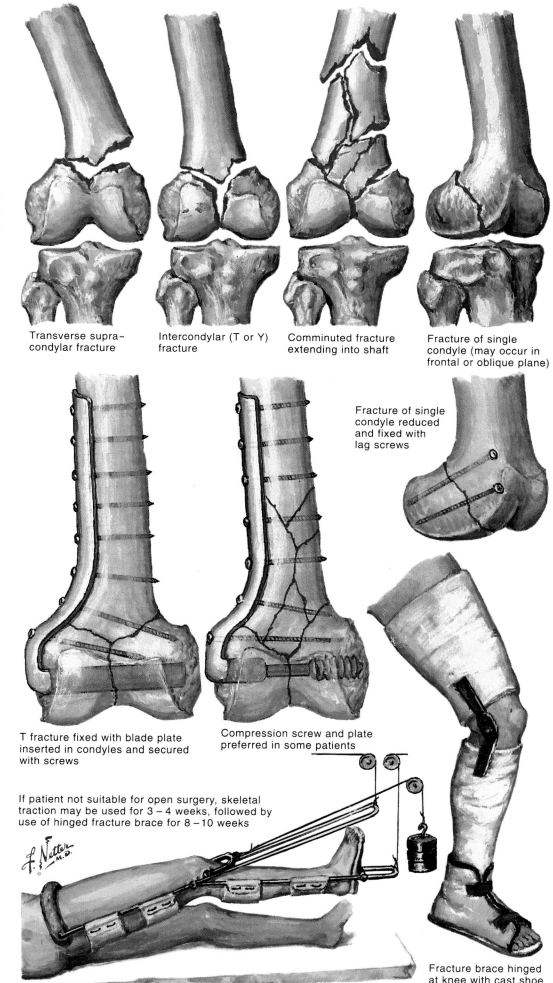

Fracture of Distal Femur

Transverse supracondylar fracture

Intercondylar (T or Y) fracture

Comminuted fracture extending into shaft

Fracture of single condyle (may occur in frontal or oblique plane)

Fracture of single condyle reduced and fixed with lag screws

T fracture fixed with blade plate inserted in condyles and secured with screws

Compression screw and plate preferred in some patients

If patient not suitable for open surgery, skeletal traction may be used for 3 – 4 weeks, followed by use of hinged fracture brace for 8 – 10 weeks

Fracture brace hinged at knee with cast shoe used after traction

Injury to Knee

The knee is a diarthrodial joint made up of the articulations between the femur, tibia, and patella. The major ligaments joining these bones are the lateral and medial collateral and the anterior and posterior cruciate. Two semilunar cartilages, the medial and lateral menisci, help stabilize the knee and dissipate forces between the femur and the tibia. The hamstring muscle group acts to flex the knee, and the quadriceps muscle group extends it. The quadriceps mechanism is complex, consisting of the quadriceps muscle group; its tendon, which inserts into the patella; the patella; the medial and lateral patellar retinacula; and the patellar ligament, which joins the patella to the tibial tuberosity.

Arthrocentesis of Knee Joint

Swelling, ecchymosis, and tenderness signal a significant injury to the knee. Clinical findings may also include joint effusion, limitation of motion, and instability. Arthrocentesis is often performed to help define the nature of the intraarticular pathology (Plate 94). A large needle (at least 18 gauge) is used via an anteromedial or anterolateral approach, with care to avoid injury to the articular cartilage.

Fluid obtained from the joint is Gram stained, cultured, and examined microscopically under polarized light to detect any crystals. Erythrocyte and leukocyte counts and glucose concentration are determined. Healthy joints usually yield less than 5 ml of fluid. Normal synovial fluid is clear and pale yellow and more viscous than water. The average number of leukocytes is about 65/mm³, and most are lymphocytes and monocytes. Acute inflammation increases the ratio of polymorphonuclear leukocytes to lymphocytes and monocytes.

Synovial effusions are categorized as group I, noninflammatory; group II, inflammatory; group III, septic; and group IV, hemorrhagic. Group I synovial fluid has high viscosity, is pale to dark yellow, and is transparent. Leukocyte count is generally under 200/mm³, of which about 25% are polymorphonuclear leukocytes. Glucose concentration is similar to that in serum. Group I fluid is typically found in joints with osteoarthritis.

Group II synovial fluid has low viscosity, may be yellow to light green, and is translucent. Leukocyte counts of 2,000 to 75,000/mm³ are common, and about 50% of the cells may be polymorphonuclear leukocytes. Glucose concentration is generally lower than that in serum. Group II synovial fluid is found in joints with rheumatoid arthritis.

Group III synovial fluid is obtained from a septic joint and has variable viscosity and color but is opaque. The leukocyte count is frequently 100,000/mm³, and polymorphonuclear leukocytes predominate (75%). The glucose level is significantly lower than that in serum. Group IV synovial fluid is bloody, has variable viscosity, and often looks like whole blood on gross examination.

Arthrocentesis of Knee Joint

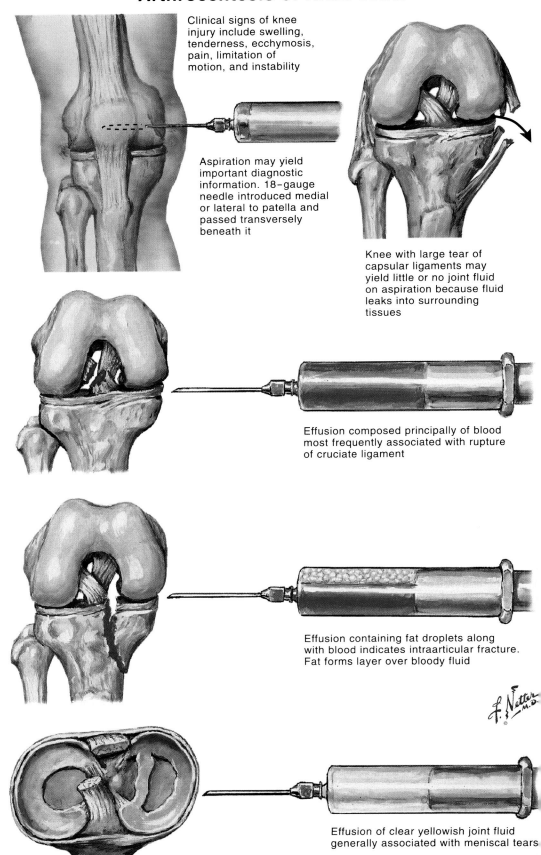

Clinical signs of knee injury include swelling, tenderness, ecchymosis, pain, limitation of motion, and instability

Aspiration may yield important diagnostic information. 18–gauge needle introduced medial or lateral to patella and passed transversely beneath it

Knee with large tear of capsular ligaments may yield little or no joint fluid on aspiration because fluid leaks into surrounding tissues

Effusion composed principally of blood most frequently associated with rupture of cruciate ligament

Effusion containing fat droplets along with blood indicates intraarticular fracture. Fat forms layer over bloody fluid

Effusion of clear yellowish joint fluid generally associated with meniscal tears

A knee joint effusion consisting principally of blood (hemarthrosis) is often associated with rupture of the anterior cruciate ligament.

An effusion containing numerous fat droplets along with blood indicates an intraarticular fracture. The volume of fat may be so great that the fat layer is visible on a lateral radiograph of the knee; after aspiration, the fat appears as a distinct layer floating on the synovial fluid and blood in the syringe. Other injuries, such as avulsion of a ligament at its insertion into bone, may produce a hemarthrosis with a few fat droplets. A large tear of the joint capsule may result in little or no detectable effusion because the blood and joint fluid leak into the periarticular tissues and thus cannot be aspirated from the joint.

Injury to Knee
(Continued)

Tears of Meniscus

Two semilunar cartilages, the medial and lateral menisci, act as surfaces for articulation and perform a cushioning function within the knee joint. The fibrocartilaginous C-shaped menisci are frequently injured, usually by a twisting trauma to the knee. Tears may occur in either meniscus or in both menisci at the same time (Plate 95). A meniscus tear becomes symptomatic if its torn portion is mobile and slides into an abnormal position between the articular surfaces of the femur and tibia. Patients with a displaced meniscus tear often report pain at the joint line and blocked extension, flexion, or both. The affected knee frequently gives way and exhibits recurrent effusions.

A bucket handle tear is a longitudinal tear through the substance of the meniscus. The torn portion remains attached to the anterior and posterior horns of the meniscus. When the unstable bucket handle portion displaces into the intercondylar notch, it blocks full extension of the knee. Patients may be able to manipulate the knee into full extension, which often occurs with a loud, audible, and palpable "clunk." This sound and the temporary resolution of symptoms indicate reduction of the bucket handle portion into its normal anatomic position.

A small radial tear initially causes very few symptoms, but if not treated, it may progress to a deeper, more symptomatic parrot beak tear. The unstable flap of meniscus may cause mechanical signs in the injured knee such as recurrent effusions, giving way, and a catching sensation. Horizontal tears of the meniscus appear to be a delamination of the substance of the meniscus. Neglected horizontal tears frequently result in an unstable flap of meniscal tissue, which can also cause mechanical signs.

When the unstable torn part of the meniscus becomes incarcerated in the area of the intercondylar notch, the knee locks. Locking of the knee can also be caused by a loose body or by the remaining stump of a torn anterior cruciate ligament. A locked knee requires urgent intervention. If it is neglected, attempts at weight bearing and knee movement cause severe, irreversible erosion of the articular cartilage surfaces of the femur and tibia. To help preserve the articular cartilage, part of the meniscus is usually removed during arthroscopy. At the time of surgery, with the patient under anesthesia, the knee may spontaneously unlock. After anesthesia is induced, the knee is examined manually to determine any ligament instability, and an arthroscopic examination is performed. If a meniscus is torn, the torn portion can often be removed using small instruments under arthroscopic guidance.

The outer one-third of the meniscus has vasculature, which permits a very small peripheral tear in this area to heal. Larger peripheral tears may be repaired arthroscopically, using percutaneously placed sutures to hold the bucket handle portion to the vascular rim.

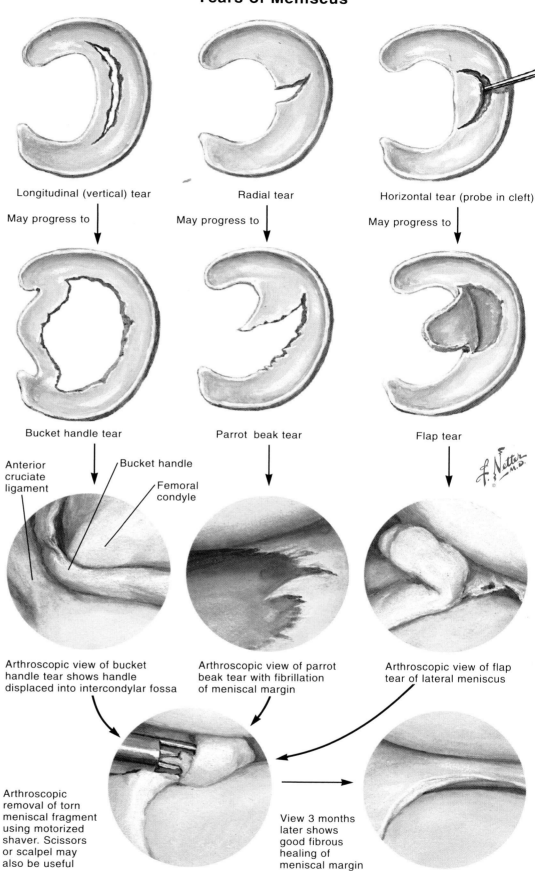

Tears of Meniscus

Longitudinal (vertical) tear
May progress to

Radial tear
May progress to

Horizontal tear (probe in cleft)
May progress to

Bucket handle tear

Parrot beak tear

Flap tear

Anterior cruciate ligament — Bucket handle — Femoral condyle

Arthroscopic view of bucket handle tear shows handle displaced into intercondylar fossa

Arthroscopic view of parrot beak tear with fibrillation of meniscal margin

Arthroscopic view of flap tear of lateral meniscus

Arthroscopic removal of torn meniscal fragment using motorized shaver. Scissors or scalpel may also be useful

View 3 months later shows good fibrous healing of meniscal margin

Rehabilitation programs after arthroscopy and partial meniscectomy generally include minimal immobilization of the knee, immediate weight bearing, and early physical therapy. Therapy consists of gait training and active and passive range-of-motion and quadriceps-strengthening exercises. Ice or heat may be applied as needed. After repair of meniscus tears, vigorous rehabilitation and range-of-motion exercises may be delayed a few weeks.

Fracture of Patella

The patella may fracture if the intrinsic strength of the patella and the extensor expansion is overcome by the pull of the quadriceps femoris muscle (Plate 96). Fractures are usually caused by

Fracture of Patella

Injury to Knee

(Continued)

indirect forces, particularly when the quadriceps mechanism contracts forcefully in an effort to extend a knee that is being forcibly flexed. The patient may stumble, feel the pain of a tear, hear a "pop," and fall as disruption of the patella occurs. Immediately after the patella fractures, as the quadriceps femoris muscle continues to contract and the knee continues to flex, the medial and lateral retinacula are torn. The degree of tearing dictates how much the patellar fragments separate. Indirect fractures are usually transverse, sometimes with comminution at the fracture site.

The patella, a sesamoid bone, is also vulnerable to injury from a direct blow. Striking the knee on an automobile dashboard or on the ground in a fall frequently results in comminuted, stellate fractures. These fractures often are nondisplaced, and the patient is able to actively extend the knee if pain is relieved. Vertical fractures of the patella occur occasionally and usually have minimal displacement.

Nondisplaced patella fractures are treated by immobilizing the knee in full extension with a long leg cast or a splint. Union occurs in about 6 weeks, after which active and gentle passive range-of-motion exercises should be instituted. Transverse fractures with displacement greater than a few millimeters require surgery. The fracture fragments are reapproximated to their anatomic positions. The medial and lateral retinacula are repaired, and the patellar fragments are held in place with a figure-of-8 tension band wire wrapped around two parallel Steinmann pins. Full knee extension should not be allowed until fracture union occurs.

A partial patellectomy is performed for fractures of the proximal or distal pole of the patella with extensive comminution of the small fragment. The object is to save at least one-half of the articular surface while excising the small comminuted fragments. The quadriceps femoris tendon or the patellar ligament is reattached to the remaining patella, and the medial and lateral retinacula are repaired. The knee is immobilized in full extension in a cast or splint for 6 weeks. After that, protected range of motion and weight bearing are allowed. A patellectomy should be considered only for severely comminuted fractures, as removal of the patella compromises the biomechanics of the quadriceps mechanism at the knee.

Osteochondral fractures are caused by a completely different mechanism. When a lateral dislocation of the patella is forcefully reduced, a bone fragment may detach from the medial facet of the patella (occasionally from the lateral femoral condyle). Clinical findings are pain along the anteromedial aspect of the knee, marked swelling, hemarthrosis, and mechanical locking and grinding in the knee. The fracture fragments may be completely cartilaginous and difficult to see on plain radiographs but may be visualized on a skyline view of the patella. The loose body is usually removed with arthroscopy. Very large fragments may be reattached to the patella.

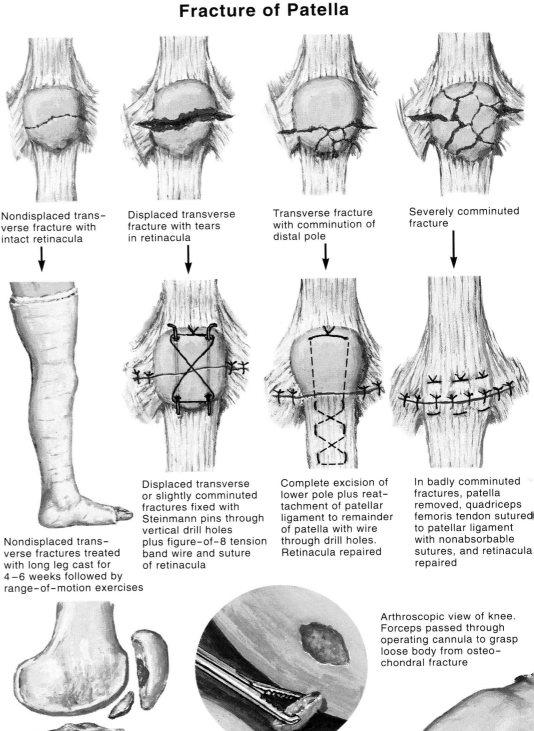

Nondisplaced transverse fracture with intact retinacula

Displaced transverse fracture with tears in retinacula

Transverse fracture with comminution of distal pole

Severely comminuted fracture

Nondisplaced transverse fractures treated with long leg cast for 4–6 weeks followed by range-of-motion exercises

Displaced transverse or slightly comminuted fractures fixed with Steinmann pins through vertical drill holes plus figure-of-8 tension band wire and suture of retinacula

Complete excision of lower pole plus reattachment of patellar ligament to remainder of patella with wire through drill holes. Retinacula repaired

In badly comminuted fractures, patella removed, quadriceps femoris tendon sutured to patellar ligament with nonabsorbable sutures, and retinacula repaired

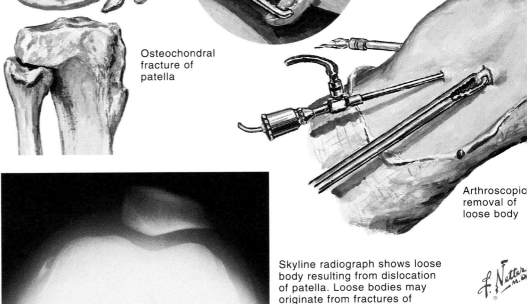

Osteochondral fracture of patella

Arthroscopic view of knee. Forceps passed through operating cannula to grasp loose body from osteochondral fracture

Arthroscopic removal of loose body

Skyline radiograph shows loose body resulting from dislocation of patella. Loose bodies may originate from fractures of femoral condyle or patella

Injury to Knee

(Continued)

Disruption of Quadriceps Femoris Tendon or Patellar Ligament

Damage to the quadriceps mechanism generally occurs when there is active contraction of the quadriceps femoris muscle against forced flexion of the knee (Plate 97). Most ruptures of this extensor mechanism occur in older patients. The tendon may be weakened by age-related degenerative changes or by pathologic changes due to psoriatic arthritis, rheumatoid arthritis, arteriosclerosis, gout, hyperparathyroidism, diabetes, chronic renal failure, or corticosteroid therapy.

At the time of injury, the patient experiences sudden pain, which may be associated with a tearing sensation about the knee. The most important finding during examination is the patient's inability to actively extend the knee fully against gravity. Also, the patient may not be able to maintain a passively extended knee against gravity. Patients with rupture of the quadriceps femoris tendon or patellar ligament without involvement of the medial or lateral retinaculum may be able to extend the injured knee actively to within 10° of full extension. When there is a widely separated tear of either tendon or ligament combined with involvement of the medial and lateral retinacula, active extension is very difficult.

Palpation of the knee reveals a hematoma, which may make examination difficult. A high-riding patella may indicate rupture of the patellar ligament, whereas a patella that is riding lower than normal suggests a rupture of the quadriceps femoris tendon. A large defect may be palpable soon after injury; if the ruptured ligament is not treated for weeks or months, the sulcus fills with scar tissue. Patients with chronic rupture of the quadriceps femoris tendon complain of giving way of the knee and marked weakness on attempting active extension.

Rupture of the quadriceps femoris tendon generally occurs at its point of insertion into the superior pole of the patella; rupture of the patellar ligament usually occurs at the inferior pole of the patella. In both cases, surgery is required to reestablish the continuity of the quadriceps mechanism. The tendon or ligament is reattached with sutures through drill holes in the patella; then, the medial and lateral retinacula are sutured. After surgery, the knee is immobilized in full extension in a cast or splint for 6 weeks.

Patients who also have chronic metabolic disorders or receive long-term corticosteroid treatment usually require a more complex repair that uses tendon, fascia, or wire to reinforce the damaged quadriceps mechanism. After postoperative immobilization for 8 to 10 weeks, patients gradually start protected range-of-motion exercises and should use a cane or walker for some time.

Rupture of the patellar ligament may also occur at its insertion on the tibia, with or without fracture of the tibial tuberosity. In children whose growth plates have not yet closed, the ligament should be sutured, since this injury may disturb

Disruption of Quadriceps Femoris Tendon or Patellar Ligament

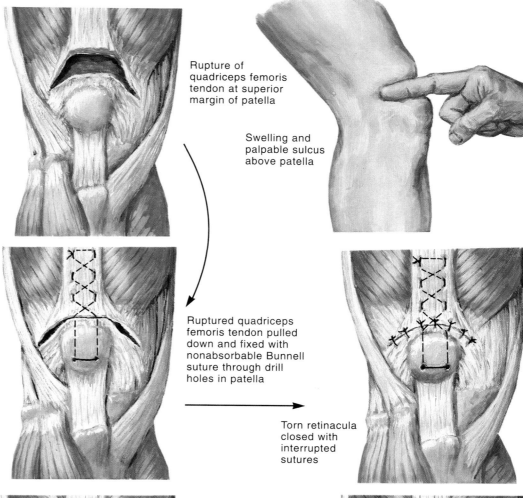

Rupture of quadriceps femoris tendon at superior margin of patella

Swelling and palpable sulcus above patella

Ruptured quadriceps femoris tendon pulled down and fixed with nonabsorbable Bunnell suture through drill holes in patella

Torn retinacula closed with interrupted sutures

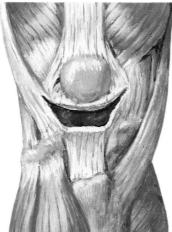

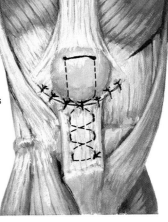

Rupture of patellar ligament at inferior margin of patella

Ruptured patellar ligament repaired with nonabsorbable Bunnell suture through drill holes in patella; torn edges of retinacula approximated with interrupted sutures

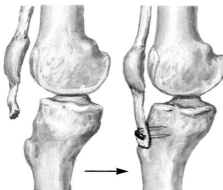
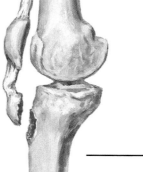
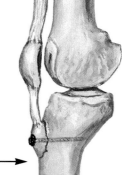

Avulsion of patellar ligament from tibial tuberosity

Repair with staple

Avulsion fracture of tibial tuberosity

Repair with screw

Injury to Knee
(Continued)

growth of the proximal tibia. In adults, avulsion of the ligament from the tibial tuberosity is repaired by suturing the avulsed ligament through drill holes in the tibia or securing it with a metal staple or screw. A displaced fracture of the tibial tuberosity may be treated with open reduction and fixation with a metal screw.

Subluxation and Dislocation of Patella

Subluxation of the patella is a common condition in which the kneecap does not track properly in the trochlear groove of the distal femur (Plate 98). Often associated with knock-knee and external tibial torsion, this condition is most commonly symptomatic in adolescent girls and young women.

A large Q angle seems to increase the patient's susceptibility to subluxation or dislocation of the patella. The Q angle is formed by the intersection of two lines drawn from the anterior superior iliac spine and the tibial tuberosity through the center of the patella.

Patients complain of anterior knee pain, particularly when climbing stairs, and giving way of the knee. Physical examination reveals tenderness along the medial aspect of the patella, patellofemoral crepitus, atrophy of the quadriceps femoris muscle (especially the oblique portion of the vastus medialis), and increased lateral mobility of the patella. A positive apprehension test may be elicited when the patient forcefully contracts the quadriceps femoris muscle and feels pain as the examiner attempts to displace the patella laterally. If the subluxation is not treated, the lateral retinaculum gradually becomes contracted, exacerbating the abnormal patellofemoral tracking.

Conservative treatment is preferred for subluxation of the patella and consists of short-arc quadriceps-strengthening exercises and use of nonsteroidal antiinflammatory drugs to control pain. The goal of exercise is to increase the tone of the oblique portion of the vastus medialis muscle to improve the mechanics of patellar tracking. To strengthen this muscle effectively, full extension of the knee must be achieved during the exercises. Compression of the patella against the femur causes pain in patients with subluxation of the patella. Reducing the amount of compression by limiting the degree of knee flexion during the exercise reduces symptoms while still rehabilitating the quadriceps muscle. An elastic strap placed about the knee at the level of the patellar ligament sometimes relieves symptoms.

When conservative treatment is not successful and a significant disability persists, a variety of surgical techniques may be used to realign the quadriceps mechanism. Patients with a normal Q angle who do not respond to conservative treatment may need a release of the lateral retinaculum, performed during arthroscopy or arthrotomy. Release of a contracted, tight lateral retinaculum allows the patella to be properly repositioned into the trochlear groove by the pull of the oblique portion of the vastus medialis muscle.

Subluxation and Dislocation of Patella

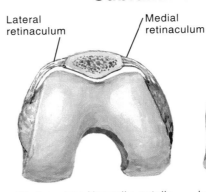
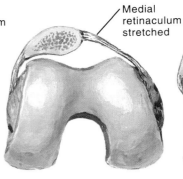
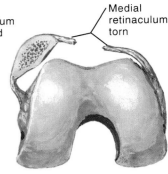

Skyline view. Normally, patella rides in groove between medial and lateral femoral condyles

In subluxation, patella deviates laterally because of weakness of vastus medialis muscle, tightness of lateral retinaculum, and high Q angle

In dislocation, patella displaced completely out of intercondylar groove

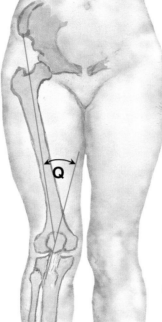

Q angle formed by intersection of lines from anterior superior iliac spine and from tibial tuberosity through midpoint of patella. Large Q angle predisposes to patellar subluxation

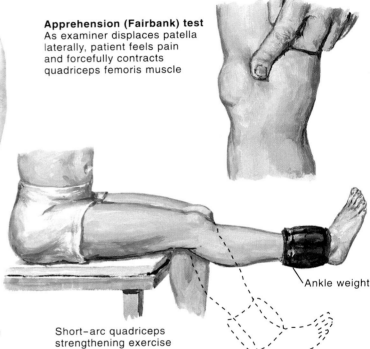

Apprehension (Fairbank) test
As examiner displaces patella laterally, patient feels pain and forcefully contracts quadriceps femoris muscle

Ankle weight

Short–arc quadriceps strengthening exercise in patients with recurrent subluxation or dislocation of patella

Surgical procedures for recurrent patellar subluxation or dislocation

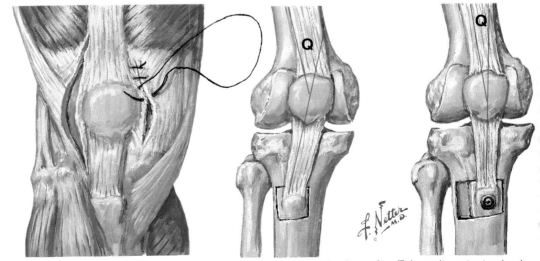

Lateral release. Lateral retinaculum incised, decreasing lateral pull on patella. Torn medial retinaculum sutured or tightened by plication

Transfer of tibial tuberosity. Tuberosity osteotomized along with attached patellar ligament. Tuberosity shifted to more medial position and fixed with screw, reducing Q angle

Sprains of Knee Ligaments

Injury to Knee
(Continued)

With arthrotomy, a medial parapatellar incision of the knee capsule can be closed in a pants-over-vest fashion and the oblique vastus medialis muscle advanced more distally and laterally. These maneuvers pull or tether the patella medially and may improve patellofemoral tracking.

Patients with an abnormally large Q angle may require release of the lateral retinaculum in conjunction with a transfer of the tibial tuberosity. Care must be taken not to transfer the tibial tuberosity distally or posteriorly.

Sprains of Knee Ligaments

Ligament injuries (sprains) of the knee are very common in athletes (Plate 99). In first-degree sprains, the ligament is stretched, with little or no tearing. These injuries produce mild point tenderness, slight hemorrhage, and swelling. Erythema may develop over the painful area but resolves in 2 or 3 weeks after injury. Joint laxity is not present, and the injury does not produce any significant long-term disability. Appropriate treatment consists of rest and muscle rehabilitation. Second-degree sprains are characterized by partial tearing of the ligament, resulting in joint laxity, localized pain, tenderness, and swelling. When stress is placed on a joint during examination, the examiner feels a definite "end point" to the joint movement. Because the ligament is only partially injured, the joint remains stable, and vigorous rehabilitation alone is sufficient treatment. Third-degree sprains produce complete rupture of a ligament, making the joint unstable. Tenderness, instability, absence of a definite end point to stress testing, and severe ecchymosis are the hallmarks of third-degree sprains. Surgical intervention may be needed.

Sprains of the tibial (medial) collateral ligament are caused by a valgus force to the knee. Patients frequently report a snapping or tearing sensation and pain on the medial aspect of the knee. If only the medial collateral ligament is injured, patients can usually continue to walk and may be able to continue the activity that caused the injury.

Physical examination reveals tenderness along the course of the tibial collateral ligament, and careful palpation can isolate the precise level of injury: at the origin of the ligament, on the medial femoral condyle, at the joint line (midsubstance), or along the long distal insertion of the ligament into the medial aspect of the tibia. Patients are more comfortable if examined lying supine on the examining table with the thigh supported. The physician cradles the lower leg in both hands off to the side of the table and alternately applies varus and valgus stresses to the knee (varus and valgus stress tests). When the leg is fully extended, the posterior cruciate ligament is the structure most responsible for medial-lateral stability. However, placing the knee in 30° flexion takes the posterior cruciate ligament "out of play" so the medial collateral ligament can be tested by applying a valgus force.

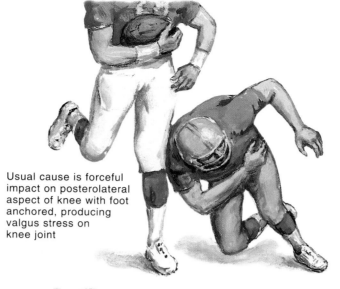

Usual cause is forceful impact on posterolateral aspect of knee with foot anchored, producing valgus stress on knee joint

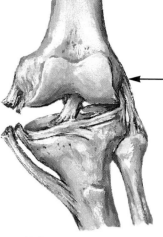

Valgus stress may rupture tibial collateral and capsular ligaments

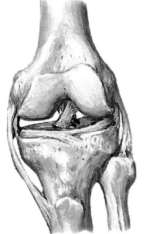

1st–degree sprain. Localized joint pain and tenderness but no joint laxity

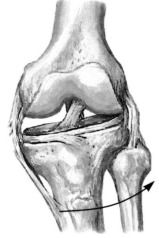

2nd–degree sprain. Detectable joint laxity plus localized pain and tenderness

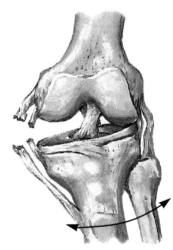

3rd–degree sprain. Complete disruption of ligaments and gross joint instability

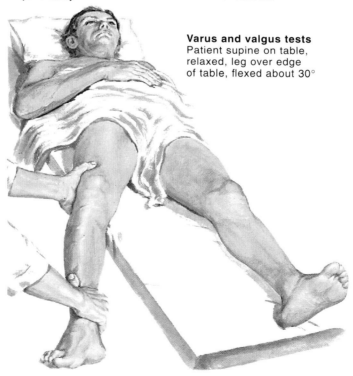

Varus and valgus tests
Patient supine on table, relaxed, leg over edge of table, flexed about 30°

With one hand fixing thigh, examiner places other hand just above ankle and applies valgus stress. Degree of mobility compared with that of uninjured side, which is tested first. For varus stress test, direction of pressure reversed

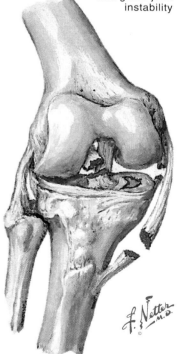

"Unhappy triad" of O'Donoghue
Rupture of tibial collateral and anterior cruciate ligaments plus tear of medial meniscus

Injury to Knee
(Continued)

Third-degree sprains of the medial collateral ligament may require direct surgical repair. However, an isolated third-degree sprain may be successfully treated by controlling swelling, increasing range of motion, and rehabilitating the quadriceps femoris and hamstring muscles.

Marked medial (valgus) laxity may indicate that the posteromedial corner of the knee capsule is also injured. Surgical repair is needed to prevent residual rotational instability. A football clipping injury may result in the "unhappy triad" of O'Donoghue, which includes ruptures of the tibial collateral and anterior cruciate ligaments plus a tear of the medial meniscus. This injury requires arthrotomy, repair of the ligaments as necessary, and repair of the medial meniscus if possible.

Rupture of Anterior Cruciate Ligament

The anterior cruciate ligament is often ruptured by an injury during vigorous athletic competition as when a player swerves, twisting the knee while the foot is firmly planted on the ground. The player hears a "pop," feels a tear and acute pain in the knee, and may not be able to continue playing. The knee may feel very unstable during weight bearing. Rupture of the anterior cruciate ligament is a common cause of acute traumatic hemarthrosis. Clinical tests to demonstrate the degree of anterior cruciate ligament instability are the Lachman, anterior drawer, and pivot shift tests.

Lachman Test. This test is simple to perform and relatively painless for the patient with an acute injury (Plate 100). The examiner compares the amount of play in the injured knee with that in the normal one to determine if abnormal motion is present. The Lachman test is performed with the knee flexed 20° to reduce the stability provided by the menisci. One of the examiner's hands stabilizes the femur while the other hand grasps the proximal tibia. With the patient relaxed, the examiner attempts to slide the proximal tibia anteriorly on the femur. An intact anterior cruciate ligament prevents the tibia from sliding forward. When the ligament is injured, the tibia is moved from its normal position and can be subluxated anteriorly during the test. The examiner must note the quality of the end point of this stress test. If there is a solid mechanical stop at the most anterior extent of tibial motion, the anterior cruciate ligament may be only partially torn. However, if the end point is soft and spongy, a complete rupture should be suspected.

The integrity of the posterior cruciate ligament must be ascertained before the result of this test can be considered valid. If the posterior cruciate ligament is ruptured, the proximal tibia sags posteriorly, and the Lachman test will seem to be positive as the posterior subluxation is reduced.

Anterior Drawer Test. The anterior drawer test is performed with the patient lying supine, resting comfortably with the knee flexed 90° (Plate 100). The patient's foot is stabilized during the test and may be held in place by the seated

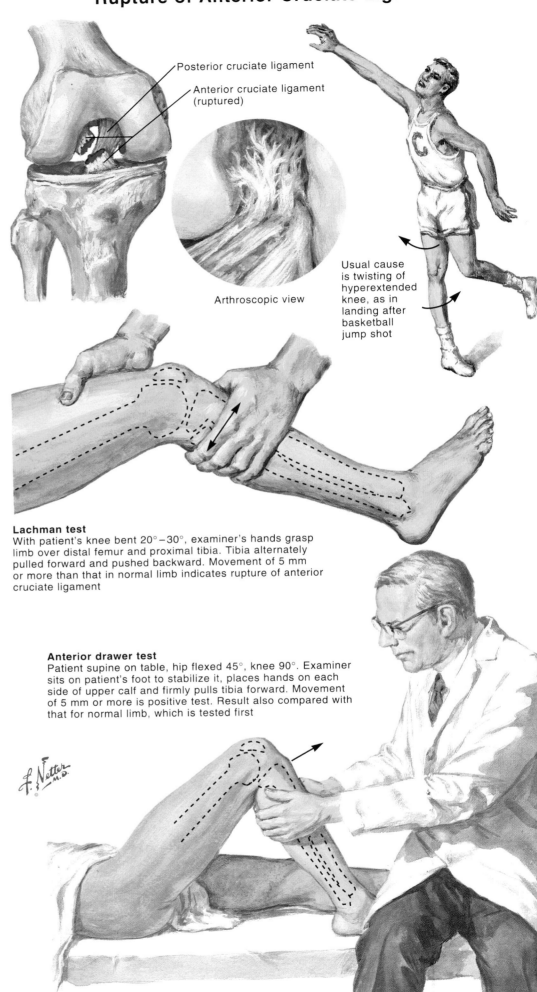

Rupture of Anterior Cruciate Ligament

Posterior cruciate ligament

Anterior cruciate ligament (ruptured)

Arthroscopic view

Usual cause is twisting of hyperextended knee, as in landing after basketball jump shot

Lachman test
With patient's knee bent 20°–30°, examiner's hands grasp limb over distal femur and proximal tibia. Tibia alternately pulled forward and pushed backward. Movement of 5 mm or more than that in normal limb indicates rupture of anterior cruciate ligament

Anterior drawer test
Patient supine on table, hip flexed 45°, knee 90°. Examiner sits on patient's foot to stabilize it, places hands on each side of upper calf and firmly pulls tibia forward. Movement of 5 mm or more is positive test. Result also compared with that for normal limb, which is tested first

Injury to Knee
(Continued)

examiner's thigh. The examiner grasps the patient's calf near the popliteal fossa with both hands and attempts to slide the tibia anteriorly. When the anterior cruciate ligament is ruptured, the tibia slides anteriorly with respect to the femur. The anterior drawer test is performed several times, with the patient's foot and leg positioned first in internal rotation, then in neutral rotation, and finally in external rotation. As in the Lachman test, the injured knee must be compared with the normal one. The anterior drawer test is useful for detecting complete ruptures of the anterior cruciate ligament but is often less sensitive than the Lachman test in diagnosing partial injuries.

Anterolateral Knee Instability

Clinically significant instability caused by injury to the anterior cruciate ligament is manifested by the giving way of the knee. Patients complain that their knee slips or slides when they turn right or left with the foot planted. This sliding reflects the tibia subluxating anteriorly on the femur.

Pivot Shift Test. The pivot shift test identifies most cases of clinically significant knee instability (Plate 101). The patient should be relaxed and lying supine. The examiner stands beside the injured leg, facing it. With one hand grasping the patient's foot, the examiner places the other hand on the lateral aspect of the knee, with the thumb underneath the head of the fibula. With the knee in full extension, a valgus force is applied at the knee while the tibia is internally rotated by the hand holding the foot. This maneuver causes the lateral tibial plateau to subluxate anteriorly on the femur. With the knee in extension, the iliotibial tract is anterior to the instantaneous center of rotation of the knee and acts as an extensor. The knee is then slowly flexed, and the subluxation becomes more apparent. At a point between 20° and 40° flexion, the iliotibial tract slides posterior to the instantaneous center of rotation of the knee and acts as a flexor, causing reduction of the tibia. The reduction is palpable, visible, and frequently audible.

One result of repeated, uncontrolled pivot shifting of the knee during daily activities is injury to the menisci. As the tibia subluxates on the femur, the lateral meniscus is carried forward and is trapped between the lateral femoral condyle and the posterior edge of the lateral tibial plateau. During reduction, compressive forces are significant in this area and may cause sudden tearing or gradual erosion of the meniscus, leading to knee locking and eventually osteoarthritis.

Other tests, such as the Losee, side-lying, and flexion-rotation drawer tests, also produce anterior subluxation of the tibia when the knee is in extension and reduction of the tibia when it is flexed 20° to 40°. All these tests are positive with instability of the anterior cruciate ligament. However, if the patient is not relaxed, the tests may produce false-negative results that obscure the degree of damage, and anesthesia is often needed for adequate examination.

Rupture of Anterior Cruciate Ligament (continued)

Pivot shift test for anterolateral knee instability

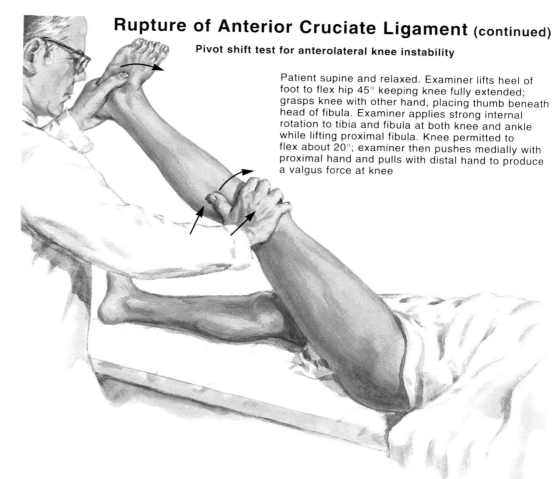

Patient supine and relaxed. Examiner lifts heel of foot to flex hip 45° keeping knee fully extended; grasps knee with other hand, placing thumb beneath head of fibula. Examiner applies strong internal rotation to tibia and fibula at both knee and ankle while lifting proximal fibula. Knee permitted to flex about 20°; examiner then pushes medially with proximal hand and pulls with distal hand to produce a valgus force at knee

As internal rotation, valgus force, and forward displacement of lateral tibial condyle maintained, knee passively flexed. If anterior subluxation of tibia (anterolateral instability) present, sudden visible, audible, and palpable reduction occurs at about 20°–40° flexion. Test positive if anterior cruciate ligament ruptured, especially if lateral capsular ligament also torn

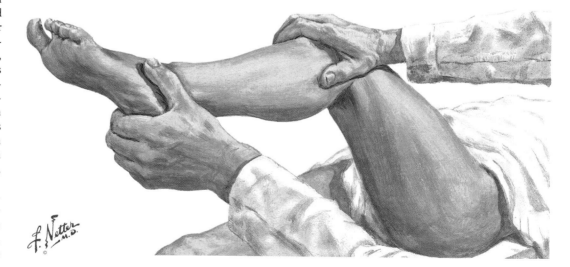

Detachment of Anterior Cruciate Ligament

Fracture of the tibial spine indicates partial or complete detachment of the anterior cruciate ligament from the tibia (Plate 102). This fracture is usually caused by hyperextension of the knee or a sudden twisting motion. If the fracture is displaced, the loose fragment may block motion and cause severe swelling and hemarthrosis. Type I fracture of the tibial spine is an incomplete fracture, whereas type II is complete but nondisplaced. Type III fractures are described as type IIIA (complete and displaced) and type IIIB (complete, displaced, and rotated out of position).

Nondisplaced fractures and those that reduce anatomically when the knee is in full extension may be treated by casting the knee in extension. Union usually occurs in 5 to 6 weeks, after which the patient begins active range-of-motion exercises and rehabilitation of the quadriceps femoris and hamstring muscles.

Surgery is indicated for type IIIA and type IIIB fractures of the tibial spine that cannot be reduced with closed methods. Any mechanical block to full extension is an indication for surgery. Reduction of the fracture may be blocked if the anterior horn of either meniscus is interposed between the displaced tibial spine and its bed. During

Rupture of Anterior Cruciate Ligament (continued)

Fracture of tibial spine may result in detachment of anterior cruciate ligament

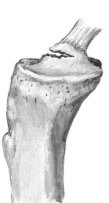

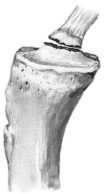

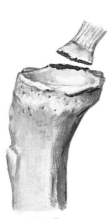

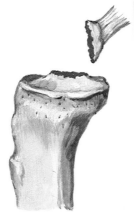

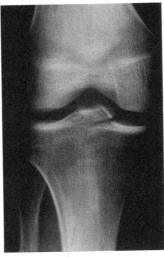

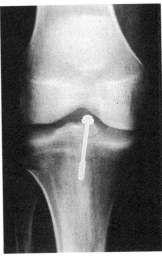

Type I. Incomplete fracture of tibial spine

Type II. Complete fracture, nondisplaced

Type IIIA. Complete fracture, displaced

Type IIIB. Complete fracture, displaced and rotated

Radiograph. Type IIIA fracture of tibial spine

Repair with long cancellous bone screw

Insall reconstruction procedure for acute midsubstance tears and chronic tears of anterior cruciate ligament with instability

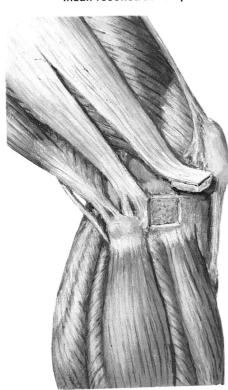

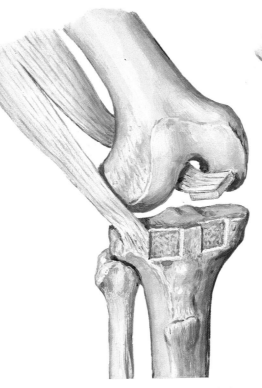

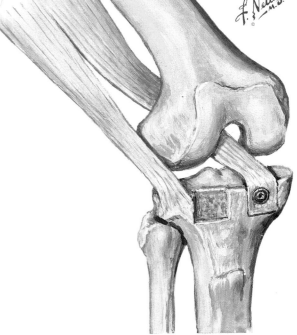

Flap fashioned and raised from anterior ⅔ of iliotibial tract along with block of bone from its attachment to tubercle of Gerdy

Flap transferred over and behind lateral femoral condyle and through intercondylar notch

Fascial flap with terminal bone fragment in newly excavated bed on anterior aspect of proximal tibia. Flap fixed with screw and washer to act as substitute for ligament

SECTION I PLATE 102   Slide 4878

Injury to Knee
(Continued)

surgery, all soft tissue is removed from the fracture site and the tibial spine is replaced in its anatomic position and fixated with sutures or a screw. Adequate and rigid internal fixation allows the patient to regain motion quickly while the injured knee is protected in a brace.

Many acute injuries of the anterior cruciate ligament do not need surgery. If the careful physical examination, using anesthesia if necessary, reveals minimal ligamentous laxity and no sign of meniscus injury, then prompt, vigorous rehabilitation is instituted. If the Lachman or anterior drawer test indicates mild ligament instability but the pivot shift test is negative and there are no other associated injuries, closed treatment with immobilization in a cast may be sufficient.

Physical therapy focuses on rehabilitation of the quadriceps and hamstring muscles. Although the knee is reasonably stable, instability may develop gradually, eventually necessitating reconstruction of the anterior cruciate ligament. Increased instability may lead to meniscus tears.

Open surgical treatment is usually indicated in patients with anterior cruciate ligament injury and a positive pivot shift test. The procedure used is dictated by the patient's life-style, expectations, and other medical conditions. Older, sedentary patients may need no surgery, whereas young, active patients should be considered for repair or reconstruction. Since instability often recurs long after repair or reconstruction of the anterior cruciate ligament, the goals of surgery are to prolong the survival of the menisci and to delay the development of osteoarthritis.

Injury to Knee
(Continued)

Significant instability may eventually develop if injury of the anterior cruciate ligament is neglected or treated conservatively. Patients whose knees give way during daily activities are candidates for delayed reconstruction of the ligament. If the instability is a problem only during intense physical activity, using a brace may provide relief.

Many techniques are used to repair or reconstruct the anterior cruciate ligament. The Insall procedure prevents anterior subluxation of the tibia on the femur (Plate 102). Rigid fixation of the transferred flap to the tibia permits early knee motion, and full weight bearing is allowed when the patient can fully extend the knee. Patients should avoid rough sports for 1 year after surgery.

Rupture of Posterior Cruciate Ligament

The posterior cruciate ligament is the chief stabilizer of the knee in full extension. The most common causes of rupture of this ligament are hyperextension of the knee and a direct blow to the anterior aspect of the flexed knee (Plate 103). Severe varus or valgus stress to the knee following injury to the collateral ligaments can cause rupture of the posterior cruciate ligament.

Posterior Drawer Test. Diagnosis is made by obtaining a complete history and performing a careful physical examination. The posterior drawer test is performed with the patient lying supine on an examining table and the knee in 90° flexion. The patient's foot is stabilized by the examiner's thigh on the table as for the anterior drawer test. The examiner uses both hands to push the proximal tibia posteriorly in an effort to displace it relative to the distal femur. By alternately pushing and pulling the tibia, the examiner can determine if the anterior cruciate ligament is intact and if the proximal tibia is moving posteriorly. The examiner must recognize the starting point of the drawer test to determine accurately which of the two cruciate ligaments is injured.

Posterior Sag Sign. With the patient supine and relaxed, a pad is placed under the distal thigh on the affected side; the heel is allowed to rest on the examining table, and the calf of the leg hangs unsupported. The examiner observes the knee from the patient's side. When a rupture of the posterior cruciate ligament is present, the proximal tibia subluxates posteriorly and the anterior surface of the proximal leg appears to sag.

A knee lacking a functioning posterior cruciate ligament may be hyperextended during examination. The examiner stands at the foot of the supine patient and simultaneously lifts both feet by the great toes, observing the amount of extension at each knee. A knee with rupture of a posterior cruciate ligament exhibits noticeable hyperextension and greater joint laxity than its normal counterpart when varus and valgus stresses are applied with the knee in full extension.

As with the anterior cruciate ligament, when avulsion of the bony attachment of the posterior cruciate ligament occurs at either end, primary

Rupture of Posterior Cruciate Ligament

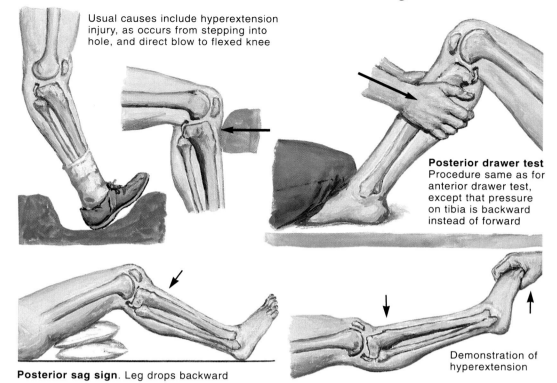

Usual causes include hyperextension injury, as occurs from stepping into hole, and direct blow to flexed knee

Posterior drawer test
Procedure same as for anterior drawer test, except that pressure on tibia is backward instead of forward

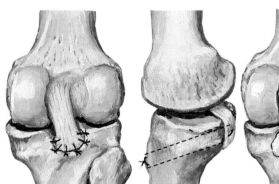

Posterior sag sign. Leg drops backward

Demonstration of hyperextension

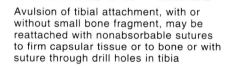

Avulsion of tibial attachment, with or without small bone fragment, may be reattached with nonabsorbable sutures to firm capsular tissue or to bone or with suture through drill holes in tibia

Large bone fragment avulsed from tibia may be fixed in place with screw

Avulsion of femoral attachment may be repaired with nonabsorbable suture through drill holes in distal femur

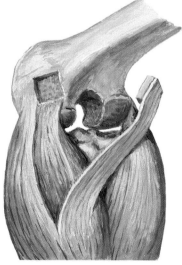

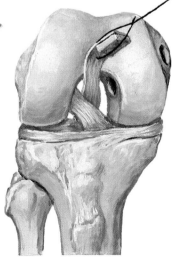

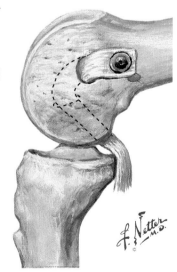

Flap formed of tendinous portion of origin of medial head of gastrocnemius muscle plus small block of bone from femoral attachment (posteromedial view)

Flap passed into intercondylar notch; tunnel drilled through medial femoral condyle. Drill guide ensures accurate placement

Flap with terminal bone block passed through tunnel and fixed with screw. Flap functions as substitute for posterior cruciate ligament

Injury to Knee
(Continued)

repair of the avulsion may be performed. If bone-to-bone repair is not possible, most surgeons elect to treat the patient without resorting to surgery. Repairs of the posterior cruciate ligament are usually less successful than those of the anterior cruciate ligament; instability often recurs after surgery, and motion is lost. Injury to the postero-lateral corner of the knee capsule predisposes to a poor surgical result when accompanied by rupture of the posterior cruciate ligament.

Only patients who have high-demand knees and severe instability are candidates for reconstruction of the posterior cruciate ligament. In one procedure, the origin of the medial head of the gastrocnemius muscle is used as a transfer. After surgery, the knee is immobilized at 30° flexion in a cast or splint for 6 to 8 weeks. Vigorous physical therapy is then instituted. Achieving full extension is very difficult after such prolonged immobilization.

Dislocation of Knee Joint

Dislocation of the knee joint must be distinguished from dislocation of the patella. Whereas a patella dislocation involves the patellofemoral joint, a knee dislocation involves the tibiofemoral articulation (Plate 104). Any dislocation is an emergency, and dislocation of the knee is no exception. Striking the knee against the dashboard during an automobile accident is the most common cause of injury, but athletic injuries are also common causes. The popliteal artery and its branches are often damaged during dislocation of the knee. Therefore, arterial injury must be suspected in every knee dislocation. Diagnosis of arterial damage frequently requires arteriography, and any necessary arterial repair should be done immediately.

Classification of knee dislocations is based on the position of the tibia in relation to the femur. In an anterior dislocation of the knee, the tibia is anterior to the femur, whereas in a posterior dislocation, the tibia is posterior to the femur. Lateral, medial, and rotational dislocations may also occur, as may combination patterns such as anterolateral and posterolateral. Associated vascular injuries are more common with anterior dislocations, whereas the peroneal nerve is more likely to be injured in posterolateral dislocations.

Diagnosis of dislocation of the knee is based on the patient's history and typical clinical findings. If the dislocation has not spontaneously reduced before the patient is examined, the diagnosis is clear because the deformity is obvious and impressive. However, spontaneous reduction of knee dislocations is common. When gross dislocation is not detected by the physical examination or radiography but there is a history of significant knee injury, a dislocation that has spontaneously reduced must be suspected. A large effusion or hemarthrosis may not develop because large tears in the joint capsule allow the fluid to escape into the soft tissues about the knee.

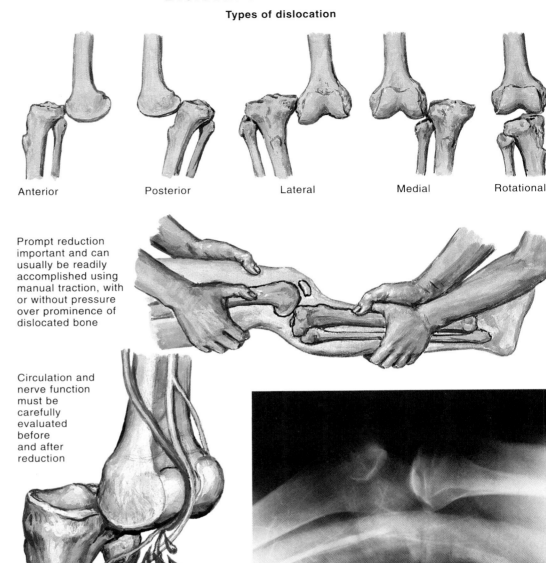

Dislocation of Knee Joint

Types of dislocation

Anterior   Posterior   Lateral   Medial   Rotational

Prompt reduction important and can usually be readily accomplished using manual traction, with or without pressure over prominence of dislocated bone

Circulation and nerve function must be carefully evaluated before and after reduction

Arteriogram shows occlusion of popliteal artery just proximal to joint in dislocation of knee

Tear or thrombosis of popliteal artery is frequent complication, requiring immediate repair or replacement. Tibial and common peroneal nerves may also be torn but usually do not require surgical repair

Compartment syndrome due to massive bleeding or ischemia is common threat. Four-compartment fasciot-omy must be done at first sign of compartment syndrome

The initial treatment of a knee dislocation is straightforward but must begin without delay. Reduction is performed using gentle longitudinal traction and is frequently accomplished with little or no sedation. If any difficulty at all is encountered, anesthesia should be induced promptly. Following reduction, the neurovascular status of the limb must be carefully monitored.

Many knee dislocations are treated with splinting or casting, but because the reduced knee is so unstable, it is difficult to keep the joint surfaces in proper apposition without internal fixation. Large Steinmann pins may be used to fixate the femur to the tibia, or early surgical repair of torn ligaments and joint capsule may be performed. Surgical repair maintains the reduction and may provide long-term stability after this devastating injury.

The trifurcation of the popliteal artery is tethered to the leg where the anterior tibial artery goes through a gap in the interosseus membrane. In anterior dislocations, stretching of the artery and vein is severe and often results in vascular injury. If the dislocation is not reduced and if the vascular supply is cut off for hours, reduction and restoration of vascular flow may be accompanied by the development of a compartment syndrome, a serious complication with often irreversible consequences (Plates 11–16). □

Fracture of Proximal Tibia Involving Articular Surface

Injury to Tibia

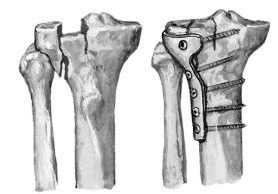

Split fracture of lateral tibial plateau.
Repair with long cancellous screws

Split fracture of lateral condyle plus depression of
tibial plateau. Repair by elevation of depressed
segment plus bone graft and buttress plate

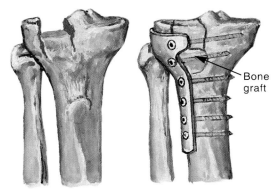
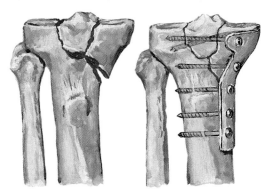

Depression of lateral tibial plateau without split
fracture. Repair by elevation of depressed segment
plus interposition of bone graft and buttress plate

Comminuted split fracture of medial tibial
plateau and tibial spine. Repair with
buttress plate

Bone
graft

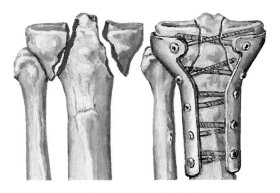
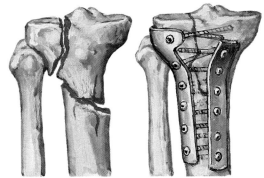

Bicondylar fracture involving both tibial plateaus
with widening. Repair with two buttress plates
and lag screws

Fracture of lateral tibial plateau with separation
of metaphyseal–diaphyseal junction. Repair with
buttress plate and anterior plate and screws

Fracture of Proximal Tibia Involving Articular Surface

Fractures of the proximal tibia that involve its articular surface at the knee are commonly referred to as fractures of the tibial plateau (Plate 105). The great majority of these fractures involve the lateral tibial plateau (condyle); isolated fractures of the medial tibial plateau and fractures of both tibial condyles occur less frequently. Fractures of both the tibial plateau and the shaft of the proximal tibia are rare injuries. Fractures of the lateral tibial plateau generally involve either cleavage of the plateau from the remaining portion of the articular surface or cleavage of the plateau with an associated depression of part of the injured plateau. Both types of fracture often require anatomic reduction of the fracture fragment to the intact portion of the articular surface.

In fractures in which the plateau has been cleaved from the remaining articular suface, stabilization can be achieved in healthy, firm bone with simple lag screws. In a depressed fracture associated with cleavage of the lateral tibial plateau, the depressed portion must be elevated to its proper position. When this articular fragment is elevated, a defect remains in the underlying cancellous bone of the tibial metaphysis. This defect must be filled with bone graft to support the fragment in its anatomic position and prevent its collapse. Fixation often involves use of a buttress plate to maintain the reduction of the split fracture of the plateau. Fractures of the medial tibial plateau often involve injury to either the tibial spine (intercondylar eminence) or the cruciate ligaments. These injuries may have associated stretching or tearing of the peroneal nerve. Peroneal nerve function must always be assessed before treatment of a displaced fracture of the medial tibial plateau.

As with many joint injuries, the joint surface must be restored, the fracture firmly stabilized, and joint motion resumed as early as possible. Plate 105 shows more complicated fractures of the proximal tibia, which require complex methods of fixation to maintain reduction and allow early joint motion.

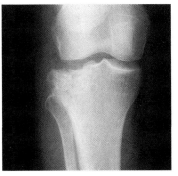
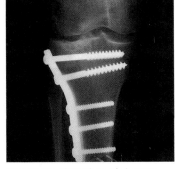

Split depression fracture of
lateral tibial plateau

Repair by elevation of depressed segment plus bone graft
and buttress plate

After surgery, the patient begins early active range-of-motion exercises, but weight bearing is delayed. When clinical and radiographic examinations demonstrate that healing is progressing normally, weight bearing can begin (usually within 10–12 weeks). If the internal fixation is not secure or the patient's bone quality is poor, internal fixation is often supplemented with a cast or functional brace, which allows early motion while providing support during healing.

Injury to Tibia
(Continued)

Fracture of Shaft of Tibia

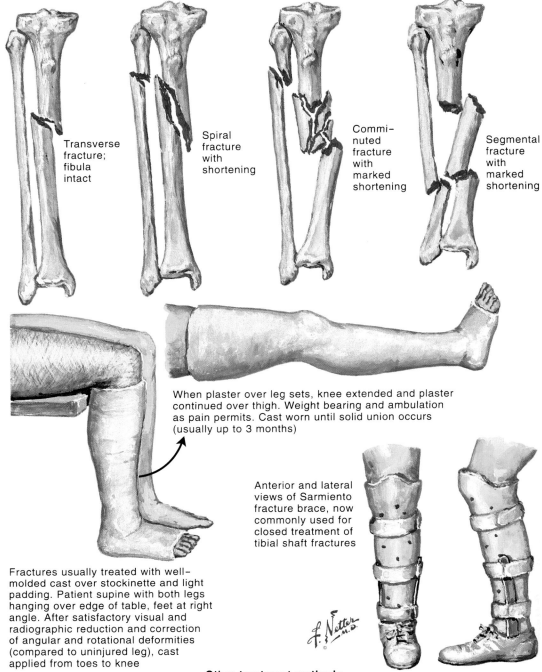

Transverse fracture; fibula intact

Spiral fracture with shortening

Comminuted fracture with marked shortening

Segmental fracture with marked shortening

When plaster over leg sets, knee extended and plaster continued over thigh. Weight bearing and ambulation as pain permits. Cast worn until solid union occurs (usually up to 3 months)

Anterior and lateral views of Sarmiento fracture brace, now commonly used for closed treatment of tibial shaft fractures

Fractures usually treated with well-molded cast over stockinette and light padding. Patient supine with both legs hanging over edge of table, feet at right angle. After satisfactory visual and radiographic reduction and correction of angular and rotational deformities (compared to uninjured leg), cast applied from toes to knee

Other treatment methods

Pins incorporated in plaster cast

External fixator device (used for open fractures to permit treatment of wound)

Intramedullary nail

Compression screws and plate

Fracture of Shaft of Tibia

Fractures of the tibial shaft are the most common fractures of a long bone (Plate 106). Because the tibia lies so close to the skin along the medial side of the leg, tibial shaft fractures are very often open injuries. Many fracture patterns are seen in the tibia. As the amount of energy causing the fracture increases, so does the complexity of the fracture. Unlike the femur, this bone is not enveloped by thick muscles, and abnormalities of healing such as delayed union, malunion, and nonunion occur more frequently.

Stable fractures of the tibial shaft (ie, fractures with little displacement and minimal comminution) are generally managed with the use of a long leg cast. When a long leg cast is used for definitive fracture treatment, it remains in place for 10 to 12 weeks. For successful treatment, the patient must be able to place weight on the injured limb to stimulate fracture healing.

Sarmiento applied the concept of early weight bearing to his development of a removable fracture brace. Treatment of a tibial shaft fracture with the Sarmiento fracture brace is preceded by placing the patient in a cast until the acute soft tissue reaction subsides. Then the fracture brace is fitted and worn until the fracture has healed sufficiently and supplementary support is no longer required.

Several other methods are used to treat tibial fractures. Treatment with pins and plaster and external fixators is generally reserved for more unstable and open tibial fractures. The external fixator allows visualization of the open fracture site while providing sufficient bone stability to allow care of the soft tissues without displacing the fracture.

Intramedullary nailing and plate fixation also have a place in the treatment of tibial fractures. These devices provide more stable internal fixation of the fracture fragments than does a cast or a functional brace. However, the risk of infection following internal fixation is increased. □

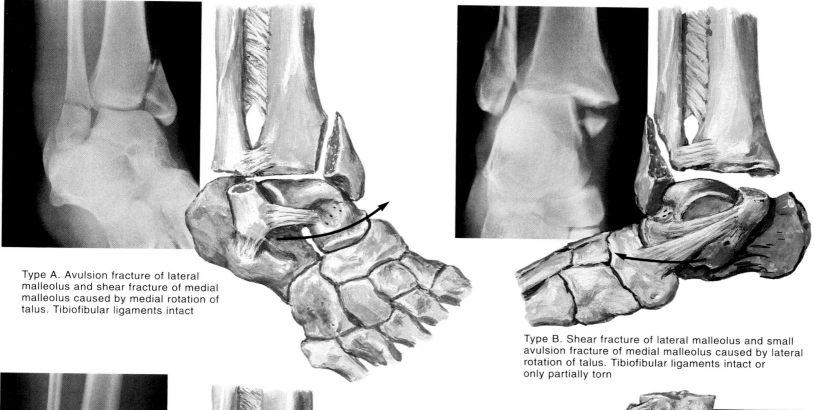

Type A. Avulsion fracture of lateral malleolus and shear fracture of medial malleolus caused by medial rotation of talus. Tibiofibular ligaments intact

Type B. Shear fracture of lateral malleolus and small avulsion fracture of medial malleolus caused by lateral rotation of talus. Tibiofibular ligaments intact or only partially torn

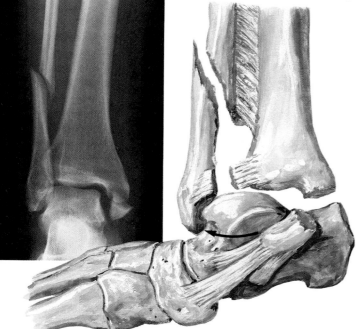

Maisonneuve fracture. Complete disruption of tibio-fibular syndesmosis with diastasis caused by external rotation of talus and transmission of force to proximal fibula, resulting in high fracture of fibula. Interosseous membrane torn longitudinally. Radiograph shows repair with long transverse screw. (These fractures easily missed on radiographs)

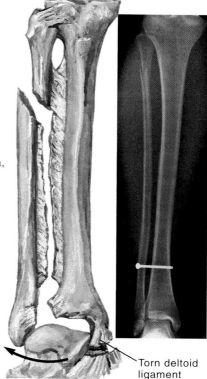

Type C. Disruption of tibiofibular ligaments with diastasis of syndesmosis caused by external rotation of talus. Force transmitted to fibula results in oblique fracture at higher level. In this case, avulsion of medial malleolus has also occurred

Torn deltoid ligament

SECTION I PLATE 107   Slide 4883

Injury to Ankle and Foot

Ankle fractures are common injuries, ranging in severity from simple, stable, nondisplaced avulsions of one malleolus to complex fracture dislocations of the joint with disruption of both malleoli and many of the supporting ligaments. A thorough understanding of the mechanisms of injury facilitates both diagnosis and treatment. Fractures of the ankle can be divided into two categories: fractures caused by rotational stresses on the talus in the ankle mortise and those caused by vertical compression of the joint.

Rotational Fracture of Ankle Mortise

The vast majority of ankle fractures are due to twisting injuries that cause the talus to rotate in the frontal plane. The talus impinges on one malleolus, causing it to fracture, and simultaneously produces tension in the ligaments of the opposite side, causing ligament disruption or avulsion fractures of that opposite malleolus. Rotational fractures are classified into three subcategories, types A, B, and C, which help the orthopedic surgeon to select the most effective means of reducing the fracture and to identify unstable fractures that require treatment with open reduction and internal fixation.

Type A Fracture. This fracture results from medial rotation of the talus in the ankle mortise (Plate 107). In the first stage of injury, the tip of the lateral malleolus or the entire lateral malleolus below the level of the tibial plafond may be avulsed. The combination of further medial rotation and displacement of the talus produces a shear fracture of the medial malleolus.

Repair of Fracture of Malleolus

Injury to Ankle and Foot
(Continued)

An isolated avulsion fracture of the tip of the lateral malleolus can be treated as an ankle sprain, with 3 to 4 weeks of immobilization in a cast, anticipating full healing and restoration of normal ankle function. Avulsion of the entire lateral malleolus can also be treated with cast immobilization if there is no significant displacement. When a lateral avulsion fracture is accompanied by a shear fracture of the medial malleolus and the fracture fragments are significantly displaced, reduction, usually combined with internal fixation of the fragments, is indicated (Plate 108).

Type B Fracture. In this type of injury, the talus rotates laterally in the ankle mortise, avulsing the deltoid ligament or all or part of the medial malleolus (Plate 107). With further lateral rotation, the talus impinges on the lateral malleolus, producing an oblique shear fracture at the level of the tibial plafond. As in type A fractures, a simple nondisplaced avulsion of a portion of the medial malleolus or an isolated tear of the deltoid ligament may be treated with cast immobilization. But when both malleoli are fractured and displaced, the fragments must be reduced to their anatomic positions. The reduction is usually maintained with internal fixation.

Type C Fracture. In both type A and type B fractures, the rotational force of the talus produces injuries of the malleoli below the level of the tibial plafond, and the interosseous membrane between the tibia and the fibula remains intact. In type C fractures, the line of injury extends proximally, disrupting part or all of the interosseous membrane and displacing the distal fibula away from its normal alignment with the tibia (Plate 107). This is the most common configuration of an unstable ankle fracture. The fibula fracture is often comminuted, and the deltoid ligament may be torn or the medial malleolus (all or part) avulsed. In addition, the posterior lip of the tibia (called the posterior malleolus) is often fractured by the pull of the posterior tibiofibular ligament as the fibula displaces laterally.

In type C fractures, the anterior tibiofibular ligament and the interosseous membrane between the tibia and the fragment of the distal fibula are also torn; these structures must be anatomically reduced to restore normal function of the ankle joint. Minimally displaced or nondisplaced type C fractures may sometimes be reduced with closed means and the reduction maintained in a long leg cast. The limb should be protected from weight bearing for at least 6 weeks; then the fracture is immobilized in a short leg walking cast for an additional 4 weeks. If anatomic reduction cannot be achieved and maintained with closed means, open reduction and internal fixation are indicated (Plate 108). The most critical step in surgical restoration of a displaced bimalleolar or trimalleolar fracture of the ankle is anatomic reduction of

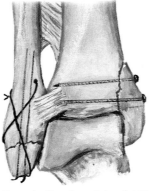

Type A. Small avulsion fracture of fibula fixated with Kirschner wires plus tension band wire; larger fracture of medial malleolus with two screws

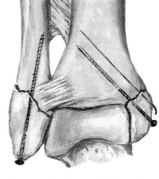

Larger fracture of lateral malleolus fixated with long, obliquely placed screw; small fracture of medial malleolus with Kirschner wire plus screw

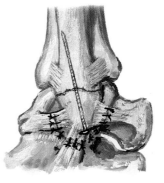

Torn lateral collateral ligament and joint capsule sutured

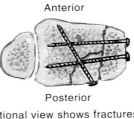

Anterior

Posterior

Sectional view shows fractures of medial malleolus and posteromedial tibia fixated with screws

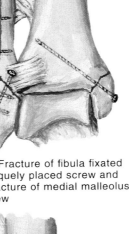

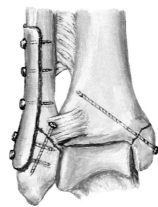

Type B. Fracture of fibula fixated with obliquely placed screw and plate; fracture of medial malleolus with screw

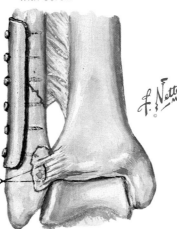

Type C. Fibula fixated with plate; small fracture of medial malleolus with Kirschner wires plus tension band wire. Tibiofibular ligaments sutured

Avulsion fracture of tibiofibular ligament fixated with wire through bone

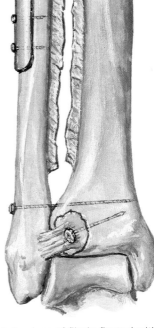

High fracture of fibula fixated with plate; avulsion of tibiofibular ligament with lag screw. Correction of diastasis with transfixion screw necessitated by extensive tear of interosseous membrane

the fibula fragments, which restores the fibula to its full length. The reduction is secured with a plate and screws. The medial malleolus fracture must also be anatomically reduced and fixated with a screw or tension band wire.

The Maisonneuve fracture is a variant of the type C fracture (Plate 107). The talus rotates laterally, usually producing an avulsion injury of the deltoid ligament. Lateral displacement of the fibula disrupts the entire interosseous membrane and causes a very high fracture of the fibula. Because patients may complain only of ankle pain and because radiographs of the ankle joint often appear normal, a fracture of the proximal fibula may be

overlooked. As in other type C fractures, disruption of the interosseous membrane makes this an unstable injury requiring restoration of the length of the fibula and fixation of the fibula to the tibia.

Vertical Compression Fracture of Ankle

Axial loading of the ankle, usually caused by a fall from a height, drives the talus upward into the articular surface of the tibia, producing a compression, or pilon, fracture (Plate 109). The ankle is usually dorsiflexed at the time of injury, and the anterior portion of the articular surface of the tibia is fractured with variable degrees of comminution. The injury causes compaction of

Vertical Compression Fracture of Ankle (Pilon Fracture)

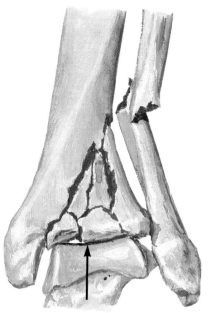

Usual cause is vertical loading of ankle joint, eg, falling from a height and landing on heel (usually with ankle dorsiflexed). Fracture and compression of articular surface of tibia plus separation of malleoli and fracture of fibula

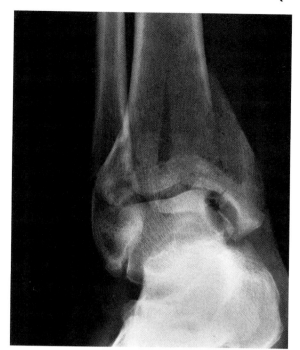

Oblique radiograph shows pilon fracture

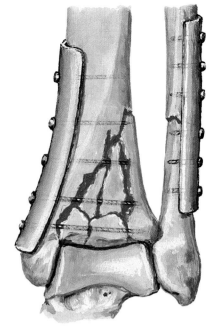

Fibula restored to correct length (determined from opposite limb) and fixed with ⅓ tubular plate. Articular surface of tibia reconstructed and stabilized with medial plate

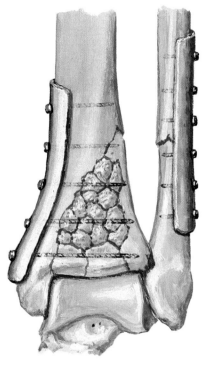

Residual bone defect filled with cancellous bone autograft from ilium

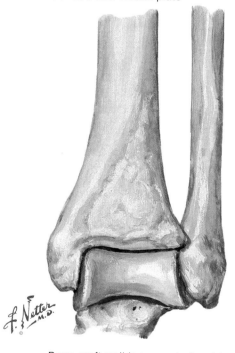

Bone graft well incorporated and fractures healed; plates removed about 1 year later. Good functional result

SECTION I PLATE 109   Slide 4885

Injury to Ankle and Foot
(*Continued*)

the cancellous (trabecular) bone of the tibial metaphysis, and the shaft of the fibula is usually fractured as well. Frequently, there is an associated fracture of the cortex of the distal tibia above the medial malleolus.

Displaced fractures require open reduction and internal fixation to restore the congruity of the articular surface of the tibia and the alignment of the malleoli. Surgical treatment of vertical compression fractures consists of four steps: (1) restoration of the correct length of the fibula, (2) reconstruction of the articular surface of the tibia, (3) stabilization of the medial aspect of the tibia with a plate and screws, and (4) grafting of the metaphysis of the tibia with autografts of cancellous bone. Rigid internal fixation and bone grafting of the fracture eliminate the need for immobilization in a cast and allow early active range of motion. The likelihood of full recovery is poor because of the extensive damage to the articular surface of the distal tibia.

Fracture of Talus

Osteochondral Fracture of Talar Dome. Fractures of the dome of the talus can occur alone or with rotational fractures of the ankle mortise (Plate 110). The fragment may be a small piece of articular cartilage of the talar dome (chondral fracture) or a larger fragment comprising both the articular surface and its underlying subchondral bone (osteochondral fracture).

The most common mechanism of injury is an inversion stress in which the lateral portion of the talus abuts the lateral malleolus, producing a shear fracture. Medial osteochondral fractures also occur, probably as a result of direct impaction of the dome of the talus against the articular surface of the tibia. A small chondral fragment devoid of bone is not visible on the routine radiograph but can be detected with magnetic resonance imaging (MRI).

Nondisplaced osteochondral fractures may heal with 6 weeks of immobilization in a cast. Displaced fracture fragments and most pure chondral fragments usually do not heal and may produce

persistent pain, swelling, catching, and locking when the patient resumes activity. If the fracture is treated soon after injury, small, displaced fragments of articular cartilage should be excised; large osteochondral fragments should be replaced in the fracture bed of the talar dome and securely fixated with pins or small screws. Loose fragments that cause persistent symptoms can be visualized and removed arthroscopically.

Fracture of Talar Neck. About one-third of talar fractures involve the talar neck and usually result from high-velocity injuries or falls from heights that cause excessive dorsiflexion of the foot. With hyperdorsiflexion, the neck of the talus

Injury to Ankle and Foot
(Continued)

fractures as it impinges against the anterior edge of the distal tibia. Further dorsiflexion leads to subluxation or dislocation of the subtalar joint. With more extreme upward force, the entire body of the talus may be extruded posteriorly out of the ankle mortise. Talar neck fractures are classified into three types: type I, nondisplaced; type II, fracture of the talar neck with subluxation or dislocation of the subtalar joint; and type III, fracture of the talar neck with dislocation of both the subtalar and tibiotalar joints.

Fracture of the talar neck often disrupts the blood supply to the body of the talus, most of which passes in retrograde fashion through the talar neck. Therefore, avascular necrosis of the body of the talus is a common complication (Plate 111). In addition, posttraumatic osteoarthritis of the subtalar joint or the tibiotalar joint is also a frequent consequence of this fracture. Avascular necrosis can be minimized with anatomic reduction of the talar neck fracture, which allows revascularization followed by creeping substitution and eventual remodeling of the body of the talus. However, during this process, which may take 2 years, the avascular talar body is susceptible to collapse, producing incongruity and subsequent arthritis of the tibiotalar joint.

Successful treatment of talar neck fractures requires prompt diagnosis and reduction of all displaced fractures and subtalar dislocations. Failure to achieve an anatomic reduction leads to persistent varus malunion of the talar neck, resulting in a varus deformity of the foot and a painful gait. The reduction is usually maintained with rigid internal fixation; open reduction and internal fixation also help prevent the later development of osteoarthritis. The talus must then be protected from weight-bearing stresses until the fracture and the talar body heal.

Fracture of Talar Processes. Fracture of either the lateral or the posterior process of the talus may be difficult to identify on radiographs, and many patients with symptoms of a simple ankle sprain may actually have sustained a fracture of a talar process (Plate 110). Failure to diagnose this fracture may lead to persistent pain and limitation of normal weight-bearing activities.

Fracture of the lateral process is best visualized radiographically on the ankle mortise view. The lateral process has two articular surfaces: one contributes a portion of the articulation with the calcaneus (subtalar joint), and the other articulates with the medial aspect of the distal fibula. Fractures that produce a large single fragment are best treated with early open reduction and internal fixation. Failure to achieve an anatomic reduction often leads to nonunion and persistent symptoms. Excision of the nonunited fragment or fragments relieves chronic pain.

Fracture of Talus

Osteochondral fracture of talar dome

If fragment small, it may be removed; if large, it should be pinned in good apposition to restore congruity of articular surface

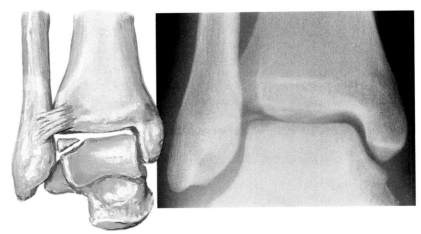

Fracture of talar neck

Usual cause is impact on anterior margin of tibia due to forceful dorsiflexion

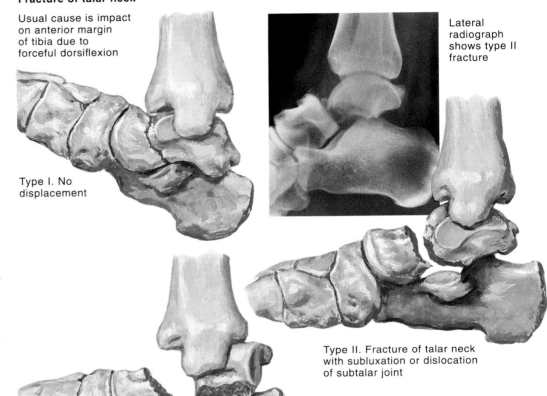

Lateral radiograph shows type II fracture

Type I. No displacement

Type II. Fracture of talar neck with subluxation or dislocation of subtalar joint

Type III. Fracture of talar neck with dislocation of subtalar and tibiotalar joints

Fracture of talar processes

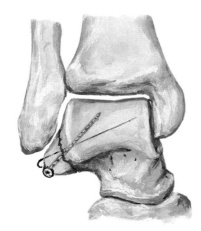

Large fracture of lateral process fixed with Kirschner wire and lag screw

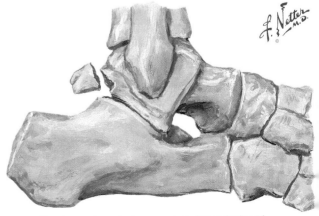

Fracture of posterior process. Irregularity of fracture line and comparison with other foot help differentiate it from congenital os trigonum

Injury to Ankle and Foot
(Continued)

Position of foot and x-ray beam for anteroposterior visualization of talar neck fracture

75°

Open repair of talar neck fracture. Anteromedial incision made with ankle in extension. Bone fragments apposed and aligned, and joints reduced. Compression screw inserted across fracture line. Alternatively, fracture fixed with two threaded pins

Intraoperative radiograph. Fixation of talar neck fracture with Kirschner wires

Anterior tibial a.

Perforating branch of peroneal a.

Anterior lateral malleolar a.

Posterior tibial a.

Dorsalis pedis a.

Anterior lateral tarsal a.

Artery of tarsal sinus

Deltoid a.

Artery of tarsal canal

Blood supply of talus. Because of profuse intraosseous anastomoses, avascular necrosis commonly occurs only when surrounding soft tissue is damaged, as in types II and III fractures of talar neck

Avascular necrosis of talar body evidenced by increased density (sclerosis) compared with other tarsal bones

Fracture of the posterior process of the talus is caused by extreme plantar flexion of the ankle, which compresses the process between the posterior lip of the tibia and the calcaneus. The os trigonum is an accessory ossicle of the foot found just behind the posterior process of the talus. On routine lateral radiographs of the foot, a fracture of the posterior process may be confused with this normally occurring accessory bone. The os trigonum is round or oval and variably sized. On radiographs, its edges appear smooth and there is a rim of dense cortical bone around its circumference. In contrast, a fragment from a posterior process fracture has a roughened and irregular surface with no dense cortical rim. Most of these fractures are nondisplaced; they can be treated with immobilization in a short leg cast and protected from weight bearing for 4 to 6 weeks. If the fracture fails to heal, the nonunited fragment should be excised.

Dislocation of Subtalar Joint and Talus

The term "subtalar dislocation" is used to describe the simultaneous dislocation of both the subtalar and the talonavicular joints (Plate 112). A medial subtalar dislocation typically results from a moderate inversion stress sustained in athletic activities that involve jumping, such as basketball. The calcaneus and the entire forefoot are rotated medially and fixated in a varus position, creating a significant deformity that has the appearance of a clubfoot. The lateral subtalar dislocation, which is less common, results in a valgus deformity of the foot, with the head of the talus prominent on the medial side.

The severe distortion of the foot that occurs with these injuries may compromise the blood supply to the forefoot. Therefore, prompt reduction is essential. Usually, reduction can be achieved with closed means, and once reduced, most subtalar dislocations are stable. Protection in a short leg, non-weight-bearing cast for 6 weeks allows healing of soft tissue and minimizes the risk of recurrent dislocation.

About 10% of medial subtalar dislocations and 20% of lateral subtalar dislocations cannot be reduced with closed manipulation. The failure of

closed reduction may be due to impaction of the articular surfaces of the talus and the navicular. A medial subtalar dislocation cannot be reduced if the head of the talus becomes trapped in the capsule of the talonavicular joint or the cruciate crural ligaments of the ankle. A lateral dislocation with entrapment of the talus by the tibialis posterior tendon around the talar neck also cannot be reduced. Open reduction is indicated to free the head of the talus from its entrapment in soft tissue. Once the reduction is achieved, it is stable and can be treated with immobilization in a cast. Long-term sequelae and recurrent dislocations are rare, but subtalar arthritis occasionally

develops, limiting joint motion. Total dislocation of the talus is rare but serious.

Extraarticular Fracture of Calcaneus

Fracture of Anterior Process. When the foot is adducted and plantar flexed, tension is placed on the bifurcate ligament, which originates at the anterior process of the calcaneus (Plate 113). This force can cause an avulsion fracture of the anterior process, producing fracture fragments that vary in size from a small chip to a very large piece extending into the calcaneocuboid joint. Significant displacement results in persistent joint incongruity and posttraumatic arthritis. Therefore, large

Dislocation of Subtalar Joint and Talus

Injury to Ankle and Foot
(Continued)

articular fragments should be reduced and pinned to restore joint congruity. Occasionally, small avulsion fractures of the anterior process fail to unite, causing persistent pain that usually responds to surgical excision of the small nonunited fragment.

Fracture of Tuberosity. The tuberosity of the calcaneus is the insertion site of the Achilles tendon. An avulsion fracture of the tuberosity may occur with forceful dorsiflexion of the foot or with a sudden contraction of the gastrocnemius and soleus muscles that exerts a powerful avulsive force on the Achilles tendon. Usually, the avulsion fracture of the tuberosity is a large, single fragment. A significantly displaced fragment must be surgically reduced and fixated to restore the functional length of the powerful Achilles tendon.

The medial process of the calcaneal tuberosity also fractures occasionally, usually as the result of a direct blow to the medial aspect of the heel. The fracture fragment is rarely displaced, and the injury heals well with 6 weeks of immobilization in a cast. Long-term sequelae are rare.

Fracture of Sustentaculum Tali. Jumping and landing on the heel with acute, severe inversion of the foot may produce an isolated fracture of the sustentaculum tali. Most of these fractures remain nondisplaced and heal well with immobilization in a cast for 6 weeks.

Fracture of Body of Calcaneus With No Involvement of Subtalar Joint. An axial load, such as jumping and landing on the heel, can drive the talus downward into the calcaneus, producing one or more fracture lines in the calcaneus body. Careful inspection of radiographs and CT scans reveals that the subtalar joint is not injured and that the fracture lines are posterior to the articular surface. Because the congruity of the subtalar joint is preserved, these fractures can be treated with closed means, and they generally heal well.

In the acute period, bed rest, elevation of the foot, and use of a compression dressing are indicated to reduce swelling. When the swelling subsides, a short leg cast is molded well around the limb, and the patient is allowed to ambulate using crutches with toe-touch weight bearing for 4 to 6 weeks. Alternatively, when the initial swelling has subsided, a compression dressing or stocking is applied, and the patient is encouraged to perform early active range-of-motion exercises for the subtalar joint to preserve function. Use of crutches for walking is mandatory until the fracture heals. Because the body of the calcaneus is composed of cancellous bone, these fractures heal rapidly.

Occasionally, these fractures cause excessive widening of the calcaneus; the increased width impinges on the peroneal tendons, leading to chronic peroneal tendonitis. If the heel is excessively widened, the medial and lateral walls of the

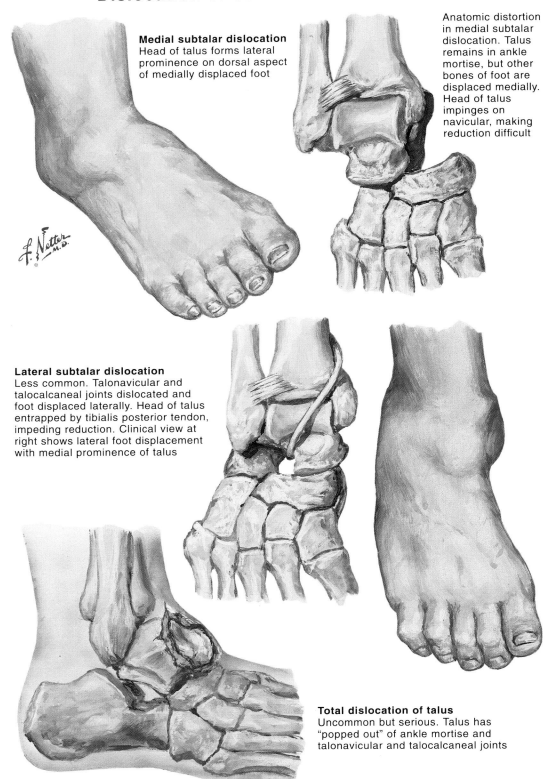

Medial subtalar dislocation
Head of talus forms lateral prominence on dorsal aspect of medially displaced foot

Anatomic distortion in medial subtalar dislocation. Talus remains in ankle mortise, but other bones of foot are displaced medially. Head of talus impinges on navicular, making reduction difficult

Lateral subtalar dislocation
Less common. Talonavicular and talocalcaneal joints dislocated and foot displaced laterally. Head of talus entrapped by tibialis posterior tendon, impeding reduction. Clinical view at right shows lateral foot displacement with medial prominence of talus

Total dislocation of talus
Uncommon but serious. Talus has "popped out" of ankle mortise and talonavicular and talocalcaneal joints

calcaneus can be compressed manually, with the patient under anesthesia.

In all extraarticular fractures of the calcaneus, preservation of the function of the subtalar joint is essential. Although the joint surface has not been damaged, severe swelling occurs, followed by scarring and contracture of soft tissue, which limit motion of the subtalar joint. Limitation of subtalar motion decreases the joint's shock-absorbing function in normal walking and running. Therefore, long periods of immobilization in a cast should be avoided, and the patient should begin active range-of-motion exercises for the subtalar joint as soon as symptoms allow.

Intraarticular Fracture of Calcaneus

Intraarticular fractures of the calcaneus make up 60% of all tarsal injuries and about 75% of all calcaneus fractures (Plate 114). In the usual mechanism of injury, the patient falls from a height and lands on the heel. The calcaneus is composed of cancellous bone that cannot withstand the impact. The talus is driven down into the calcaneus, producing an intraarticular fracture of the subtalar joint. Because associated fractures of the ankle, leg, or even lumbar spine are not uncommon, patients with fractures of the calcaneus must be examined for these associated injuries.

Extraarticular Fracture of Calcaneus

Injury to Ankle and Foot
(Continued)

The most common pattern of intraarticular fracture of the calcaneus has two fracture lines. The primary fracture line runs across the posterior facet of the subtalar joint, producing two large fragments, the anteromedial and the posterolateral. Often, one of two types of secondary fracture lines develops as well. If the secondary fracture line extends from the subtalar joint back through the tuberosity of the calcaneus, a tongue-type fracture is produced. In contrast, if the secondary fracture line extends from the subtalar joint to the dorsal surface of the tuberosity, a joint depression–type fracture results.

As the talus is further depressed into the body of the calcaneus, the fracture fragments rotate, producing incongruity of the posterior facet of the subtalar joint and distortion of the lateral profile of the calcaneus. The Böhler angle is used to measure the configuration of the calcaneus. This angle normally ranges between 25° and 40° and is determined by the intersection of a first line drawn through the anterior process and the highest point on the posterior facet of the calcaneus and a second line drawn parallel to the superior cortex of the tuberosity of the calcaneus. In displaced fractures, this angle decreases to 0° or even a negative number. Closed or open reduction should restore the Böhler angle to normal.

The subtalar joint is the shock absorber of gait. Without its normal function, walking on irregular or rough surfaces is difficult. Therefore, if the congruity of the joint is disrupted by a fracture of the calcaneus, it must be restored. However, because the calcaneus is composed of cancellous bone, reduction of the fracture fragments into their anatomic positions is often difficult. Occasionally, a displaced tongue-type fracture can be reduced using the Essex-Lopresti technique. A Steinmann pin is driven into the displaced tongue fragment, and the fragment is rotated back into an anatomic position; the Steinmann pin is then driven across the primary fracture line, holding the fragment of the tuberosity in the reduced position.

An alternative method of aligning the subtalar joint consists of open reduction and internal fixation. The fracture is usually approached from the lateral side, where both the tongue fragment and the joint depression fragment can be identified and rotated back into proper position. Sometimes, a medial incision is also necessary.

A second objective of open reduction and internal fixation is to restore the normal width of the heel. In most of these fractures, the heel is compressed and the walls of the calcaneus displaced outward, particularly on the lateral side. The displacement of fracture fragments can cause both persistent impingement on the peroneal tendons and chronic peroneal tendonitis. Therefore, at the time of open reduction and internal fixation, the

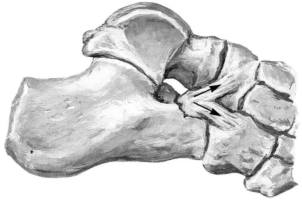

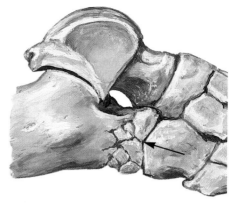

Avulsion fracture of anterior process of calcaneus caused by tension on bifurcate ligament

Comminuted fracture of anterior process of calcaneus due to compression by cuboid in forceful abduction of forefoot

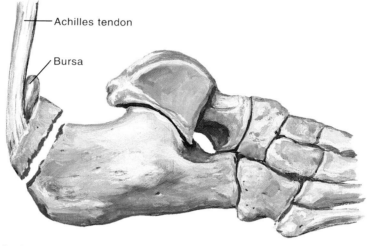

Achilles tendon

Bursa

Avulsion fracture of tuberosity of calcaneus due to sudden, violent contraction of Achilles tendon

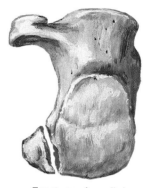

Fracture of medial process of tuberosity of calcaneus

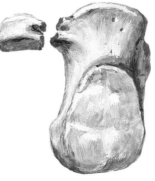

Fracture of sustentaculum tali

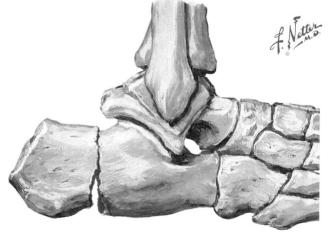

Fracture of body of calcaneus with no involvement of subtalar articulation

normal height of the heel should also be restored and the width of the tuberosity reduced to normal. Reduction often leaves a large osseous defect in the body of the calcaneus, which must be filled with bone graft. The fracture fragments should be maintained in place with screws or staples or both. Although open reduction and internal fixation of severely comminuted fractures can be difficult, every attempt must be made to restore the congruity of the subtalar joint, achieve stable internal fixation, and allow early active range of motion of the subtalar joint.

Long-term complications of intraarticular fractures of the calcaneus include the development of degenerative osteoarthritis of the subtalar or calcaneocuboid joint, painful bone spurs of the calcaneus, and persistent peroneal tendonitis. The pain of peroneal tendonitis can sometimes be relieved by excising the protruding lateral wall of the calcaneus to allow adequate gliding space for the peroneal tendons behind and beneath the lateral malleolus. Prominent bone spurs, particularly on the lateral aspect, can be removed to relieve local irritation. Isolated osteoarthritis of the subtalar joint is best treated with arthrodesis. If arthritis in the calcaneocuboid joint is also present, a triple arthrodesis of the subtalar, calcaneocuboid, and talonavicular joints is indicated.

Injury to Ankle and Foot

(Continued)

Injury to Midtarsal Joint Complex

The midtarsal joint complex, or Chopart joint, refers to the confluence of the talonavicular and calcaneocuboid joints (Plate 115). These two joints work together to allow supination and pronation of the midfoot as well as a moderate amount of dorsiflexion and plantar flexion.

An avulsion fracture of the navicular tuberosity can result from the powerful pull of the tibialis posterior tendon at its insertion on the tuberosity. This fracture is usually nondisplaced or minimally displaced and heals with simple immobilization in a cast. Substantial displacement requires surgical reduction and fixation to restore the important function of the tibialis posterior tendon.

The most common mechanism of injury in the midfoot region is a longitudinally applied force that produces either a compression fracture of the cuboid or a vertical fracture of the body of the navicular. Rarely, the entire midtarsal joint complex is dislocated, with the forefoot displaced plantarly. Such dislocations are commonly associated with avulsion fractures or compression fractures of the adjacent bones. Prompt reduction of any dislocation is essential because of the potential for compression or disruption of the vessels to the forefoot. Because many of these fractures are intraarticular, there is significant risk of late posttraumatic osteoarthritis if adequate reduction and fixation are not achieved soon after the injury. Persistent pain and swelling after healing may necessitate fusion to relieve symptoms in the arthritic joints.

Injury to Tarsometatarsal Joint Complex

The tarsometatarsal joint complex, or Lisfranc joint, is susceptible to injury by direct, indirect, and crushing forces (Plate 115). A great variety of injuries can occur, and only rarely is one of the five joints injured alone. Although relatively little motion normally occurs at the Lisfranc joint, dislocation or fracture dislocation often leads to posttraumatic osteoarthritis with significant and persistent pain.

Dislocations of the bases of the metatarsals typically result from an axial load applied to a foot in extreme plantar flexion. The base of the second metatarsal is recessed more proximally than the bases of the other four metatarsals. This configuration gives some stability to this joint complex and helps resist abduction and adduction forces. On the plantar aspect, a thick ligament complex ties the bases of the metatarsals together. Dorsally, however, the ligament complex is relatively weak, and most dislocations of the metatarsal bases occur dorsally. Direct crushing blows to the midfoot can injure the tarsometatarsal joint, usually fracturing the base of the second metatarsal and dislocating or subluxating one or all of the other tarsometatarsal joints.

Intraarticular Fracture of Calcaneus

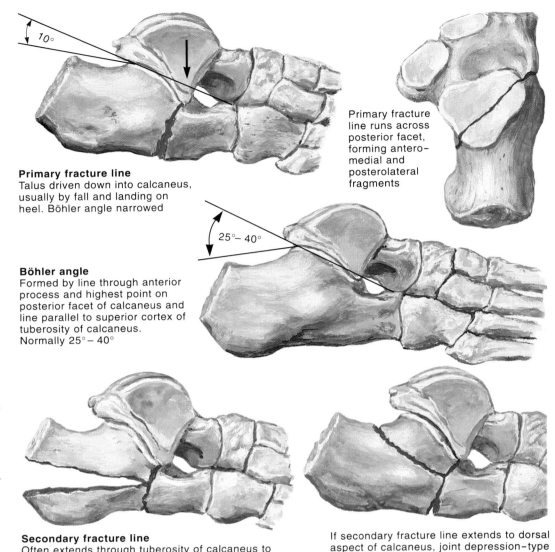

Primary fracture line
Talus driven down into calcaneus, usually by fall and landing on heel. Böhler angle narrowed

Primary fracture line runs across posterior facet, forming antero-medial and posterolateral fragments

Böhler angle
Formed by line through anterior process and highest point on posterior facet of calcaneus and line parallel to superior cortex of tuberosity of calcaneus. Normally 25°–40°

Secondary fracture line
Often extends through tuberosity of calcaneus to produce tongue–type fracture

If secondary fracture line extends to dorsal aspect of calcaneus, joint depression–type fracture results

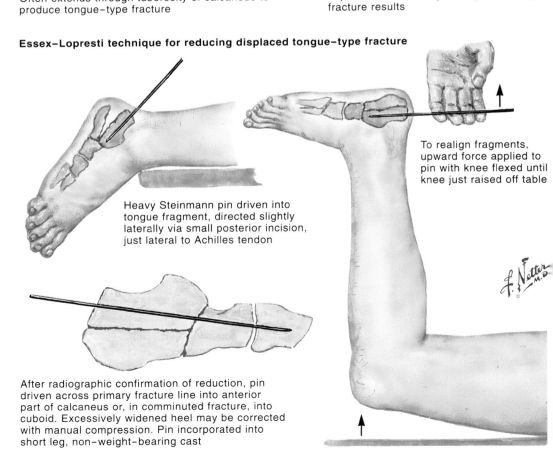

Essex–Lopresti technique for reducing displaced tongue–type fracture

Heavy Steinmann pin driven into tongue fragment, directed slightly laterally via small posterior incision, just lateral to Achilles tendon

To realign fragments, upward force applied to pin with knee flexed until knee just raised off table

After radiographic confirmation of reduction, pin driven across primary fracture line into anterior part of calcaneus or, in comminuted fracture, into cuboid. Excessively widened heel may be corrected with manual compression. Pin incorporated into short leg, non–weight–bearing cast

Injury to Ankle and Foot
(Continued)

A variety of classifications have been used to describe the injury patterns in the tarsometatarsal joint. One common system categorizes Lisfranc joint injuries into homolateral, isolated, and divergent dislocations. In the homolateral dislocation, all five metatarsals are displaced in the same direction, usually laterally. Fracture of the base of the second metatarsal usually occurs along with dislocation of the other four joints. In an isolated dislocation, one metatarsal (usually the first) is displaced from the others. In a divergent dislocation, the force of injury is applied between the first and second rays, resulting in medial displacement of the first metatarsal, fracture of the base of the second metatarsal, and lateral displacement of the four lateral metatarsals. In addition to these frontal plane deformities, the metatarsal bases are often displaced dorsally. Occasionally, the path of injury extends more proximally with dislocation or subluxation of an intercuneiform joint or an associated fracture of the cuboid or the navicular.

Tenderness, swelling, or any deformity in the region of the tarsometatarsal joint mandates a careful inspection of the radiographs to identify any degree of displacement in the frontal or sagittal plane. Because of the high incidence of posttraumatic osteoarthritis following injury to this joint, complex anatomic reduction is always essential. The keys to a satisfactory reduction are (1) perfect alignment of the medial edge of the base of the second metatarsal with the medial edge of the middle cuneiform, (2) alignment of the base of the fourth metatarsal with the medial articular surface of the cuboid, and (3) no significant residual dorsal displacement of the metatarsal bases.

Although adequate reduction can often be achieved with toe traction, the reduction is frequently unstable, with displacement recurring once traction is released. Treatment usually comprises closed reduction and percutaneous Kirschner wire fixation of the unstable metatarsals. The wires are kept in place for 6 weeks until the soft tissues and the fracture of the base of the second metatarsal heal. Sometimes, adequate closed reduction cannot be achieved because fragments of a comminuted fracture are interposed at the base of the second metatarsal. In this case, open reduction is necessary to remove the incarcerated fragments and allow reduction of the shaft of the second metatarsal. The alignment of the second metatarsal is the critical element in a satisfactory restoration of the entire joint complex.

Late posttraumatic osteoarthritis is a common complication of injuries of the Lisfranc joint. Persistent pain in this region is best treated with arthrodesis of the entire joint complex.

Injury to Midtarsal (Chopart) Joint Complex

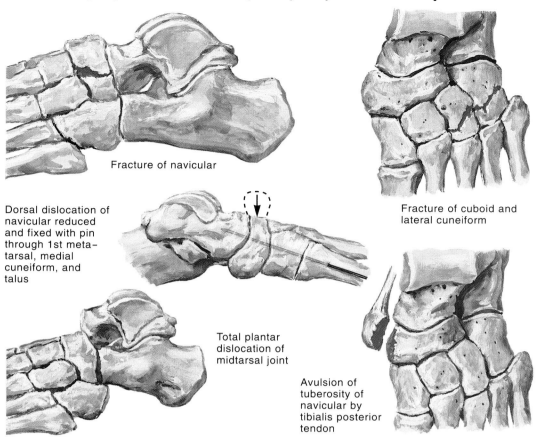

Fracture of navicular

Dorsal dislocation of navicular reduced and fixed with pin through 1st metatarsal, medial cuneiform, and talus

Fracture of cuboid and lateral cuneiform

Total plantar dislocation of midtarsal joint

Avulsion of tuberosity of navicular by tibialis posterior tendon

Injury to Tarsometatarsal (Lisfranc) Joint Complex

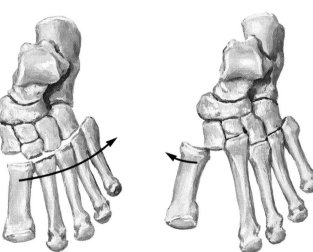

Homolateral dislocation. All five metatarsals displaced in same direction. Fracture of base of 2nd metatarsal

Isolated dislocation. One or two metatarsals displaced; others in normal position

Divergent dislocation. 1st metatarsal displaced medially, others superolaterally

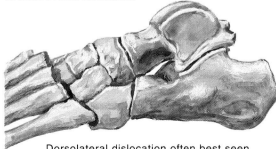

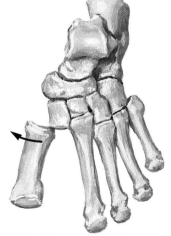

Dorsolateral dislocation often best seen in lateral view

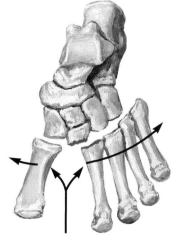

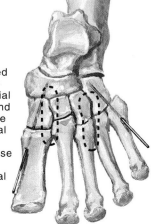

Tarsometatarsal dislocation reduced and fixed with two smooth pins. Medial edge of base of 2nd metatarsal must be aligned with medial edge of middle cuneiform, and base of 4th metatarsal aligned with medial edge of cuboid

Injury to Metatarsals and Phalanges

Injury to Ankle and Foot
(Continued)

Injury to Metatarsals and Phalanges

Fracture of Metatarsal Shaft. A direct blow to the forefoot is the usual cause of fractures of the metatarsal shaft (Plate 116). Fortunately, most of these fractures are not significantly displaced and therefore can be treated effectively with immobilization in a short leg walking cast for about 6 weeks.

If the fracture fragments are significantly displaced, the metatarsal head shifts dorsally or plantarly, disturbing its weight-bearing function. When the metatarsal head is significantly displaced plantarly, a painful callus develops under it, and if it is significantly displaced dorsally, excessive loads on the remaining metatarsal heads produce painful calluses under them. In these cases, a closed or open reduction of the fracture is needed to restore the proper position of the metatarsal head and preserve its weight-bearing function. Fractures of the metatarsal shaft heal rapidly, and with adequate reduction, long-term sequelae are not common.

Fracture of Base of Fifth Metatarsal. The most common fracture of the base of the fifth metatarsal is the simple avulsion fracture of a small fragment of bone. This fragment rarely displaces significantly, and the fracture usually heals well in 3 to 4 weeks with supportive casting.

A fracture of the proximal portion of the shaft of the fifth metatarsal is distinctly different from the avulsion fracture of the tuberosity. This injury, common in runners and high-performance athletes, is often believed to be a stress fracture. It does not heal rapidly and in many patients fails to heal, resulting in a persistently painful nonunion. The initial treatment consists of cast immobilization and avoidance of weight bearing for 6 weeks. If evidence of healing is not visible on the radiograph after 6 weeks, internal fixation with screws or bone grafting or both may be necessary.

Fracture of Sesamoid Bones. Direct trauma or repetitive stresses can fracture either of the two sesamoids underneath the head of the first metatarsal. This injury is most commonly seen in athletes and dancers, who apply repetitive stresses to the flexor tendon complex in which the sesamoid bones lie. The initial symptom is persistent pain over the area of the sesamoid, and radiographs reveal a fresh fracture or fragmentation of the sesamoid into several separate pieces.

Fractures of the sesamoid heal slowly, and healing requires the elimination of repetitive stresses, usually with use of a short leg cast and protective toe plate for 2 months or longer. Occasionally, the fragmented sesamoid does not heal, necessitating surgical excision to relieve the pain. Excision of the sesamoid is a last resort, however, as it may disrupt the critical function of the flexor tendons.

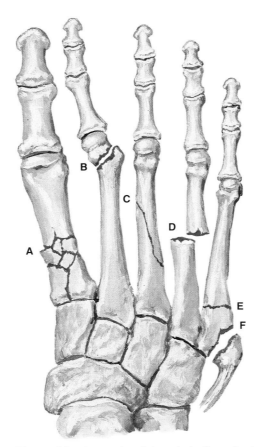

Types of fractures of metatarsal: A. Comminuted fracture. B. Displaced neck fracture. C. Oblique fracture. D. Displaced transverse fracture. E. Fracture of base of 5th metatarsal. F. Avulsion of tuberosity of 5th metatarsal

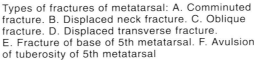

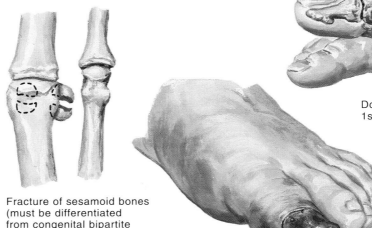

Fracture of sesamoid bones (must be differentiated from congenital bipartite sesamoid bones)

Crush injury of great toe

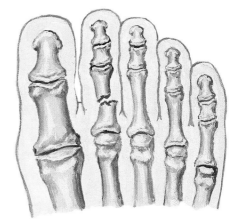

Fracture of proximal phalanx

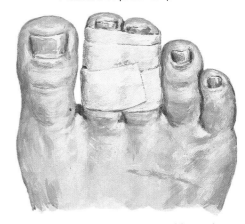

Fracture of phalanx splinted by taping to adjacent toe (buddy taping)

Dorsal dislocation of 1st metatarsophalangeal joint

Fracture of Toes. Toe fractures are common injuries, and most heal well without later complications. Initially, they are extremely painful and may be disabling for the first 3 to 4 weeks. Nondisplaced or minimally displaced toe fractures can usually be adequately treated with buddy taping. The patient should use analgesic medications, crutches, and supportive shoes until the pain subsides. Displaced fractures of the toes can be reduced with longitudinal traction. Since most reductions are stable, they can be maintained with buddy taping. Only rarely are fractures of the phalanges unstable and in need of fixation with percutaneous Kirschner wires.

Injury to First Metatarsophalangeal Joint. Sprain or frank dislocation of the first metatarsophalangeal joint is common, particularly in athletes and ballet dancers. Repeated hyperdorsiflexion of the first metatarsophalangeal joint eventually leads to disruption of the plantar capsule of the joint, causing persistent pain and preventing the patient from running or participating in athletic or dance activities. A frank dislocation or sprain requires splinting to allow the damaged plantar capsule to heal. With cast immobilization for about 4 weeks, the soft tissues heal satisfactorily and the patient can resume running, jumping, or dancing. □

Microsurgical Instrumentation for Replantation

Replantation

Replantation is defined as the reattachment of a completely severed part. The first successful replantation of an above-elbow amputation was reported in 1962 by Malt and McLehman. In 1965, Komatsu and Tamai reported the successful replantation of a thumb. The development of this type of microsurgery has been greatly aided by advances in optical instrumentation and especially in the manufacture of needles and sutures fine enough to repair vessels 1 mm in diameter (Plate 117).

Replantation is not suitable or possible for all patients with amputations. Great care must be given to the assessment of patients and their requirements. The surgical technique is exacting and the postoperative care prolonged and difficult. However, with an experienced team and a well-informed and motivated patient, the procedure can produce good functional and cosmetic results.

Amputations and replantations are categorized as major or minor. A major amputation involves muscle and is treated differently from a minor amputation, which involves tendons but no muscle. Because both types of amputation require great expertise and special surgical techniques, patients with amputations should be referred to centers where such resources are available.

Indications

The decision to undertake replantation of a severed part is influenced by many factors, especially the level and mechanism of the amputation and, equally important, the needs and desires of the patient. There are no hard-and-fast rules to help in this decision. The patient and the family must be fully informed about the possible outcomes and consequences of replantation in terms of hospitalization, postoperative care, and physical therapy.

In a child, replantation of any amputation should probably be attempted. In adults, replantation is indicated for amputation of the thumb, multiple digits, hand, distal forearm, or single digit distal to the insertion of the flexor digitorum superficialis tendon. Replantation should be considered whenever the amputated part is crucial to hand function or when good functional restoration of the part can be expected.

Contraindications

The only absolute contraindication to replantation is a health condition, either a preexisting illness or associated injuries, that precludes a prolonged surgical procedure. Treatment of other severe injuries, which often accompany a major amputation, obviously takes priority over the replantation effort. Relative contraindications are numerous and can be either patient related or injury related.

Systemic Illness. Diabetes, renal failure in a patient treated with dialysis, generalized vascular disorders of the upper limb, and advanced connective tissue disease all reduce the likelihood of a successful outcome because of associated microvascular damage and possible vessel thrombosis.

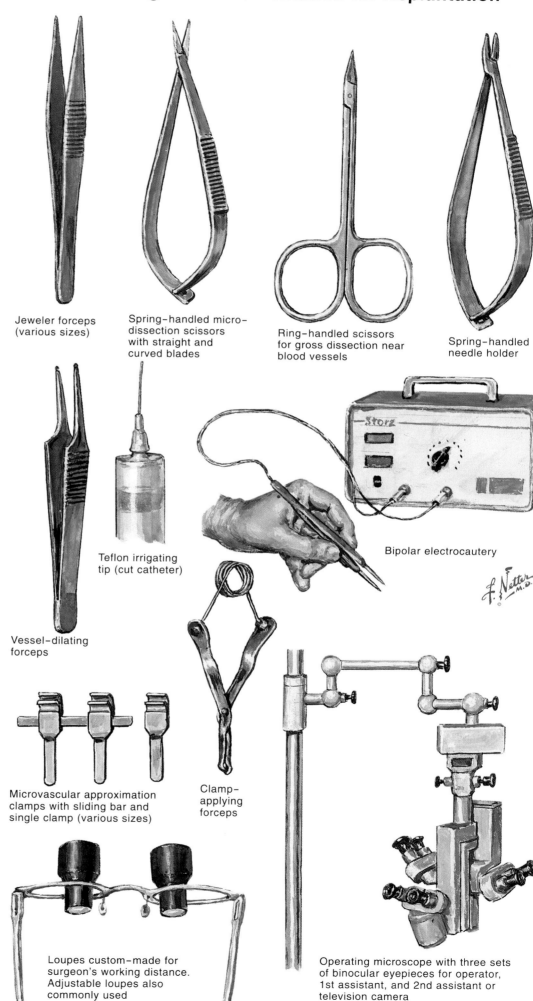

Jeweler forceps
(various sizes)

Spring–handled micro-
dissection scissors
with straight and
curved blades

Ring–handled scissors
for gross dissection near
blood vessels

Spring–handled
needle holder

Teflon irrigating
tip (cut catheter)

Bipolar electrocautery

Vessel–dilating
forceps

Microvascular approximation
clamps with sliding bar and
single clamp (various sizes)

Clamp–
applying
forceps

Loupes custom–made for
surgeon's working distance.
Adjustable loupes also
commonly used

Operating microscope with three sets
of binocular eyepieces for operator,
1st assistant, and 2nd assistant or
television camera

Debridement, Incisions, and Repair of Bone in Replantation of Digit

Replantation
(Continued)

Multiple Level Injury. Replantation is rarely successful when there is widespread vascular damage due to multiple level injury. If the injury is both above and below the elbow, however, every attempt should be made to save the elbow because the presence of the joint improves the function of a prosthesis.

Extreme Contamination. Replantation is contraindicated when both the stump and the amputated part have been inoculated with soil bacteria (particularly with *Clostridium* species). This degree of contamination is common in some farm injuries and in war injuries.

Age. The patient's age alone is not a contraindication to replantation, but it must be taken into account. Although the tiny size of infants' vessels reduces the chance that the replanted part will survive, the function gained by a successful replantation is often quite good. In elderly persons, useful or functional recovery is not a realistic expectation. Even in patients with mild degenerative joint disease, postoperative edema and the required postoperative splinting lead to stiffness in the whole hand. Therefore, replantation in an elderly patient must be carefully considered.

Amputation of Single Digit. Replantation of a finger amputated proximal to the insertion of the flexor digitorum superficialis tendon on the middle phalanx may be contraindicated because motion is limited by the severe scarring and tendon adhesions that develop after replantation. The index finger is not an essential finger; if the return of function or sensation after replantation is poor, the patient may prefer to use the normal adjacent middle finger for tasks usually accomplished with the index finger. A stiff little finger does not flex well in power grip, often catching in clothing. The benefits of replantation of either of these digits must therefore be carefully assessed.

Avulsion. The likelihood of successful replantation of digits or limbs torn from the body is poor because of the extent of injury and the amount of dissection needed to escape the zone of injury. A red line on the skin overlying the neurovascular bundle of a digit suggests an extensive avulsion of these structures and a poor chance of recovery. Ring avulsions are the most difficult avulsion injuries to replant. Even major vessel repair may not revascularize the devascularized flexor tendons and proximal interphalangeal joint, and although the finger may be successfully replanted, it often becomes stiff and atrophic. A revision amputation may be a better treatment choice, especially in the older patient.

Prolonged Ischemia. Either warm (32°C) or cold (5°–10°C) ischemia seriously reduces the likelihood of a successful replantation. Unfortunately, studies have not yet shown what duration of warm or cold ischemia is critical. Most amputated parts sustain some warm ischemia until medical help arrives. Once the replantation procedure begins, the part goes through a second period of warm

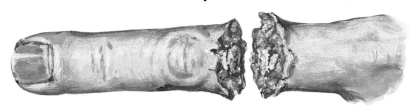

Digit traumatically amputated through proximal phalanx (before debridement)

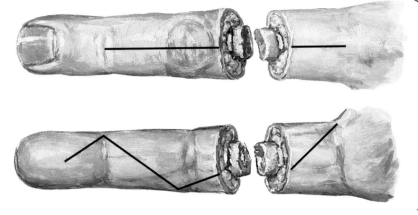

Debridement
Proximal and distal ends of amputation site cleaned and debrided, removing all nonviable tissue. Bone ends not yet shortened.
Incisions: longitudinal on dorsal surface, zigzag on volar surface

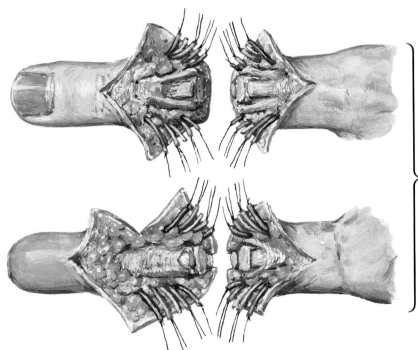

Trimming of bone
Bone ends trimmed, flaps reflected, and structures to be joined identified and marked with sutures (one for veins and nerves, two for arteries)

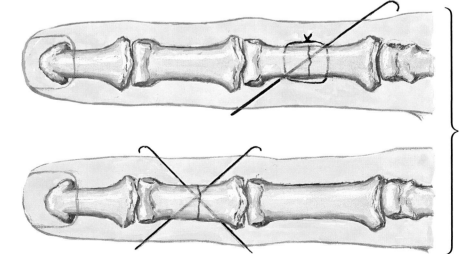

Repair of bone
Bone fixed with Kirschner wire inserted diagonally plus interosseous wire to prevent rotational displacement. Sometimes, crossed Kirschner wires preferred

Repair of Tendon

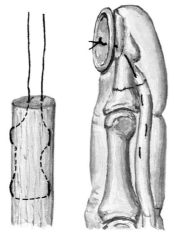

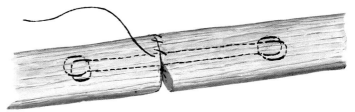

Replantation
(Continued)

ischemia until vascular continuity is restored. Cooling (cold ischemia) to about 10°C clearly helps to preserve the amputated part. Given adequate cooling, major replantations have been successfully performed 8 to 16 hours after amputation, and minor replantations have been successful even after 18 to 30 hours.

Amputation of Proximal Forearm. Replantation of the proximal forearm usually functions poorly because debridement of the dead and contused tissue often removes the neurovascular pedicles to the forearm musculature.

Preoperative Management

Treatment at the scene of the accident and at first medical contact strongly affects the outcome of later replantation. Improper handling of the amputated part or stump can seriously compromise the final result. The initial assessment of the patient's status must exclude any life-threatening injuries, particularly if a major amputation is involved. The patient must be hemodynamically stable before either transportation or replantation is attempted.

Once the patient's safety is ensured, the stump is cleaned of gross contamination and protected with a sterile compression bandage. Bleeding after amputation is rarely a problem because fully transected vessels usually contract. If bleeding persists, however, it should never be stopped with the blind application of a hemostat, as this may further damage the neurovascular structures. Elevation of the stump usually stops the bleeding. A tourniquet should not be used because unregulated pressure increases the risk of ischemia and vascular damage.

The severed part is cleaned of any gross contamination and foreign material and cooled to reduce its metabolic rate. A severed digit should be wrapped in moist gauze and placed in a watertight plastic bag, which is then immersed in ice water. The amputated part must not be allowed to come into direct contact with any ice, and dry ice should never be used. Properly cooled, a digit can be successfully replanted within 30 hours of amputation.

With a major amputation, preparation of the severed part is even more important. The amputated part is cleaned of all gross contamination, wrapped in a moist towel, and placed in a plastic bag. The part should be rapidly cooled to 10°C by immersing the plastic bag in ice water for 20 to 60 minutes. The part is then placed in an insulated container (but not in contact with the ice) and maintained at 10°C. Thus prepared, the amputated part is clearly labeled and rapidly transported to the replantation center.

Cold ischemia can preserve muscle up to 8 to 12 hours, after which irreversible changes may occur. Warm ischemia, which results from improper cooling, can lead to irreversible changes in as little as 4 to 6 hours, thus preventing successful replantation. Several attempts have been

For tears of flexor digitorum profundus tendon at distal phalanx, tendon advanced and reinserted using pullout wire through nail tied over button

Round or oval tendons repaired with 4 – 0 polyester Kessler core suture with knot in gap, followed by circumferential repair with running epitenon suture of 6 – 0 or 7 – 0 nylon

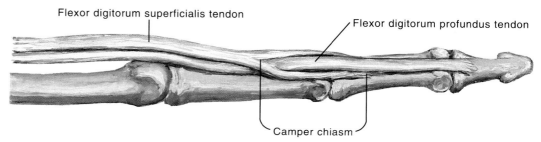

Flat tendons repaired with central core suture, followed by running epitenon suture

Flexor digitorum superficialis tendon

Flexor digitorum profundus tendon

Camper chiasm

Flexor digitorum superficialis tendon runs volar to flexor digitorum profundus tendon but splits over proximal phalanx to allow passage of flexor digitorum profundus tendon. Two slips of flexor digitorum superficialis tendon unite and interlace at insertion on middle phalanx dorsal to flexor digitorum profundus tendon. In injury involving zone of divided flexor digitorum superficialis tendon (Camper chiasm), one, two, or three tendon slips may be divided and require careful suturing

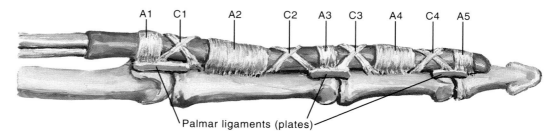

A1 C1   A2   C2   A3   C3   A4   C4   A5

Palmar ligaments (plates)

Flexor digitorum superficialis and profundus tendons are encased in synovial sheath bound to bones of digits by fibrous sheaths made up of alternating strong annular (A) and weaker cruciate (C) pulleys. When sheath must be opened to repair severed tendon, opening should be made in zones of cruciate pulleys because annular pulleys difficult to repair

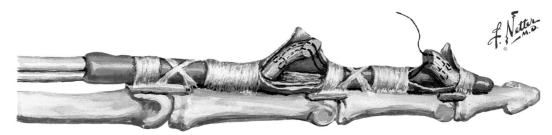

Pulley system must be preserved. If synovial sheath must be incised to repair flexor tendons, small funnel–shaped openings made in cruciate pulley area and subsequently meticulously repaired to prevent catching during gliding of tendons

Repair of Blood Vessels and Nerves

Replantation
(Continued)

made to reduce ischemia time by perfusing the amputated limb with various substances such as oxygenated fluorocarbon solutions. At present, the most reliable fluid appears to be autologous arterial blood mixed with heparin. Perfusion plus cooling may make major replantations possible as much as 12 to 16 hours following injury.

In the emergency room, tetanus prophylaxis and a broad-spectrum antibiotic are administered as soon as possible. A complete history is obtained and a physical examination carried out. Treatment options are thoroughly discussed with the patient and family. The decision to replant or to revise the amputation is based on the patient's wishes, age, health, and occupation; the type and level of the amputation; ischemia time; associated injuries; and the surgeon's experience.

Technique for Minor Replantation

Repair of Bone and Tendon. Ideally, every replantation center should have two surgical teams available at all times. Once the decision to undertake replantation is made, the severed part is taken to the operating room. While one team prepares the patient for surgery, the other team thoroughly debrides the amputated part, viewing it under magnification (Plate 118). All devitalized and heavily contaminated tissue is excised, including the smallest margin of skin compatible with adequate debridement, frayed tendon ends, and comminuted bone fragments. Frayed tendon ends are excised because the damage to the exposed tendon surfaces greatly increases the risk that adhesions will subsequently form and restrict motion.

Bone is trimmed to (1) remove avascular bone that could initiate the development of osteomyelitis; (2) provide flat, congruent surfaces for stable bone fixation; and (3) provide the necessary skeletal shortening to facilitate tension-free vessel anastomoses and nerve coaptations after debridement. At the digital or metacarpal level, the bone may be shortened about 1 cm. In the arm or forearm, the amount of bone shortening may be as much as 2 to 4 cm.

A severed part can be handled more easily while it is detached from the body. An interosseous wire or a Kirschner wire can be placed in the bone of the amputated part to facilitate later fixation. A tendon suture of the Kirchmayr type (modified Kessler) can also be inserted at this time. The distal arteries, veins, and nerves are identified and tagged with fine sutures. Skin incisions are usually needed to expose these structures. The volar aspect of the finger is usually opened with a Brunner zigzag incision. A straight midline incision is made on the dorsal aspect. Only full-thickness skin flaps are reflected; the subcutaneous tissue and veins are left intact for later dissection under microscopic visualization.

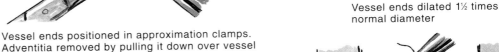

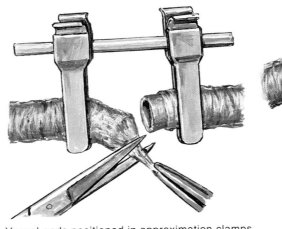

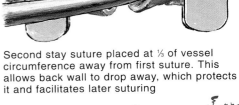

Blood cleared from vessel ends by jet of saline

Vessel ends dilated 1½ times normal diameter

Vessel ends positioned in approximation clamps. Adventitia removed by pulling it down over vessel end, cutting it, and letting it retract

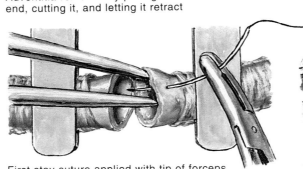

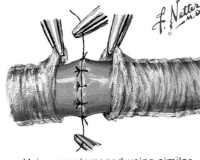

First stay suture applied with tip of forceps in lumen to protect back wall from needle and to provide counter pressure

Second stay suture placed at ⅓ of vessel circumference away from first suture. This allows back wall to drop away, which protects it and facilitates later suturing

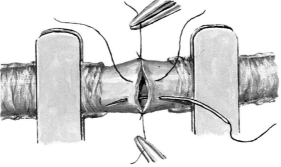

Gaps between stay sutures closed with interrupted sutures. Vessel turned over for suturing back wall. For large arteries, running suture may be used, carefully avoiding purse-stringing. In areas where clamp does not fit, back wall repaired first, with top of vessel and lumen in view at all times

Veins anastomosed using similar technique; because they are very fragile, veins must be handled with great care. Clamps may be used but very cautiously

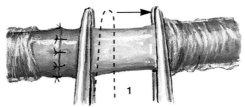

Test for patency and security of anastomosis. 1. Nontoothed jeweler forceps applied just downstream of suture line. Second forceps applied just distal to first and slid farther downstream to milk blood from intervening segment. 2. First forceps removed to allow flow of blood into empty segment; leaks noted

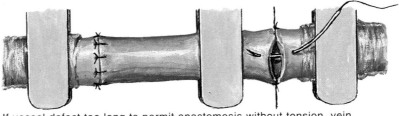

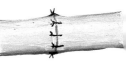

If vessel defect too long to permit anastomosis without tension, vein graft may be interposed. Graft harvested from dorsum of finger or volar aspect of wrist; for vein replantations in lower limb of structures larger than digit, graft obtained from saphenous vein

Since digital nerves contain only sensory fibers, they are repaired with simple sutures through epineurium only

Postoperative Dressing and Monitoring of Blood Flow

Replantation
(Continued)

While the amputated part is being prepared, the patient is transferred to the operating room and regional anesthesia is administered (preferably an axillary block). Regional anesthesia provides some sympathetic blockade and vasodilation as well as pain relief. The arm is cleaned with antiseptics, draped, and exsanguinated. The surgeon thoroughly debrides the stump, shortening the bone and tendon to permit easier anastomosis of vessels and coaptation of nerves. Use of a tourniquet facilitates the debridement. Once corresponding structures in the stump and the amputated part have been identified, replantation is begun. Because stability is essential for the vascular reconstruction, bone fixation is carried out first.

The technique of bone fixation should be appropriate for the type and level of amputation and provide stable fixation for early mobilization. Fixation devices include interosseous wires, Kirschner wires, and compression plates.

Replantation at the phalangeal level can be secured with interosseous wires with or without the added stability of a Kirschner wire; some surgeons prefer to use crossed Kirschner wires. Replantations at the joint level require a removable fixation device if the joint is to be preserved; otherwise, any standard technique for arthrodesis of small joints is suitable. At the metacarpal or more proximal level, a compression plate is preferred. If contamination is significant, however, an external fixator should be used to reduce the risk of infection. If possible, the periosteum is repaired to help bone healing and minimize adhesions to the flexor and extensor tendons. Kirchmayr (Kessler) sutures are used to repair flexor tendons, and interrupted figure-of-8 sutures are used for extensor tendons (Plate 119).

Repair of Blood Vessels and Nerves. After repair of bone and tendon, microvascular clamps are applied to the prepared arteries and veins, the tourniquet is released, and the blood flow is noted (Plate 120). This is the only way to assess arterial inflow. If arterial bleeding from the stump is not pulsatile after the arterial clamp is released, further resection of the artery is required to bypass the zone of injury. The distal artery and vein must be resected to remove all damaged tissue. Vein grafts are inserted to bridge the gap produced by the resection if the vessels cannot be anastomosed without tension. When used for repairing arteries, vein grafts are reversed so that valves do not impede the flow of blood. Repairing rather than resecting injured and compromised vessels to avoid use of vein grafts almost always ends in failure because thrombosis occurs almost immediately in these injured vessels.

The surgeon's preference dictates whether repair of the arterial or the venous system is carried out first. Generally, the arteries are repaired first to reduce ischemia time and to allow the surgeon to assess the adequacy of the venous debridement and determine which veins are best suited for repair.

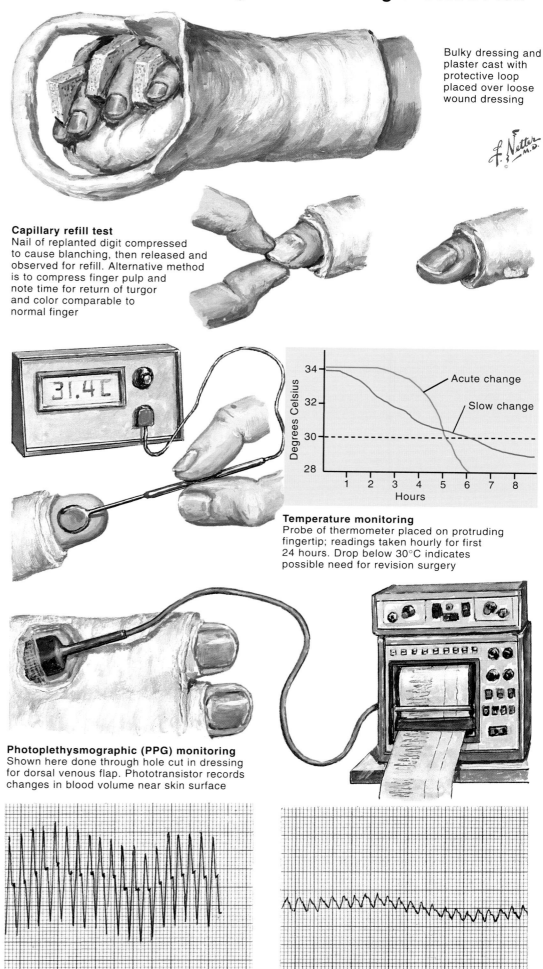

Bulky dressing and plaster cast with protective loop placed over loose wound dressing

Capillary refill test
Nail of replanted digit compressed to cause blanching, then released and observed for refill. Alternative method is to compress finger pulp and note time for return of turgor and color comparable to normal finger

31.4C

Temperature monitoring
Probe of thermometer placed on protruding fingertip; readings taken hourly for first 24 hours. Drop below 30°C indicates possible need for revision surgery

Acute change
Slow change

Photoplethysmographic (PPG) monitoring
Shown here done through hole cut in dressing for dorsal venous flap. Phototransistor records changes in blood volume near skin surface

Normal PPG tracing

Tracing shows occluded blood supply

Replantation
(Continued)

Ideally, both arteries and at least three veins are repaired in each digit.

Once the finger is revascularized, the nerves are repaired in standard fashion. Then the skin is loosely approximated to avoid constriction of the vasculature when postoperative edema develops. Skin grafts or flap coverage should be used if primary closure is not possible.

Replantation of multiple digits is carried out in a similar sequence. One finger is completed at a time, while the other fingers are kept cold. If all the fingers are replanted together (ie, bone fixation completed, then all tendons sutured, then blood vessels and nerves repaired), the prolonged duration of warm ischemia under the microscope lights may compromise the final result.

Postoperative Dressing. Following replantation of fingers, a bulky dressing is applied to splint and protect the finger and hand in a position that enhances mobility (Plate 121), taking into account the delicate nature of the surgical repairs. The ideal position for postoperative immobilization is with the metacarpophalangeal joints in 70° flexion, interphalangeal joints in neutral position, and thumb in maximal volar abduction. If this position is not possible, the alternative position used should come as close as possible to the ideal yet not stress or compress the vascular repairs. The dressing should be applied to allow easy visual inspection and temperature monitoring of the finger yet guard against excessive manipulation of the finger itself.

Technique for Major Replantation

The presence of ischemic muscle in the amputated part necessitates certain modifications in technique. Muscle is sensitive to ischemia, quickly building up high concentrations of extracellular potassium, lactic acid, and myoglobin, which can lead to life-threatening complications.

As with minor replantation, the severed part is prepared while the patient is being assessed. The devitalized tissue is excised, the neurovascular structures are identified and tagged, and the bone is shortened. Because forearm muscles receive the blood supply through the proximal half, any forearm muscle present in the severed distal forearm must be excised because it may not revascularize following major vessel repair. Similarly, amputations at the metacarpal level necessitate resection of the distal, avascular intrinsic muscles (Plate 122).

Traumatic amputations at or proximal to the forearm level are usually the result of very violent trauma, and the zone of injury is thus more extensive than in minor amputations (Plate 123). Consequently, more bone (2–4 cm) must be resected than for finger replantations. For amputations through the wrist joint, however, the smallest possible amount of bone should be resected to preserve either midcarpal or radiocarpal wrist motion. In wrist replantation, bone fixation is carried out with either interosseous or Kirschner

Replantation of Avulsed Thumb

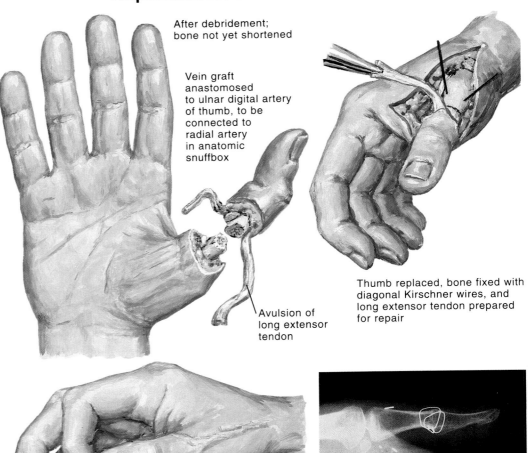

After debridement; bone not yet shortened

Vein graft anastomosed to ulnar digital artery of thumb, to be connected to radial artery in anatomic snuffbox

Avulsion of long extensor tendon

Thumb replaced, bone fixed with diagonal Kirschner wires, and long extensor tendon prepared for repair

Good functional result. Thumb readily opposes to index finger despite shortening

Postoperative radiograph. Arthrodesis of interphalangeal joint of thumb often indicated in such cases

Replantation of Midpalm

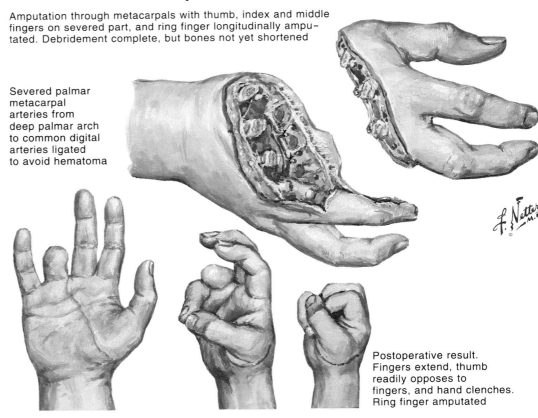

Amputation through metacarpals with thumb, index and middle fingers on severed part, and ring finger longitudinally amputated. Debridement complete, but bones not yet shortened

Severed palmar metacarpal arteries from deep palmar arch to common digital arteries ligated to avoid hematoma

Postoperative result. Fingers extend, thumb readily opposes to fingers, and hand clenches. Ring finger amputated

Replantation
(Continued)

wires to stabilize the residual carpus. As with minor replantations, much of the bone fixation in the amputated part can be performed while the patient is being assessed and prepared for surgery.

Once the patient is resuscitated, an axillary block is performed; with very proximal replantations, general anesthesia is often required. The stump is debrided and the bone shortened. If ischemia time is prolonged, a shunt is placed between the proximal and distal arteries and veins to perfuse the limb as soon as possible. The first venous effluent from the amputated limb must be discarded because it contains high levels of potassium, lactic acid, and myoglobin. The metabolic imbalance produced by these toxins is responsible for the acute tubular necrosis seen with myoglobinuria and for the occasional deaths associated with major replantation. To help prevent such metabolic imbalance, the patient must be kept well resuscitated and well hydrated to maintain a high urinary output.

Once vascular continuity is established, bone fixation is performed with compression plates or external fixation device. Muscles and tendons are repaired first, followed by arteries, veins, and nerves, using appropriate grafts as needed. Ideally, at least two veins are repaired for every arterial anastomosis. Skin closure is then attempted; if swelling or extensive debridement precludes primary skin closure, skin grafts or flaps are needed. If the total ischemia time is prolonged, fasciotomies of distal muscle compartments are usually performed. The fasciotomy wounds are covered with split-thickness skin grafts.

A loose, bulky dressing and a splint are applied. Positioning of the hand after major replantation is determined by the associated nerve injury. All amputations proximal to the wrist transect both the median and ulnar nerves, resulting in a potential claw deformity (intrinsic minus hand). Allowing the hand to contract in this manner compromises functional recovery, and the hand should therefore be placed in the safe, intrinsic plus position (ie, with the metacarpophalangeal joints in 70° flexion, interphalangeal joints in neutral position, and thumb in maximal volar abduction). The hand must be accessible for visual inspection and temperature monitoring in the postoperative period.

Special Techniques

Vein Graft. The need for vein grafts is so common in replantation that their use can often be anticipated. They can be harvested early, following the initial debridement. Vein grafts may be stored under refrigeration for later use if vascular thrombosis occurs in the postoperative period.

Vein grafts are obtained from many possible sites, depending on the size needed. For distal amputations, the grafts are most often taken from the volar aspect of the forearm just proximal to the wrist or from the medial aspect of the proximal forearm if nerve grafts are also needed. For replantation of a single finger, the best donor site

Replantation of Forearm

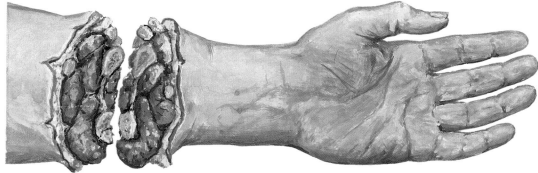

Amputated part and stump before debridement

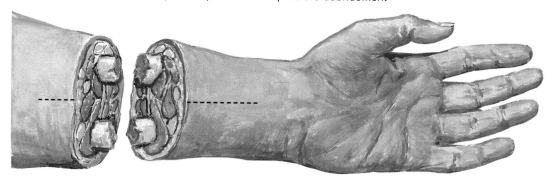

After debridement and clean resection; bones not yet shortened. Broken lines indicate longitudinal incisions

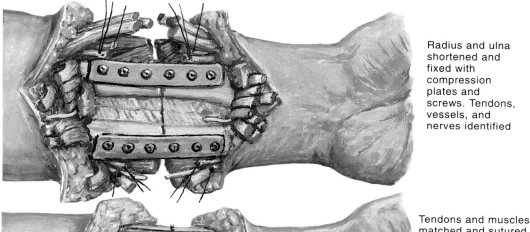

Radius and ulna shortened and fixed with compression plates and screws. Tendons, vessels, and nerves identified

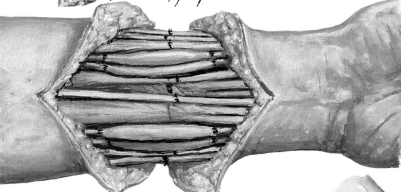

Tendons and muscles matched and sutured. Vessels and nerves also repaired. Note vein grafts attached to radial and ulnar arteries and veins, which were too short for direct anastomosis

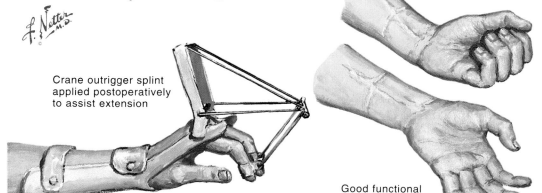

Crane outrigger splint applied postoperatively to assist extension

Good functional result

Replantation
(Continued)

is the dorsal aspect of an adjacent uninjured finger; for major replantations, the contralateral arm or the legs. Vein harvesting is best performed under tourniquet control, with care to ligate or clip side branches, avoid damage to the intima, and clearly mark the proximal and distal ends to ensure correct orientation of the graft. The graft must be inserted under adequate tension without twisting or kinking, which could lead to vascular occlusion. The orientation of the graft is reversed when used for the reconstruction of arteries.

Nerve Graft. Although required less often than vein grafts, nerve grafts are useful for one-stage reconstructions (Plate 123). The grafts are usually harvested from the medial or lateral antebrachial cutaneous nerves or from the sural nerve.

Skin Graft. Skin grafts are used when closure with available skin is not possible or would lead to vascular compromise. If possible, the vascular anastomoses should be covered with local flaps, and the intervening areas covered with split-thickness skin grafts taken from any appropriate area. A tie-over dressing may be used, with care taken to avoid pressure on underlying vessels.

Venous Flap. A common result after replantation of a digit is a dorsal skin defect with lack of venous drainage from the replanted part. This problem may be solved with the use of a flow-through venous flap harvested from an adjacent finger (Plate 124). The flap consists of full-thickness skin, subcutaneous tissue, and veins, much the same as the flap elevated for a cross-finger flap. The veins are harvested beyond the borders of the skin flap and used to reconstruct venous drainage from the amputated finger. The skin is kept alive by the venous flow through the flap.

Free Flap. After major replantation, the degree of trauma frequently necessitates extensive debridement that leaves a large soft tissue defect, exposing repairs of bone, tendon, and neurovascular structures. This soft tissue defect must be covered to prevent desiccation of the underlying structures, osteomyelitis, vascular thrombosis, and compromised function. The donor site of the flap is determined by the site and size of the defect. For amputations of the hand and distal forearm, a lateral arm flap from the same arm provides extensive skin and fascia and some bone on a single pedicle without sacrificing an artery. For injuries of the arm and upper forearm, suitable flaps can be taken from the latissimus dorsi muscle or the scapula. The lateral arm flap and the scapula flap provide good cutaneous coverage of limited size (Plates 124–125). A larger defect requires the bulk of a muscle such as the latissimus dorsi muscle, which can be taken as free flap, with or without overlying skin, or as a pedicle transfer (elevated and relocated without transecting its pedicle) for upper arm defects. The muscle can also be used as an innervated flap to replace a muscle group lost in the injury.

Venous Flap for Defect After Replantation of Thumb

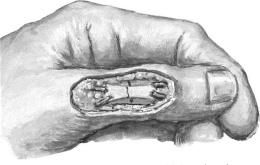
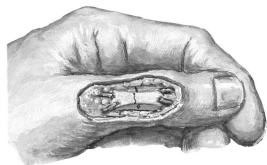

Flap of skin and subcutaneous tissue with veins extending proximally and distally removed from normal finger, using flat rubber template as guide

Defect after thumb replantation. Veins cleanly dissected for anastomosis to veins of flap

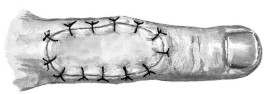

Undersurface of flap shows veins to be anastomosed. Veins normally extend beyond skin margin

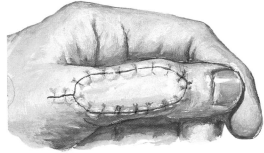

Donor site covered with split–thickness skin graft from forearm

Flap transferred to defect, veins anastomosed proximally and distally, and skin sutured

Free Vascularized Scapular Flap After Replantation of Forearm

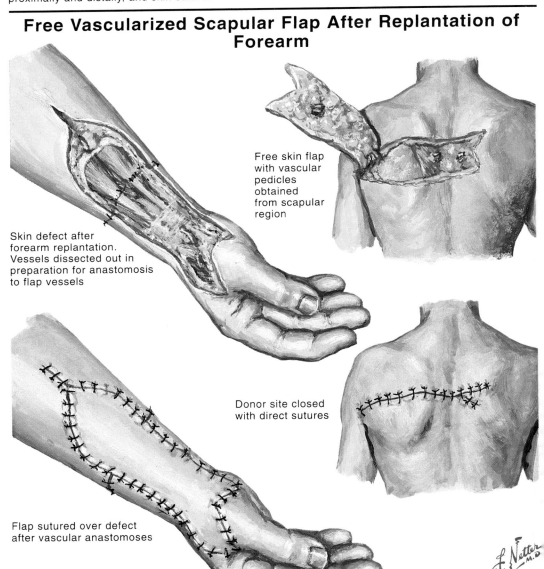

Skin defect after forearm replantation. Vessels dissected out in preparation for anastomosis to flap vessels

Free skin flap with vascular pedicles obtained from scapular region

Donor site closed with direct sutures

Flap sutured over defect after vascular anastomoses

Lateral Arm Flap for Defect of Thumb Web

Replantation
(Continued)

Occasionally, bone loss is so excessive that not enough of it is left for revascularization. The lost bone can be replaced with a vascularized bone graft from the humerus with a lateral arm flap, from the iliac crest with a groin flap, or from the fibula with a peroneal flap. The goal of this type of one-stage surgery is to repair or replace all damaged or lost tissues in one procedure. Before this major surgery is attempted, the relative risks and benefits must be assessed carefully. The risks of infection and vascular thrombosis resulting in loss of the flap or limb are high. When successful, however, this type of reconstruction yields rewarding benefits.

Postoperative Management

Early Management. Postoperative management of patients with either major or minor replantation must be carried out by an experienced staff. The initial management involves reducing the risk of vascular thrombosis and monitoring the replanted part to detect occlusion at the site of the anastomoses (Plate 121). Proper hydration of the patient, a warm environment, adequate analgesia, and a ban on smoking help prevent peripheral vasospasm and hypotension. Most patients are given aspirin, heparin, and low-molecular-weight dextran in single or combination doses; in some centers, prostaglandins and urokinase are also administered.

The monitoring of a replantation is best performed visually. Although a temperature probe, photoplethysmograph, or laser Doppler can play a useful role, clinical examination provides the most information. A finger that becomes pale and cool and loses tissue turgor has sustained an arterial occlusion, whereas venous occlusion in a finger is indicated by swelling, congestion, and bleeding dark blood on needle prick. A finger with venous occlusion is often warm until arterial compromise occurs; a digit with arterial occlusion may appear blue because of blood stasis but is not congested, as with venous occlusion.

Hourly temperature measurements are taken in the first 48 hours following surgery and then at increasing intervals until discharge. Temperature monitoring evaluates both the absolute temperature of the digit and its temperature relative to the adjacent normal digits. In general, a drop in absolute temperature to below 30°C or a sudden drop greater than 2.5°C suggests arterial occlusion. Venous occlusion is often evidenced by a slow decline in temperature and may be detected late.

Early vascular compromise, which may be due to poor surgical technique or inadequate resection of damaged vessels, requires surgical treatment. If vascular compromise is detected and the digit can be saved, the patient is returned to the operating room and surgical repairs are carried out.

The patient is observed for 5 to 7 days, after which smaller dressings are applied, a protective splint is added, and the patient is discharged.

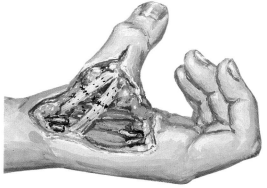

Defect after thumb replantation. Recipient vessels carefully dissected to receive flap vessels

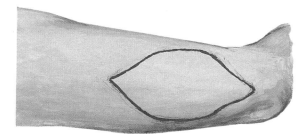

Skin flap marked on arm using template

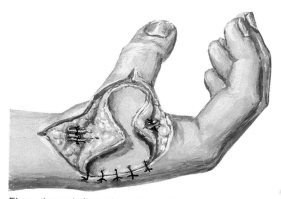

Flow–through flap placed in defect; vessels anastomosed proximally and distally to revascularize thumb

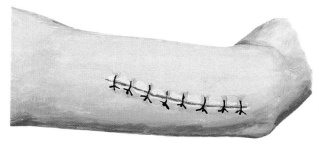

Repair of donor site with direct sutures

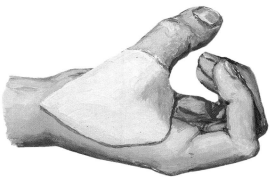

Template of flat, thin rubber fashioned to conform to defect

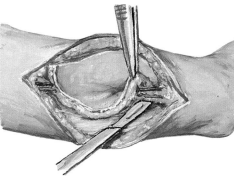

Flap with adequate subcutaneous tissue dissected free with vascular pedicles at both ends

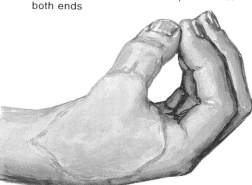

After healing, good cosmetic and functional results

Postoperative care of patients with major replantations includes additional monitoring to ensure good urinary output and avoid tubular necrosis. Because the risk of infection is higher in these patients, intravenous antibiotics are administered for a longer period, and the patient usually remains in the hospital for 10 to 14 days.

Late Management. Care after discharge from the hospital consists of regular physical therapy and use of splints and braces to maximize function and prevent contracture and stiffness in the uninvolved parts of the hand. Because cold intolerance is common, the hand must be protected from cold at all times. Passive mobilization is initially preferred because of injury to both the flexor and the extensor structures, with emphasis on protecting the thinner, flat extensor tendons.

After major amputations, hand splinting is essential while awaiting recovery of the nerves. A crane outrigger splint protects the extensor tendons until function of the intrinsic muscles returns (Plate 123). This device consists of a removable forearm-based splint that holds the thumb abducted and provides a dorsal block to metacarpophalangeal extension while allowing full finger flexion. Elastic bands attached to the crane outrigger provide assisted extension to the interphalangeal joints, thus protecting repairs to the extensor tendon

Transfer of Great Toe to Thumb

Replantation

(Continued)

while allowing mobilization of the fingers. The crane portion of the splint helps to minimize the force placed on the repaired flexor tendons.

Secondary Reconstruction

One-stage reconstruction (primary repair or grafting of all divided structures) is the preferred treatment because it avoids scarring from additional surgical procedures and because the patient can concentrate on rehabilitation following surgery. However, some procedures cannot be effectively completed at the time of replantation. Rarely, a replanted part is stiff, painful, useless, and ugly, and the patient may benefit from reamputation. Secondary reconstruction is much more common after major replantations than after minor replantations. The most common secondary procedures are bone grafting to treat a nonunion, soft tissue surgery to correct scar deformity at the amputation site, tenolysis to restore motion, and nerve grafting to improve sensation. Most often, however, patients require muscle and tendon transfers to restore function following poor recovery after nerve repair.

A toe-to-hand transfer is recommended when an additional digit would significantly improve hand function (Plate 126). Because the transplanted toe never functions as well as the original finger, patients must first appreciate the deficit created by the missing finger before they can accept the reconstructed digit.

Results

Results of replantation must be interpreted with great care and compared not to normal function but to function with the best prostheses. Replantations often survive, but the more important outcome—subsequent hand and limb function—is not well reported. For example, the person who cannot return to work because a replanted finger is stiff and painful has a much greater disability than someone who has a well-performed revision amputation and can return to work 4 weeks after surgery.

Generally, functional recovery is determined by nerve regeneration, which tends to be better in patients less than 35 years of age with more distal amputation sites. However, good recovery is often seen in young patients with more proximal amputations. Regarding nerve regeneration, different parts of the hand have different functional requirements. For example, the thumb and index finger require good sensation and stability, whereas the three ulnar digits require motion for power grip and are less involved in sensation. A comparison of functional assessments of replantations is difficult because patients' needs with respect to mobility and stability vary. However, most patients are satisfied with the replanted part and report that they would choose the procedure again. □

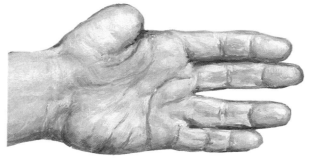

Hand with stump of previously amputated thumb

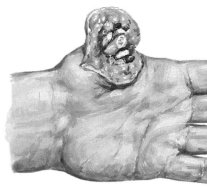

Incision, reflection of skin flap, and identification of structures

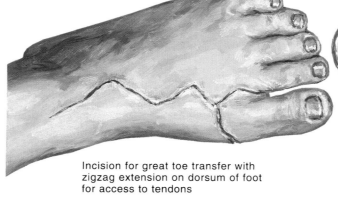

Incision for great toe transfer with zigzag extension on dorsum of foot for access to tendons

Amputated toe with tendons and neurovascular bundles left long

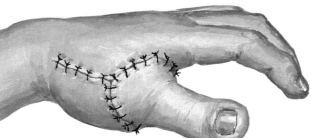

Great toe transplanted. Bone, tendons, vessels, and nerves united, and skin loosely closed. Skin graft not needed in this patient

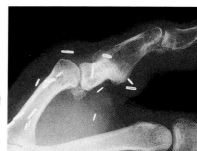

Postoperative radiograph

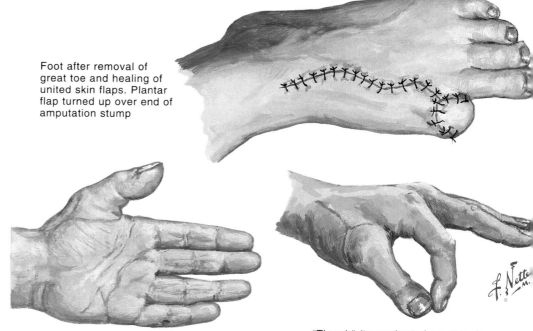

Foot after removal of great toe and healing of united skin flaps. Plantar flap turned up over end of amputation stump

Hand after healing; fingers in extension

"Thumb" (transplanted great toe) opposed to index finger

Fractures in Children

Fractures in children are particularly common because children are very active, frequently participating in high-energy activities (especially athletics), and because growing children are often awkward and clumsy. Therefore, a fracture should be suspected whenever a child injures a limb.

Children's bones differ from those of adults in several ways. The long bones in children contain at least one growth plate (physis), which is responsible for the growth in length of the limb as the child matures; damage to the growth plate can retard growth. Also, in comparison with adult bone, bones in children are relatively flexible and deform to a greater degree before fracturing. Although complete fractures can and do occur frequently, a bending or twisting force on a long bone often produces an incomplete fracture. Fractures also heal more quickly in children than in adults—fractures of the growth plate within 3 to 4 weeks and fractures of the shaft (diaphyseal fractures) within 6 weeks. The normal vigorous periosteal reaction in children produces abundant callus. Nonunion is rare.

Fractures in children, particularly those near a joint, often remodel, a phenomenon not seen in adults. Thus, many angular deformities straighten out as the child matures. Less remodeling occurs in fractures in the middle of the shaft and none in rotational deformities.

Because children's bones have this potential for rapid healing and remodeling, open reduction and internal fixation are rarely needed for fractures of the shaft. Surgery is usually reserved for significant intraarticular displacement, persistent malalignment of the growth plate, and gross and irreducible deformity.

In growing children, fractures in the shaft of a long bone may stimulate the nearby growth plate, producing a temporary overgrowth of the limb. Because this occurs most commonly in the femur, fractures of the shaft are often allowed to overlap and heal with a slight limb shortening to compensate for the anticipated overgrowth.

Incomplete Fracture

Incomplete fractures such as greenstick, bending, or torus fractures occur frequently in children (Plate 127). In the greenstick fracture, a bending force causes the bone to fail partially but not break completely. The cortex on the concave side remains intact, whereas on the convex side, the cortex fractures. The characteristic radiographic appearance is very similar to the breaking pattern of a green stick. The bending, or bowing, fracture, another incomplete diaphyseal fracture in children, is also caused by a bending force. There is plastic deformation of the bone as the bending force is applied. Microfractures occur in the cortex, but radiographs show no evidence of cortical disruption. Moderate bending of 10° to 15° may occur, often producing a significant clinical deformity. The torus, or buckle, fracture is due to compressive forces that cause the cortex to buckle.

Incomplete Fracture in Children

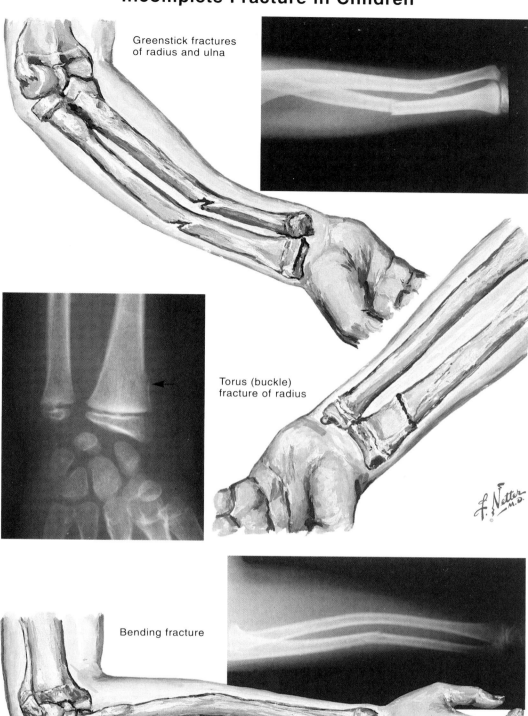

Greenstick fractures of radius and ulna

Torus (buckle) fracture of radius

Bending fracture

When a greenstick or bending fracture produces a significant deformity, closed reduction should be carried out to restore proper limb alignment. The greenstick fracture is usually easy to reduce; the bending fracture, however, may require considerable force to restore the bent bone to its normal alignment. Torus fractures are stable and usually nondisplaced. They do not require reduction because they rarely produce significant deformity. Once reduced, incomplete fractures require immobilization in a plaster cast to maintain alignment until fracture healing occurs. Torus fractures heal in about 3 weeks, whereas greenstick and bending fractures take 6 to 8 weeks.

Injury to Growth Plate

The cartilaginous growth plate (physis) in the bones of children is very susceptible to injury because it is weaker than the adjacent bone. Growth plate injuries are classified into six types according to the modified Salter-Harris classification (Plate 128). This classification aids in the choice of reduction methods and provides a rough prognosis for the injury. Although injuries to the growth plate usually heal fairly rapidly, all should be followed for at least 1 year to ensure that shortening or angular deformities do not develop and that the growth plate continues to function normally.

Fractures in Children

(Continued)

Type I Injury. In this fracture pattern, the epiphysis is separated from the shaft of the bone through the growth plate. This cartilaginous injury is most commonly seen in the newborn or the very young child. The periosteum surrounding the growth plate is usually disrupted but occasionally remains intact. The epiphysis may not yet be calcified, and thus the fracture and displacement may not be detected on radiographs.

Type II Injury. Ninety percent of growth plate fractures are Salter-Harris type II. The fracture passes across the growth plate but then extends into the metaphyseal bone, creating a small triangular fragment of metaphysis that displaces with the epiphyseal fragment. Usually, the periosteum on the side adjacent to the metaphyseal fragment remains intact and can be used as a hinge to facilitate reduction of displaced fractures. With adequate reduction and immobilization for 3 to 4 weeks, virtually all type I and type II fractures heal satisfactorily. The proliferating cells that produce longitudinal growth of the limb are usually not damaged.

Type III Injury. The uncommon type III injury is an intraarticular fracture that originates on the articular surface, extends through the epiphysis, and then passes across the growth plate and out to the periphery of the bone. Open reduction and internal fixation are often needed to restore joint congruity. Failure to restore normal joint alignment leads to persistent incongruity, predisposing to later development of osteoarthritis.

Type IV Injury. This fracture is usually caused by an axial load or a shear stress in which the fracture line originates on the articular surface and extends directly across the growth plate into the metaphysis. Because of the high risk of complications from malunion, open reduction and internal fixation are nearly always indicated. It is most important to achieve alignment of the growth plate; otherwise, a bone bridge may develop across the growth plate, preventing further longitudinal growth of that segment of the bone.

Type V Injury. Forced abduction or adduction of the limb or application of an axial load to the limb may produce severe compression of the growth plate, disrupting its architecture and destroying its ability to produce longitudinal limb growth. Type V fractures are rarely displaced and are thus very difficult to diagnose on initial radiographs. If the entire growth plate is damaged, growth ceases at this site. If only a portion of the growth plate is damaged, growth stops in that

Injury to Growth Plate (Salter–Harris Classification, Rang Modification)

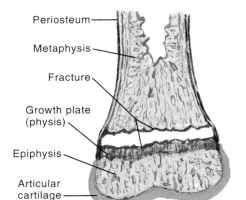

Periosteum
Metaphysis
Fracture
Growth plate (physis)
Epiphysis
Articular cartilage

Type I. Complete separation of epiphysis from shaft through calcified cartilage (growth zone) of growth plate. No bone actually fractured; periosteum may remain intact. Most common in newborns and young children

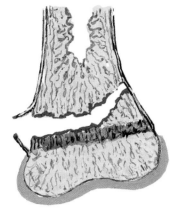

Type II. Most common. Line of separation extends partially across deep layer of growth plate and extends through metaphysis, leaving triangular portion of metaphysis attached to epiphyseal fragment

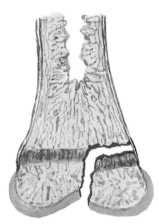

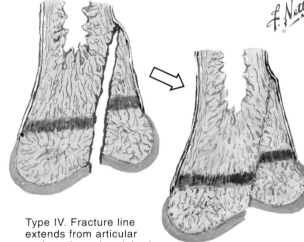

Type III. Uncommon. Intra-articular fracture through epiphysis, across deep zone of growth plate to periphery. Open reduction and fixation often necessary

Type IV. Fracture line extends from articular surface through epiphysis, growth plate, and metaphysis. If fractured segment not perfectly realigned with open reduction, osseous bridge across growth plate may occur, resulting in partial growth arrest and joint angulation

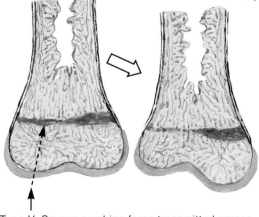

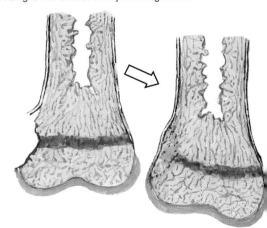

Type V. Severe crushing force transmitted across epiphysis to portion of growth plate by abduction or adduction stress or axial load. Minimal or no displacement makes radiographic diagnosis difficult; growth plate may nevertheless be damaged, resulting in partial growth arrest or shortening and angular deformity

Type VI. Portion of growth plate sheared or cut off. Raw surface heals by forming bone bridge across growth plate, limiting growth on injured side and resulting in angular deformity

portion but continues in the remainder of the growth plate, resulting in an angular deformity.

Type VI Injury. In the type VI fracture pattern, identified by Rang, a portion of the growth plate is sheared off or cut off as a result of a direct

blow or a skiving injury. New bone forms to heal the raw surface, creating a bridge across the growth plate, which inhibits further growth in that area. The asymmetric growth arrest may produce an angular deformity.

Fractures in Children
(Continued)

Fracture of Clavicle and Humerus

Fracture of Clavicle. One of the most common injuries in childhood, a clavicle fracture usually results from a fall on the outstretched hand, when the force of impact is transmitted through the limb up to the clavicle (Plate 129). Young children with a fracture of the clavicle hold the entire upper limb protectively at their side. Clavicle fractures are rarely open injuries, although the fragments may tent the skin over the shoulder region. The subclavian vessels and brachial plexus lie just beneath the clavicle but are rarely injured. Nevertheless, a careful examination to identify any injury must be carried out. During treatment of the fracture, care must be taken to ensure that these structures are not injured and that they continue to function properly.

The clavicle often breaks in a greenstick pattern, but occasionally, the fracture is complete, with overriding fracture fragments. Both types of fracture are treated with a figure-of-8 bandage, which holds both shoulders in abduction to maintain the length of the clavicle and the alignment of the fracture fragments. Moderate, persistent overriding of the fracture fragments is acceptable. Stability of the fracture occurs in 3 to 4 weeks, and the fracture virtually always heals without long-term residual problems. Abundant callus forms around the fracture, frequently producing a bump that may persist for some time. With growth, remodeling eliminates most of the deformity, particularly in young children.

Fracture of Proximal Humerus. Fractures of the growth plate of the proximal humerus occur in children of all ages. In newborns, fractures are usually Salter-Harris type I injuries, whereas in older children, they are almost invariably Salter-Harris type II (Plate 128). If the fracture is complete, the strong pull on the fracture fragments by the large muscles of the shoulder often produces angulation and displacement.

Severely displaced fractures can be reduced with closed manipulation, but anatomic reduction is often difficult to maintain. Because of the proximity of this fracture to the shoulder joint, which is a universal joint, some angulation (as much as 45°) and displacement are acceptable because remodeling usually reverses any persistent angular deformity. Once an acceptable reduction has been achieved, most of these fractures can be immobilized with a modified Velpeau bandage made of stockinette. Open reduction and pin fixation are reserved for severely angulated or grossly displaced fractures.

Fracture of Shaft of Humerus. Fractures of the humeral shaft are rare in children and are less likely to remodel than fractures of the proximal humerus. It is therefore important to achieve good

Fracture of Clavicle in Children

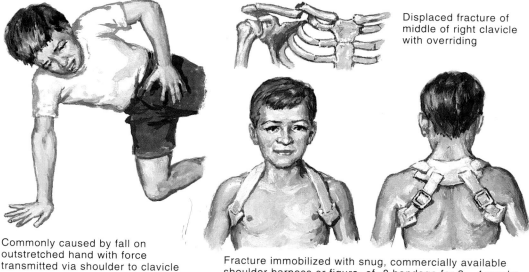

Commonly caused by fall on outstretched hand with force transmitted via shoulder to clavicle

Displaced fracture of middle of right clavicle with overriding

Fracture immobilized with snug, commercially available shoulder harness or figure-of-8 bandage for 3 – 4 weeks

Fracture of Proximal Humerus in Children

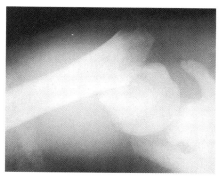
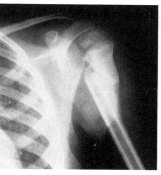
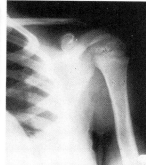

Displaced fracture of proximal humerus

Persistent malalignment despite reduction by traction and manipulation

Remodeling over months resulted in relatively normal alignment and full shoulder joint motion

After reduction by manual traction and manipulation, fracture treated with modified Velpeau bandage made of stockinette

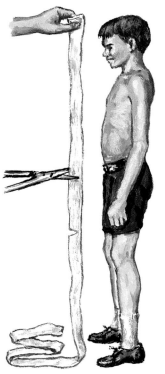
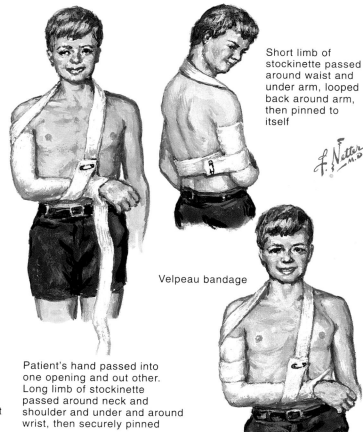

Short limb of stockinette passed around waist and under arm, looped back around arm, then pinned to itself

Velpeau bandage

Stockinette segment ⅓ longer than patient's height. Two openings ⅓ diameter of stockinette cut at about ⅓ length of stockinette

Patient's hand passed into one opening and out other. Long limb of stockinette passed around neck and shoulder and under and around wrist, then securely pinned

Supracondylar Fracture of Humerus in Children

Fractures in Children

(Continued)

alignment and to eliminate any rotational deformity with closed reduction. As with a fracture of the humeral shaft in adults, reduction must be gentle to minimize the risk of entrapment of the radial nerve in the fracture site. In most instances, closed reduction can be maintained with a sugar tong splint (Plate 40).

Supracondylar Fracture of Humerus

A supracondylar fracture of the humerus is one of the most dangerous fractures in childhood, occurring most commonly in the latter part of the first decade. It usually results from a fall on the outstretched hand (Plate 130).

The fracture line extends transversely across the distal humerus just proximal to the epicondyles. In 95% of supracondylar fractures, the humeral shaft fragment is displaced anteriorly, and the distal fragment is both angulated and displaced posteriorly; this fracture pattern is called an extension-type injury because it occurs with the limb outstretched. With significant displacement, the sharp spike of the proximal fragment displaces anteriorly, impinging on the critical neurovascular structures at the elbow, particularly the median nerve and brachial artery. As a result, displaced fractures are associated with a risk of neurovascular injury, with a 7% incidence of nerve injuries. Occasionally, the brachial artery is impaled by a bone spike; more commonly, severe swelling often accompanies this injury, causing vascular compression. Thus, there is a significant risk of ischemia of the limb distal to the fracture, necessitating prompt reduction and secure stabilization of the fracture. Vascular decompression or repair or both are sometimes needed.

The first focus of management is on reduction of the displaced fracture fragments to alleviate any nerve or vessel compression. This reduction must be accomplished promptly and with the patient under general anesthesia. Longitudinal traction applied to the distal fragment combined with manipulation usually results in a satisfactory reduction, but maintaining an adequate reduction is often difficult. After reduction, extension-type supracondylar fractures remain stable only with the elbow flexed greater than 90°. However, flexion of the elbow to this extent often compresses the vessels in the antecubital fossa, obliterating the radial pulse and jeopardizing the circulation to the distal limb.

When the fracture is satisfactorily aligned with closed reduction and the radial pulse can be maintained with the elbow flexed more than 90°, the upper limb is immobilized in a posterior plaster slab combined with a figure-of-8 plaster cast around the elbow. A collar and cuff is added to keep the patient's hand close to the chin so as to maintain the elbow in extreme flexion. Following

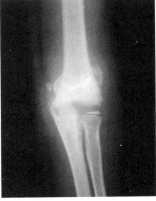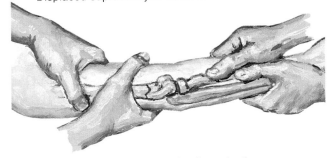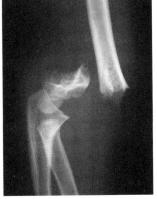

Injury to brachial artery and median nerve by fracture may lead to Volkmann contracture

Anteroposterior (left) and lateral (right) radiographs. Displaced supracondylar fracture

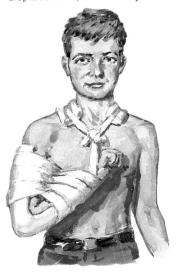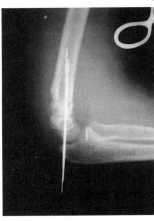

With patient under general anesthesia, reduction accomplished with traction and countertraction, plus gentle manipulative correction of medial or lateral displacement, followed by flexion of elbow beyond 90°

Percutaneous pinning indicated if reduction difficult to maintain with closed method

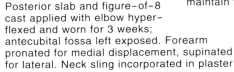

Posterior slab and figure-of-8 cast applied with elbow hyperflexed and worn for 3 weeks; antecubital fossa left exposed. Forearm pronated for medial displacement, supinated for lateral. Neck sling incorporated in plaster

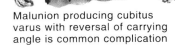

Malunion producing cubitus varus with reversal of carrying angle is common complication

closed reduction and cast immobilization, the peripheral pulse and capillary refill are monitored closely, particularly in the first 48 hours after injury, to ensure that adequate circulation is maintained to the distal limb.

Because it is often hard to maintain an adequate reduction with simple casting techniques, many surgeons advocate percutaneous pin fixation under image intensification or even open reduction and internal fixation of displaced supracondylar fractures. These methods secure and maintain adequate reduction and stability of the fracture without the need to keep the elbow acutely flexed. Following open reduction and internal fixation or

percutaneous pinning, careful monitoring of the peripheral circulation is still necessary to avoid ischemia of the distal limb.

Complications from supracondylar fractures are frequent and varied. The most important are loss of peripheral nerve function and Volkmann contracture of the forearm musculature secondary to laceration or compression of the brachial artery. Residual deformity due to inadequate reduction of the fracture is another frequent complication. The most common residual deformity is cubitus varus (gunstock deformity), a medial and varus rotation of the distal fracture fragment that persists after fracture healing.

Fractures in Children

(Continued)

Injury to Elbow

Diagnosis of elbow injury in a child is often difficult, and radiographs are particularly confusing because of the presence of the growth plates and the relatively late ossification of some of the epiphyses in the elbow region (Plate 131). Simple elbow sprains are very rare in children, and elbow pain following injury mandates careful clinical and radiographic examination of the joint. Comparison radiographs of the uninjured elbow often help in identifying subtle fracture lines and displaced fracture fragments.

Avulsion of Medial Epicondyle of Humerus. This injury is one of the most common elbow injuries in children. It results from a valgus stress applied to the elbow and is frequently associated with lateral dislocation of this joint. Dislocation causes the strong ulnar collateral ligament to pull the epicondyle fragment free from the humerus. During reduction of the dislocation, the fragment sometimes becomes trapped in the elbow joint. If not incarcerated in the joint, the fragment may be slightly displaced or rotated more than 1 cm away from the distal humerus. A significantly displaced fragment is sometimes easily palpable and freely movable on the medial aspect of the elbow joint.

Nondisplaced and minimally displaced fractures heal well with simple splint immobilization. A displaced fragment trapped in the joint as a result of an elbow dislocation requires open reduction to restore joint congruity and stability. Significantly displaced fragments outside the joint may not heal, and some surgeons recommend open reduction and internal fixation. However, even if the fragment fails to unite, long-term complications are few.

Dislocation of Elbow. This uncommon childhood injury is usually seen in boys between 13 and 15 years of age and is frequently associated with athletic injuries. Most elbow dislocations are posterior. Associated avulsion fractures of the elbow, particularly avulsion fracture of the medial epicondyle, are not uncommon. With adequate anesthesia, most elbow dislocations can be reduced easily. Maintaining the elbow in a flexed position for 3 to 4 weeks usually allows full healing with little risk of recurrent dislocation.

Fracture of Lateral Condyle. If not reduced well and securely fixed, this type of fracture tends to lead to significant long-term problems. Growth arrest of the lateral humerus produces a progressive valgus deformity of the joint, which in turn may lead to ulnar nerve palsy later in life. Nondisplaced fractures of the lateral condyle can be treated with immobilization in a cast. However, because of a significant risk of late displacement of the fracture, the patient must be monitored with frequent radiographic examinations during the 2 weeks following injury. Significantly displaced fractures require reduction and pin fixation

Elbow Injury in Children

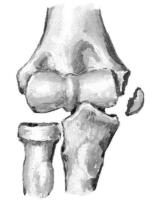

Avulsion of medial epicondyle of humerus

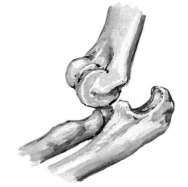

Posterior dislocation of elbow joint

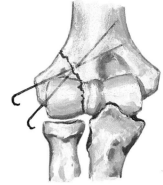

Open reduction and pinning of fracture of lateral condyle

Subluxation of radial head

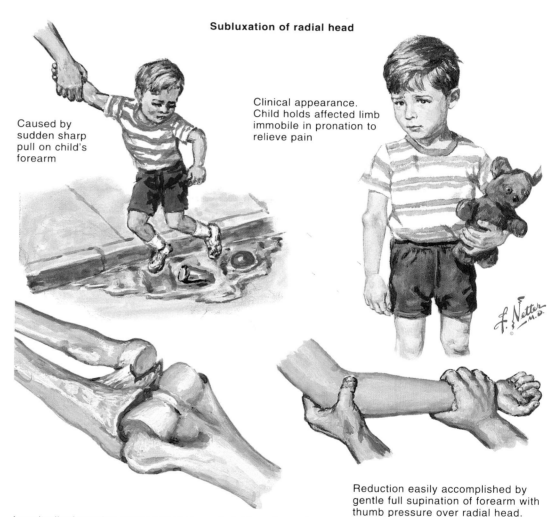

Caused by sudden sharp pull on child's forearm

Clinical appearance. Child holds affected limb immobile in pronation to relieve pain

Longitudinal traction causes tearing or stretching of annular ligament of radius, permitting radial head to subluxate and ligament to prolapse into radiohumeral joint

Reduction easily accomplished by gentle full supination of forearm with thumb pressure over radial head. "Click" may be felt or heard as radial head goes back into place; pain promptly and completely relieved

to maintain a satisfactory reduction and avoid the deformity and neurologic complications associated with this injury.

Subluxation of Radial Head. This injury, also known as nursemaid elbow, is common in children between 2 and 4 years of age and results from longitudinal traction applied to the limb. Clinical findings are characteristic: the injured limb hangs dependent, the forearm is pronated, and any attempt to flex the elbow or supinate the forearm produces significant pain. Radiographs do not show any significant bone abnormality about the elbow. Physical examination almost always reveals localized tenderness over the radial head.

In most patients, reduction can be achieved by complete supination of the forearm. Although this causes a moment of fairly severe pain, supination causes the radial head to slide back into its normal position, and frequently a "click" is felt as the annular ligament slides back around the radial neck. Reduction brings almost immediate and complete relief of pain, and within a few moments, the child begins to use the elbow. If the closed reduction is successful, immobilization is not necessary. The physician should explain the cause of the subluxation to the child's parents and tell them to avoid longitudinal traction on the limb. The risk of recurrent subluxation is minimal.

Fracture of Forearm Bones in Children

Fracture of distal forearm

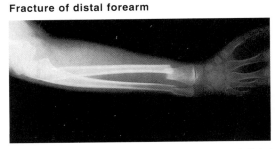

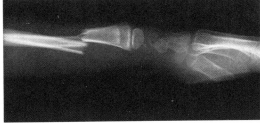

Anteroposterior radiograph shows fracture of distal radius and ulna in child

In lateral radiograph, dorsal displacement and overriding more apparent

Fractures in Children

(Continued)

Fracture of Forearm Bones

Fractures of the bones of the forearm are quite common in children. A fall on the outstretched hand is the most common cause, and the break can occur anywhere along the radius or ulna or both (Plate 132).

Fracture of Radial Head or Neck. During a fall on the outstretched hand, the radial head or neck may fracture as it impacts against the capitulum of the humerus. Significant angulation of the radial head fragment may occur, and if the angulation is greater than 30°, the fracture should be reduced with closed manipulation. Reduction is achieved using digital pressure over the angulated head while alternatively supinating and pronating the forearm. Although closed reduction is sufficient for most fractures, severely displaced or angulated fractures of the radial head require open reduction and internal fixation. Even completely displaced fragments should be reduced and fixed in place. In a growing child, the radial head should never be excised because excision always leads to significant loss of elbow function.

Fracture of Shaft and Growth Plate. Fracture of the shafts of both bones is one of the most common patterns of injury in the forearm. Shaft fractures of both forearm bones range from incomplete greenstick fractures to complete fractures with severe angulation. Fractures of the growth plate of the distal radius are particularly common, and the injury is usually a Salter-Harris type II fracture (Plate 128). Almost all fractures of both bones of the forearm can be treated with closed reduction and cast immobilization. Most fractures have a significant potential for remodeling, particularly those at or near the distal end.

Monteggia Fracture. A fracture of the shaft of the ulna associated with a dislocation of the radial head is known as the Monteggia fracture. The most common configuration consists of anterior angulation of the ulnar fracture combined with anterior dislocation of the radial head. Other directions of the angulation and displacement may be posterior, medial, or lateral. The dislocation of the radial head is easily overlooked in the clinical evaluation, and the examiner should always suspect an injury to the proximal or distal joint when a fracture of one of the paired forearm bones is detected. Thus, when a forearm bone is fractured, radiographs of the elbow and wrist must be obtained to make sure that the alignment of these joints is normal. In children, most Monteggia fractures can be reduced with closed means; a satisfactory reduction can be maintained with the elbow flexed at least 90° and immobilized in a long arm cast.

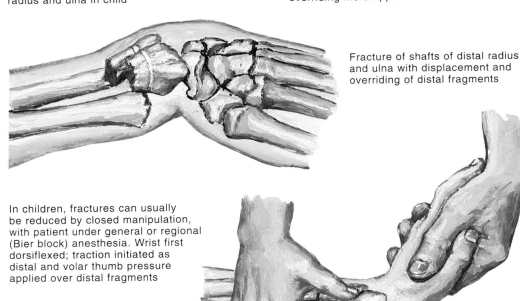

Fracture of shafts of distal radius and ulna with displacement and overriding of distal fragments

In children, fractures can usually be reduced by closed manipulation, with patient under general or regional (Bier block) anesthesia. Wrist first dorsiflexed; traction initiated as distal and volar thumb pressure applied over distal fragments

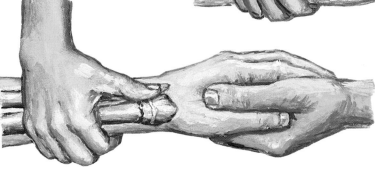

With pressure and traction maintained, wrist gently straightened

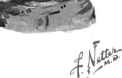

Long arm cast applied and worn for 6 weeks with sling

Monteggia fracture

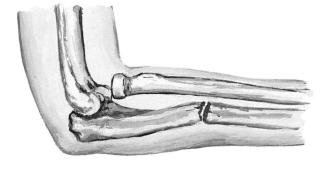

Fracture of shaft of ulna with dislocation of proximal radioulnar joint (Monteggia fracture) not uncommon in children. May result in serious disability if dislocation of radial head not recognized and promptly corrected. Monteggia fractures in children, unlike those in adults, can usually be reduced with gentle traction plus manual pressure over radial head and over angulation of ulna. Cast applied with elbow acutely flexed

Fractures in Children

(Continued)

Fracture of Femur

Fracture of Proximal Femur. In children, fractures of the proximal femur usually result from high-velocity trauma such as a fall from a height or a vehicular accident (Plate 133). The injury may occur in the femoral neck or intertrochanteric region or through the growth plate. Although rare in children, a fracture of the proximal femur may lead to significant complications that can result in permanent disability. These complications include (1) avascular necrosis of the femoral head, which develops in 40% of patients and if not treated can result in collapse of the femoral head and later osteoarthritis; (2) nonunion, which occurs in 5% to 10% of patients; and (3) malunion in intertrochanteric and femoral neck fractures, with residual varus deformity. Because of these common risks, many surgeons advocate open reduction and internal fixation to secure an anatomic reduction of proximal femur fractures in children.

Fracture of Femoral Shaft. These fractures occur often in children as a result of falls or high-velocity injuries. Treatment depends on the age of the child. In infants and children less than 2 years of age, closed reduction is performed with the child under anesthesia, and a spica cast is applied either immediately or 1 or 2 days after fracture. In young children, bone has a significant ability to remodel moderate angular deformities that may develop during cast immobilization, and extreme limb shortening is rare in this age group.

Children between 2 and 10 years of age can be treated with early application of a spica cast unless the fracture fragments override greater than 2 cm. In young children with significant shortening of the limb at the fracture site, the best treatment includes a period of skin traction to maintain adequate limb length until early callus formation occurs, followed by application of a spica cast about 2 to 3 weeks after injury. A diaphyseal fracture in a child in this age group produces increased blood flow to the adjacent growth plate, which causes a transient period of increased growth. Fractures of the femoral shaft often stimulate rapid growth in the epiphysis of the distal femur, resulting in approximately 1 cm of overgrowth. Therefore, it is quite acceptable—and indeed often preferable—to allow the fracture fragments to overlap about 1 cm, which compensates for the anticipated overgrowth.

In children between 10 and 16 years of age, skeletal traction is usually needed to achieve satisfactory alignment and minimize overriding of the fracture fragments until callus forms at about 3 weeks. A cast is then applied and is worn until fracture healing is complete. Some surgeons prefer closed femoral nailing to ensure good alignment, which eliminates the need to depend on remodeling to achieve adequate fracture alignment and limb function. There is a slight risk of infection with this technique, but early closed nailing allows adolescents to be mobilized early and to walk using crutches within a few days after injury.

Fracture of Femur in Children

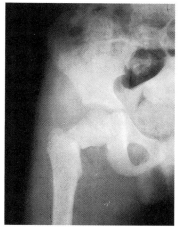

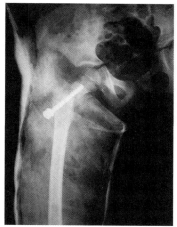

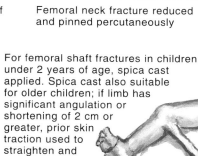

Avascular necrosis of femoral head following fracture of neck

Radiograph shows fracture of femoral neck

Femoral neck fracture reduced and pinned percutaneously

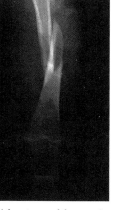

Spiral fracture of femoral shaft

For femoral shaft fractures in children under 2 years of age, spica cast applied. Spica cast also suitable for older children; if limb has significant angulation or shortening of 2 cm or greater, prior skin traction used to straighten and lengthen limb

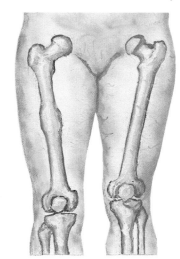

Russell skin traction with balanced suspension

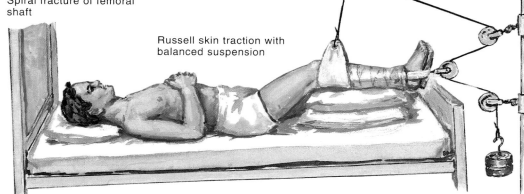

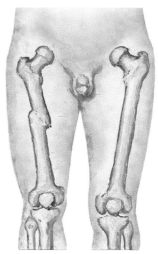

Fracture of right femoral shaft that has been allowed to heal with slight shortening

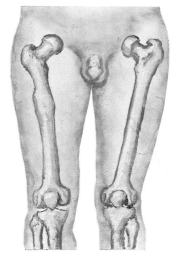

Same child, 2 years later. Good remodeling. Femurs of equal length because of more rapid growth of fractured bone

Patient with femoral shaft fracture that healed with no shortening, but subsequent overgrowth resulted in limb length discrepancy

Fractures in Children
(Continued)

Fracture of Tibia

Children have strong ligaments, and ligament injuries about the knee are not common. Consequently, injuries that commonly produce ligament damage in adults are more likely to cause fractures, particularly growth plate injuries, in growing children (Plate 134).

Avulsion of Anterior Tibial Spine. Avulsion of the anterior tibial spine (intercondylar eminence) is one of the most common knee injuries in children. Excessive tension on the anterior cruciate ligament, which inserts into the anterior tibial spine, results in an intraarticular fracture. The fragment of tibial spine may be nondisplaced, or it may be displaced substantially from its bed. Nondisplaced or minimally displaced fractures can be treated by immobilizing the knee in full extension in a long leg cast. Full extension of the knee joint tends to reduce the fragment and hold it in position during healing. Significantly displaced fractures, however, require open anatomic reduction and fixation to ensure restoration of knee stability.

Fracture of Shaft and Metaphysis. Occurring fairly often in children, fractures of the tibial shaft are usually amenable to closed reduction and casting. Once satisfactory reduction is achieved, healing usually proceeds well with few or no long-term complications. One complication unique to children occurs following fracture of the proximal tibial metaphysis. This fracture usually appears to be benign, with little or no angulation, but after healing has occurred, the limb tends to develop a progressive valgus angulation. The cause of this deformity is not certain, but the angulation may be due to overgrowth of the tibia without concomitant overgrowth of the fibula. Fortunately, as the child continues to grow, the valgus deformity partially corrects. The recommended treatment consists of closed reduction and cast immobilization followed by close observation.

Injury to Growth Plate. The growth plate (physis) of the distal tibia is very susceptible to injury. Twisting injuries, similar to those seen in adults, produce a variety of fracture patterns unique to the child's ankle because of the presence of the open growth plate. The Tillaux fracture, a Salter-Harris type III injury of the distal tibia, is common in children 12 to 15 years of age. An external rotation injury to the ankle joint avulses the anterolateral portion of the epiphysis. Significantly displaced fragments require anatomic reduction and fixation to restore satisfactory function of the ankle joint.

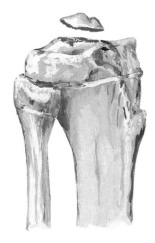

Fracture of anterior tibial spine

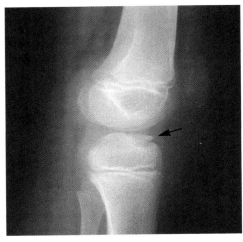

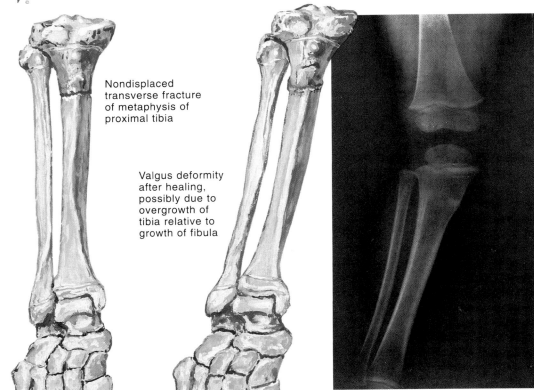

Nondisplaced transverse fracture of metaphysis of proximal tibia

Valgus deformity after healing, possibly due to overgrowth of tibia relative to growth of fibula

Anteroposterior radiograph. Healed transverse fracture with valgus deformity

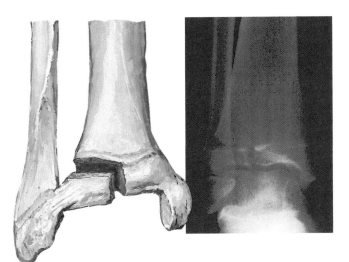

Tillaux (Salter–Harris type III) fracture of distal tibia. Fracture line extends partially across growth plate and vertically through epiphysis. Medial portion of growth plate and epiphysis remain intact

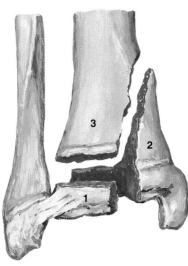

Triplane fracture. Three fragments: 1. Anterior portion of epiphysis of distal tibia. 2. Postero-medial portion of epiphysis with attached spike of metaphysis. 3. Shaft of tibia

Fractures in Children
(Continued)

Fracture in Abused Children

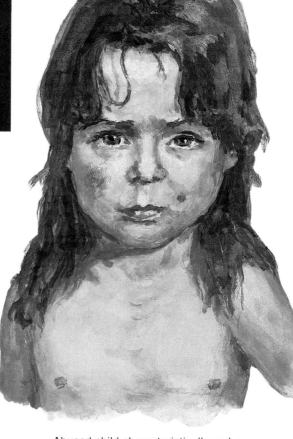

Radiograph shows fracture of proximal right femur for which patient was brought to hospital. Healing fracture of growth plate of distal femur noted, arousing suspicion of child abuse

Abused child characteristically sad or withdrawn. Signs such as poor skin and hair care or malnutrition should increase suspicion

Further examination may reveal bruises, welts, or cigarette burns in various stages of healing on other parts of body

The triplane fracture has the appearance of Salter-Harris types II and III fractures on antero-posterior and lateral radiographs. Commonly, the three fracture fragments are (1) the anterolateral portion of the epiphysis of the distal tibia (similar to the Tillaux fragment), (2) the tibial shaft, and (3) the large posterior fragment comprising the posterior and medial portions of the epiphysis plus a large metaphyseal fragment of variable size. Triplane fractures require anatomic reduction of the articular surface to ensure satisfactory function of the ankle joint after the fracture heals.

Fracture in Abused Children

Child abuse is unfortunately all too common, particularly in children less than 3 years of age (Plate 135). In approximately 30% to 50% of cases of child abuse, the first injury that is encountered is a fracture. Although the diagnosis of child abuse can be extremely difficult, several signs and circumstances should arouse suspicion when the physician examines a young child with a fracture.

The most important clues to an abuse-related injury are a history that is inconsistent with the type of fracture and discrepancies in the histories provided by parents or care givers. A significant delay in seeking medical attention may also be a sign of abuse. Any child with a fracture and other signs of maltreatment, such as malnutrition, poor skin hygiene, or other signs of neglect, should be considered a possible victim of abuse.

Abused children are frequently withdrawn and inordinately quiet despite the presence of a painful fracture. Examination of abused children frequently reveals multiple fractures, often in various stages of healing. For this reason, a radiographic skeletal survey should be obtained for every child suspected of being abused. The physical and radiographic examinations should look for evidence of trauma in various locations on the body and in different stages of healing. No fracture is diagnostic of abuse, but epiphyseal separations are especially common in abused children. Fractures of the shafts of long bones and rib fractures occur as well.

Abused children who are returned to the home face a significant risk of repeated abuse. Therefore, whenever child abuse is suspected, it should be reported to the local child protective authorities. Accusations of abuse should not be made witout significant evidence. This evidence can be provided by careful examination of the child, documentation of injuries, and investigation of the family situation by skilled social workers. When a physician suspects child abuse, the best course is to admit the child to the hospital for further evaluation and protection while appropriate authorities investigate the cause of the injuries. □

Stress and Pathologic Fractures

Stress Fracture

Stress fractures are a common problem. Although most are often considered a disorder of young athletes, they can occur at any age. A stress, or fatigue, fracture is the final stage of a broader condition called stress injury of bone. The initial event, a stress reaction, is not visible on radiographs and is therefore very difficult to diagnose. Stress reaction can evolve into the true stress fracture, which is evident both clinically and radiographically.

Bone that is subjected to new, repetitive stresses remodels to accommodate to those stresses (Plate 136). According to Wolff law, bone adapts by first resorbing trabeculae and then forming new trabeculae along the stress lines (see CIBA COLLECTION, Volume 8/I, page 187). The most vulnerable period during this remodeling is between 7 and 21 days, when the old trabeculae have been resorbed but the new ones have not yet been laid down. If bending stresses continue to be applied, focal microfractures occur. This stage of injury is described as the stress reaction.

Because microfractures are painful, the patient may seek medical attention. At this stage, the only clinical findings are localized swelling and point tenderness. Radiographs are normal. If the patient avoids the specific stress that has caused the injury, the stress reaction usually resolves. However, if the repetitive loads continue, the microfractures coalesce to form a complete fracture line—the stress fracture. The formation of a complete fracture induces the full fracture repair process.

Stress injury is precipitated by participation in new forms of activity, increased participation in established activities and overtraining, or change in the environment in which the person participates. The change may be as minor as a new pair of athletic shoes or a change in the direction of the regular jogging route. Stress injury is also common after foot surgery. For example, after bunionectomy, weight-bearing stresses are often transferred to the second metatarsal and may lead to stress fracture.

Although any bone can be affected, stress injuries are most common in the lower limb. Overall, the metatarsals are the most common site. In joggers, stress fractures often occur in the fibula, 2 or 3 inches above the ankle mortise. Stress fracture of the calcaneus is a common cause of chronic heel pain. Fortunately, stress fractures in these sites are unlikely to displace or cause serious long-term problems even if diagnosis is delayed. This is not true of all stress fractures, however. Persistently painful nonunions may result from stress fractures of the navicular, the sesamoid bones of the great toe, and the proximal shaft of the fifth metatarsal.

Stress Fracture

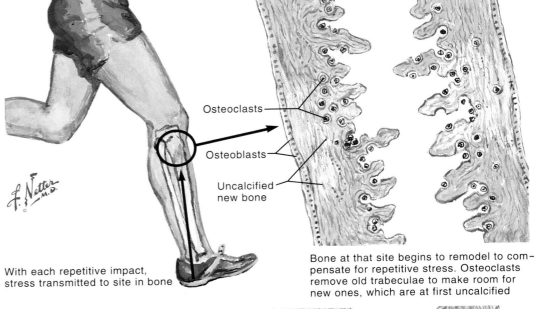

With each repetitive impact, stress transmitted to site in bone

Bone at that site begins to remodel to compensate for repetitive stress. Osteoclasts remove old trabeculae to make room for new ones, which are at first uncalcified

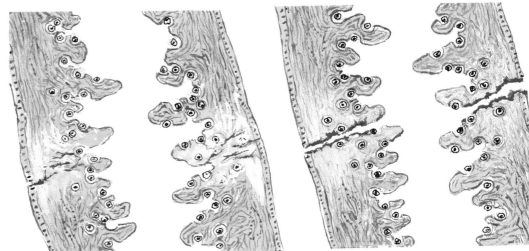

During remodeling period, bone weakens. As stress repeatedly applied, microfractures (stress reaction) occur, characterized by bone pain

In response to further repetitive stress, microfractures coalesce to form complete fracture through both cortices

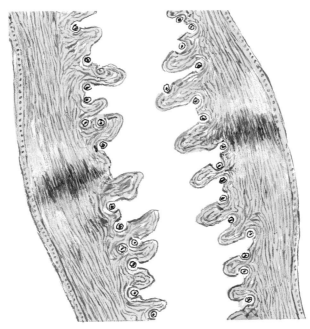

If fracture protected from further stress, normal fracture healing occurs

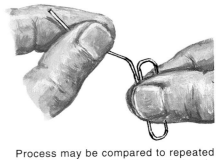

Process may be compared to repeated bending of paper clip. No single bend sufficient to break wire, but repeated bending results in metal fatigue and finally a break

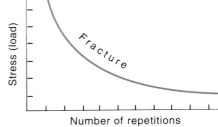

Fatigue fracture is product of magnitude of applied stress multiplied by number of repetitions

Stress and Pathologic Fractures

Stress Fracture (continued)

Stress fracture of the femoral neck is a serious problem in persons of all age groups, from military recruits to older persons with osteoporosis. The stress fracture may occur on the inferior or superior aspect of the femoral neck, where tension distracts the two fracture fragments. Although a resorptive process may occur on the inferior aspect, the more common injury is an impacted fracture with dense, new bone formation. In all stress fractures of the femoral neck, continued weight bearing may displace the fracture fragments. As with other displaced fractures of the femoral neck, there is a 25% incidence of avascular necrosis of the femoral head with an equal incidence of nonunion.

The initial diagnosis of stress injury is often difficult and is based primarily on clinical findings (Plate 137). The most important symptoms are point tenderness and pain that occurs with activity and subsides with rest. Swelling may also be present. Radiographs are not useful in the early stage, because the fracture line is not visible before the microfractures have coalesced. Technetium 99m bone scans show increased radioisotope uptake in the early stage of stress injury. Magnetic resonance imaging is fairly sensitive early in stress injury, showing a decreased signal on T^1-weighted images at the site of the stress fracture.

If the injury is identified in the stress reaction phase, simply eliminating the repetitive loads for 10 days to 2 weeks is often sufficient treatment. If the injury has progressed to a complete stress fracture, the full process of fracture healing with callus formation occurs. This repair process takes 6 to 12 weeks and sometimes longer. Most stress fractures do not require treatment with a cast but must be protected from excessive stresses. Patients whose injuries are detected in the stress reaction stage return to normal activity much faster than those with full-blown stress fractures.

Some stress fractures in the foot, particularly those involving the navicular and the proximal shaft of the fifth metatarsal, require cast immobilization and complete elimination of weight bearing for 6 to 8 weeks. Surgical treatment with open reduction and internal fixation is required

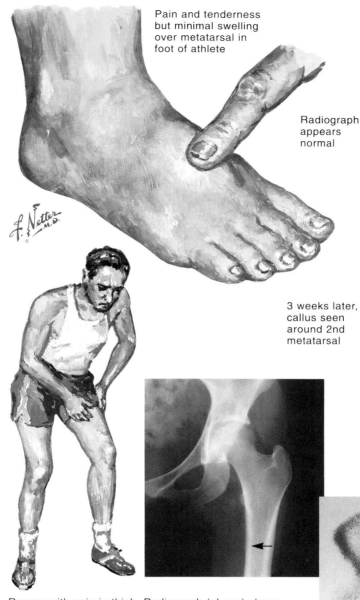

Pain and tenderness but minimal swelling over metatarsal in foot of athlete

Radiograph appears normal

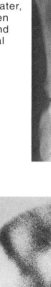

3 weeks later, callus seen around 2nd metatarsal

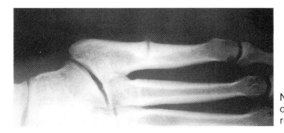

Runner with pain in thigh. Radiograph (above) shows questionable periosteal reaction (arrow). Technetium 99m bone scan (right) reveals increased uptake in same area

Nonunion of stress fracture of shaft of 5th metatarsal. May require open repair with bone graft and screw fixation

for all displaced stress fractures of the femoral neck. Even if the fracture is not displaced, internal fixation is advisable to prevent further fatigue failure and the consequent serious complications.

Pathologic Fracture

Primary bone tumors, metastatic bone tumors, and a variety of diseases can weaken bone, making it more susceptible to fracture. A fracture through such a weakened bone is called a pathologic fracture (Plate 138).

When a patient presents with a fracture caused by a trivial injury, the examiner should suspect that the fractured bone has been weakened by a pathologic process. The diagnosis may be obvious in patients with chronic, widespread metastatic or metabolic disease. Sometimes, a pathologic fracture is the first manifestation of certain pathologic processes of bone, particularly primary bone tumors and even metastatic tumors. Careful inspection of the radiographs often reveals the destructive process that has predisposed the bone to fracture.

Primary Bone Tumor. Primary bone tumors are relatively rare and most are benign. Fractures through benign bone tumors usually heal, but after the fracture is fully healed, surgical treatment of the benign tumor may be necessary.

Stress and Pathologic Fractures
(Continued)

Pathologic Fracture

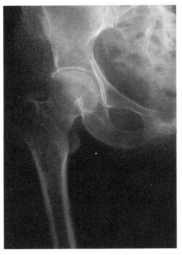

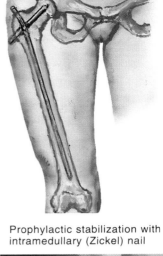

Radiograph of impending fracture of femur due to tumor

Prophylactic stabilization with intramedullary (Zickel) nail

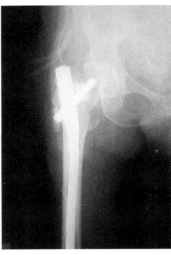

Internal fixation with Zickel nail

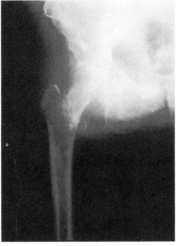

Pathologic fracture of proximal femur due to primary bone tumor

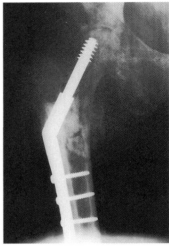

Same fracture after open reduction and internal fixation with cement and compression screw and plate

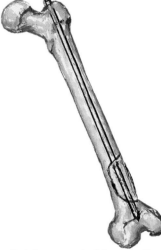

Reinforcement of femur with intramedullary rod and cement after removal of tumor of distal femoral shaft

Pathologic fractures through primary malignant bone tumors, such as osteosarcoma, may adversely affect the management of both the fracture and the tumor: the malignant process may impair fracture healing, and the fracture releases tumor cells, contaminating the local soft tissues. Local contamination can significantly compromise the surgeon's ability to resect the tumor successfully.

Metastatic Disease. Pathologic fracture secondary to metastatic disease is a more common problem than fracture due to a primary tumor. In as much as 25% of patients with pathologic fractures due to cancer, the fracture itself is the first sign of disease. Therefore, any radiographic evidence of a lytic process at the fracture site must alert the physician to the possibility of a metastatic malignancy. Metastases to the skeleton are very common—70% of patients who die of cancer have metastatic skeletal lesions. However, only a small proportion of these metastases weaken the bone sufficiently to result in fracture.

The breast, lung, kidney, colon, thyroid, and prostate are common sites of origin of metastatic bone lesions. Multiple myeloma, although a primary bone tumor, should be managed as a metastatic bone lesion because it also produces multiple lytic lesions.

Although many physicians feel that a pathologic fracture secondary to metastatic disease is a terminal event, about 40% of patients survive for 6 months and about 30% survive for 1 year or longer. Treatment, therefore, should be aimed at improving the quality of life for these patients during their remaining time. A pathologic fracture that causes significant pain or loss of function should be treated aggressively to decrease pain and restore as much function as possible. Heppenstall identified four goals of early and aggressive surgery for pathologic fractures: (1) to afford adequate pain relief, (2) to increase functional mobility, (3) to facilitate nursing care, and (4) to improve the patient's attitude. Early surgical stabilization using internal fixation devices, often combined with methylmethacrylate cement, can promptly restore function and relieve pain.

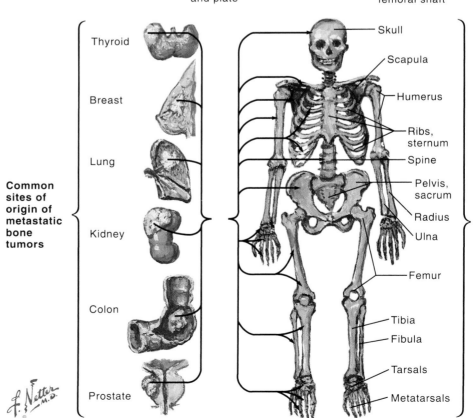

Common sites of origin of metastatic bone tumors

Thyroid

Breast

Lung

Kidney

Colon

Prostate

Skull

Scapula

Humerus

Ribs, sternum

Spine

Pelvis, sacrum

Radius

Ulna

Femur

Tibia

Fibula

Tarsals

Metatarsals

Common sites of metastatic bone tumors

Stress and Pathologic Fractures

(Continued)

Some specific metastatic bone lesions should be treated prophylactically with internal fixation if there is a substantial and immediate likelihood of fracture. Lesions that involve more than 50% of the diameter of the major long bones, particularly the humerus, femur, and tibia, significantly increase the risk of fracture. Prophylactic stabilization, usually using a blind intramedullary nailing technique, is relatively simple. In addition to preventing later fracture, prophylactic fixation often relieves pain as well.

Metabolic Disease. The most common metabolic bone disease that predisposes to pathologic fracture is osteoporosis. Indeed, a fracture is frequently the first clinical sign of this disease. The incidence of fractures of the distal radius, proximal humerus, proximal femur, and vertebral bodies increases markedly with age, and the fractures often result from very minor trauma. A fracture in an osteoporotic bone retains its capacity to heal and is treated in the same way as a fracture of a normal bone. Because many patients with osteoporosis are elderly and debilitated, treatment emphasizes prompt mobilization to avoid prolonged bed rest and help prevent joint stiffness, pneumonia, pressure sores, and urinary tract infections.

The osteoporotic thoracolumbar spine is particularly vulnerable to fracture. Movements such as twisting or leaning forward to raise a window may be enough to cause a fracture. The resulting injuries range in severity from a very mild indentation fracture of the vertebral body to a near-complete collapse of one or more vertebrae. Usually, the presenting symptom of a vertebral compression, or crush, fracture is pain in the area of the fracture that radiates along the dermatomal distribution of the affected spinal segment. Percussion over the injured vertebra elicits tenderness. Involvement of multiple vertebrae produces a significant kyphosis (dowager hump).

Treatment of vertebral compression fractures focuses on adequate pain relief to allow continued mobility. Prolonged immobilization only exacerbates the osteoporosis and increases the risk of pneumonia. Management to prevent further fractures includes minimizing the risk of falls, dietary supplementation with calcium, a regular exercise program, and hormone replacement therapy in some patients. Despite preventive treatment, many patients with a vertebral compression fracture remain at risk for further vertebral collapse and fractures of a long bone. (For a more extensive discussion of osteoporosis, see CIBA COLLECTION, Volume 8/I, pages 216–227.)

Osteogenesis imperfecta and other congenital disorders of bone such as renal rickets (renal osteodystrophy) may profoundly affect the structure

Pathologic Fracture (continued)

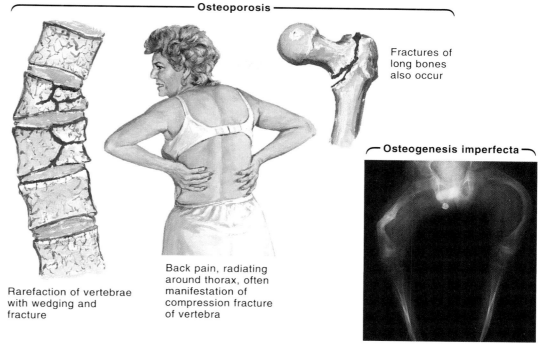

— Osteoporosis —

Rarefaction of vertebrae with wedging and fracture

Back pain, radiating around thorax, often manifestation of compression fracture of vertebra

Fractures of long bones also occur

— Osteogenesis imperfecta —

Radiograph shows multiple and recurrent fractures and deformities

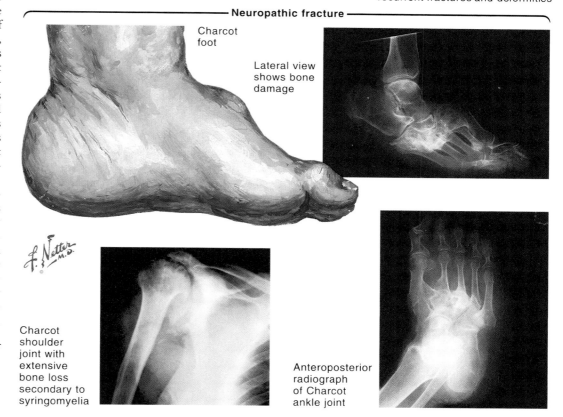

— Neuropathic fracture —

Charcot foot

Lateral view shows bone damage

Charcot shoulder joint with extensive bone loss secondary to syringomyelia

Anteroposterior radiograph of Charcot ankle joint

of the skeleton in growing children, making it quite susceptible to pathologic fractures (see CIBA COLLECTION, Volume 8/I, pages 205–214 and 229–231).

Neuropathic Disease. Some chronic neurologic disorders, such as tabes dorsalis, diabetes mellitus, and leprosy, also predispose to pathologic fractures near joints. Charcot originally described this process in 1868, and it is still called Charcot arthropathy.

The common denominator in all these disorders is a significant decrease or a complete absence of pain sensation combined with the continued use of the insensate limb. Because patients lack

protective sensation, they ignore trivial injuries such as minor fractures or sprains. Patients continue to stress the injured area rather than protecting it to allow the normal reparative processes to heal the injury. Continued use creates excessive motion at the site of injury and abundant callus forms. However, the fracture often fails to heal, and marked disruption of the injured joint occurs. The patient with a peripheral neuropathy who is injured must be forced to protect the injured limb from all stresses until healing is complete. Otherwise, the osseous structures will collapse, resulting in severe deformity and substantial loss of function. □

Complications of Fracture

Neurovascular Complications of Fractures

A major objective in the management of fractures and dislocations is to avoid as many complications as possible. The principles of fracture treatment direct the surgeon to reduce the fracture and immobilize it, with either a cast or internal fixation devices, to allow natural healing to occur. A variety of complications, either as a consequence of the injury itself or as a consequence of treatment, can produce serious and permanent problems. Acute complications such as damage to nerves and blood vessels, adult respiratory distress syndrome, and infection usually arise from the injury itself. Complications also develop during the healing process and may lead to irreparable loss of function. Chronic complications include failure of union, deformities, osteoarthritis, joint stiffness, implant failure, and reflex sympathetic dystrophy.

Neurovascular Injury

Displacement of fracture fragments or bone ends at a dislocated joint often produces compression or laceration of adjacent vessels and nerves (Plate 140). Critical neurovascular structures (eg, the brachial plexus) lie deep in the limb, close to the skeleton, which protects them from injuries. A fracture or dislocation makes nerves or vessels vulnerable to injury from sharp bone fragments or from entrapment in the fracture site.

Neurovascular complications must be identified by careful examination immediately after the injury and after any manipulation of the injured limb. Some complications are not immediately evident but do appear 24 to 48 hours after injury. Reexamination and monitoring are essential both during this period and while circular compression dressings and casts are in place. Prompt and sometimes aggressive treatment is required to restore function and prevent permanent loss.

Radial Nerve Palsy. The radial nerve is commonly damaged in fractures of the distal shaft of the humerus. Normally protected in the spiral groove on the humeral shaft, the nerve is easily impaled by a fracture fragment or entrapped in the fracture site. Aggressive manipulation of the fracture during closed reduction may also result in nerve entrapment. Wrist drop is a common long-term consequence of this injury.

Sciatic Nerve Palsy. Nerves and vessels at or near joints are particularly vulnerable to injury. The neurovascular structures are more securely tethered to the soft tissues around the joints than elsewhere and are less likely to escape injury when significant joint displacement occurs. For example, the sciatic nerve is often injured in posterior dislocation of the hip, resulting in sciatic nerve palsy and foot drop. Generally, the nerve is simply stretched or contused by direct impingement of the femoral head. Immediate reduction of the dislocation relieves pressure on the nerve, and about 60% of patients recover completely; the other 40% experience variable loss of nerve function.

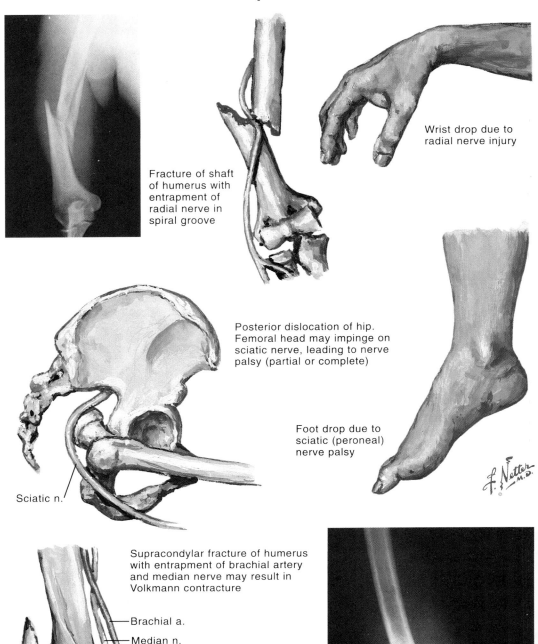

Fracture of shaft of humerus with entrapment of radial nerve in spiral groove

Wrist drop due to radial nerve injury

Posterior dislocation of hip. Femoral head may impinge on sciatic nerve, leading to nerve palsy (partial or complete)

Sciatic n.

Foot drop due to sciatic (peroneal) nerve palsy

Supracondylar fracture of humerus with entrapment of brachial artery and median nerve may result in Volkmann contracture

Brachial a.

Median n.

Radial a.

Ulnar a.

Neurovascular Injury to Elbow. A musculoskeletal injury that is frequently associated with neurovascular injury is the supracondylar fracture of the humerus. It is most common in children between 5 and 10 years of age and usually results from a fall on the outstretched hand. In the most common type of fracture, hyperextension injury, the humeral shaft fragment is displaced anteriorly, impinging on the critical neurovascular structures in front of the elbow. The radial and median nerves are both particularly susceptible to direct injury from the displaced fracture fragment, and the brachial artery may be lacerated or entrapped in the fracture site at the time of injury or during closed reduction. Distal neurovascular function must be assessed critically, and manipulative reduction must be very careful and gentle.

Compartment Syndrome. Direct damage to an artery or severe swelling in a muscle compartment can lead to the development of compartment syndrome and Volkmann contracture. This serious outcome is common after any fracture in which bleeding and swelling are extreme. Compartment syndromes can occur with open as well as with closed fractures and may also be caused by a circular cast. Failure to identify compartment syndrome early may lead to permanent loss of limb function (Plates 11–16).

Complications of Fracture
(Continued)

Adult Respiratory Distress Syndrome
(Fat Embolism Syndrome)

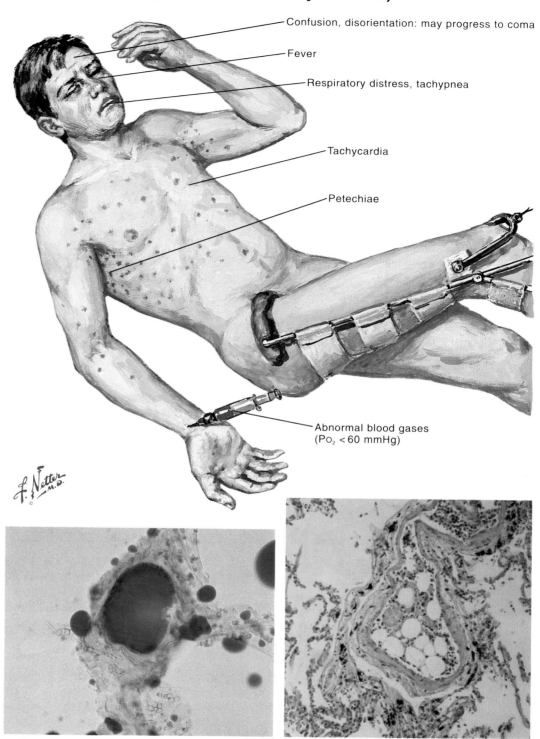

Confusion, disorientation: may progress to coma

Fever

Respiratory distress, tachypnea

Tachycardia

Petechiae

Abnormal blood gases
(Po₂ < 60 mmHg)

Fat emboli in lung (stained red with Sudan III). Pulmonary edema visible

Bone marrow embolus in lung

Adult Respiratory Distress Syndrome

Respiratory failure often develops 24 to 72 hours after severe musculoskeletal injury. The precise pathogenesis of the syndrome is not fully understood, and many etiologic factors play a role in its development, including pulmonary embolism, aspiration of gastric contents, pulmonary edema due to fluid overload or heart failure, atelectasis, and pneumonia. Whereas all these conditions may occur following trauma, a specific pattern of pulmonary deficit called adult respiratory distress syndrome (ARDS), or fat embolism syndrome, has been linked to fractures of long bones (Plate 141). However, although the syndrome is more common after fractures of the long bones, it has been reported following fracture in nearly every bone.

Adult respiratory distress syndrome is characterized by the sudden onset of respiratory insufficiency and extreme arterial hypoxia in the immediate postinjury period. Clinical manifestations include fever, tachycardia, tachypnea, and mental confusion. Arterial oxygen tension falls below 60 mmHg. Airway resistance increases, lung compliance progressively decreases, and pulmonary arteriovenous shunting becomes evident. Petechiae often develop, especially in the axillae.

Occasionally, marrow emboli have been identified in the lungs of patients, leading to the term "fat embolism syndrome," but ARDS may also develop in the absence of fracture marrow emboli. Recent studies have demonstrated the release of free fatty acids into the bloodstream, which produces characteristic pulmonary changes: congestion, atelectasis, venous and capillary engorgement, and interstitial edema. These pulmonary changes prevent the exchange of oxygen across the alveolocapillary membrane, resulting in profound systemic hypoxia. As a consequence, the patient becomes progressively more hypoxic and may die if the disorder is not treated aggressively. When ARDS is suspected, arterial oxygen tension should be determined. Arterial oxygen tension less than 60 mmHg confirms the diagnosis.

Extensive clinical evidence demonstrates that ARDS can be prevented, or at least minimized, by mobilizing the patient early and avoiding prolonged bed rest and traction. These precautions require immobilization of the fracture as soon as possible after the injury, often with open reduction and internal fixation. This is particularly important in patients with multiple injuries. A good example of this preventive approach is the nailing of femoral shaft fractures. This procedure allows the patient to be mobilized immediately after fracture fixation, minimizing bed rest and eliminating the need for skeletal traction.

If promptly recognized and treated vigorously, the pulmonary changes of ARDS are usually fully reversible. Failure to treat the patient aggressively may be fatal. Treatment focuses on correcting the hypoxemia and maintaining arterial oxygen tension greater than 70 mmHg until the pulmonary lesions resolve. Treatment may be required for 2 days to 3 weeks, depending on the severity of the pulmonary lesions. High-concentration oxygen should be administered, but if oxygen delivered with a face mask does not restore the arterial oxygen tension to the desired level, mechanical ventilation with a closed system should be instituted. Positive end expiratory pressure may be necessary to drive sufficient oxygen across the alveolocapillary membrane for adequate arterial oxygenation. Even at this stage, fracture fixation to allow mobilization of the patient combined with vigorous respiratory therapy may help reverse the pulmonary insufficiency.

Complications of Fracture
(Continued)

Infection

A fracture or dislocation becomes contaminated, and thus potentially infected, any time the protective layers of soft tissue enclosing the injury hematoma are violated. The hematoma is an excellent medium for the growth of bacteria, resulting in acute cellulitis or abscess or leading to a chronic deep infection of the bone (osteomyelitis). To help prevent infection, all skeletal injuries should be classified as open or closed immediately after injury. In an open fracture, the overlying skin has been penetrated, and therefore the fracture hematoma may be contaminated.

Classification of Open Fracture. Open fractures are graded by the severity of soft tissue damage, fracture pattern, and degree of contamination, as defined by Gustilo and Anderson (Plate 142). In type I open fractures, the wound is less than 1 cm in length and is free of contamination. Type II fractures have a wound greater than 1 cm in length, and the soft tissues are not extensively stripped from the bone. In type IIIA fractures, the wound is large, but soft tissue coverage remains adequate. In type IIIB fractures, the wound is large, the periosteum is stripped from the bone, and the bone is exposed. Type IIIC fractures have a large wound with significant arterial injury that requires surgical repair.

This classification system correlates the risk of infection with the severity of the wound. Gustilo and colleagues noted that the incidence of infection was 1% for type I fractures, 1.8% for type II fractures, and 20.8% for type III fractures.

Contamination of Open Injury. The most important factors contributing to wound infection of an open fracture are the degree of contamination and the severity of the injury. However, even a type I wound may become infected if not adequately cleaned and treated. The potential for infection due to various strains of *Clostridium* (eg, tetanus and gas gangrene, Plate 144) always exists, regardless of the severity of the wound, because clostridia are ubiquitous, and every contaminated wound may contain them.

Injuries at high risk for infection include wounds contaminated by manure or standing water (which often contains clostridia) and wounds caused by high-velocity mechanism, such as a gunshot wound. An open fracture of the toe caused by a lawn mower blade is a very high risk wound.

Classification of Open Fractures

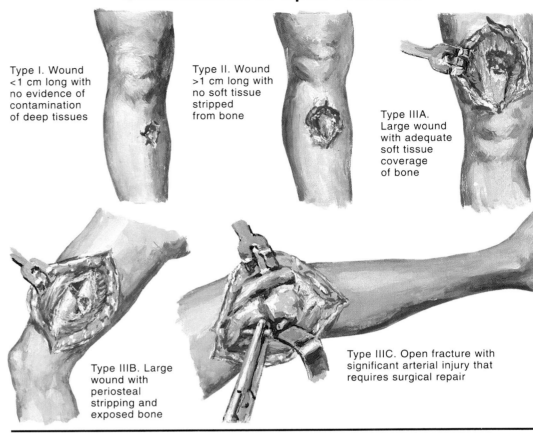

Type I. Wound <1 cm long with no evidence of contamination of deep tissues

Type II. Wound >1 cm long with no soft tissue stripped from bone

Type IIIA. Large wound with adequate soft tissue coverage of bone

Type IIIB. Large wound with periosteal stripping and exposed bone

Type IIIC. Open fracture with significant arterial injury that requires surgical repair

Open Injury With High Risk for Infection

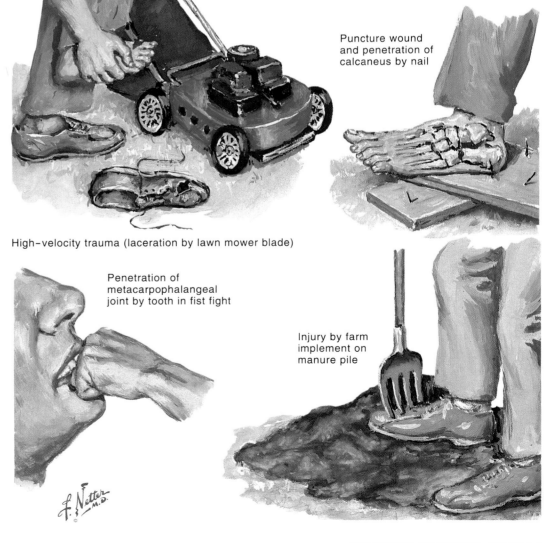

High-velocity trauma (laceration by lawn mower blade)

Puncture wound and penetration of calcaneus by nail

Penetration of metacarpophalangeal joint by tooth in fist fight

Injury by farm implement on manure pile

Complications of Fracture

(Continued)

The high velocity of the blade edge imparts tremendous energy, increasing soft tissue damage and the risk of contamination. Even in some wounds that appear trivial (such as a puncture in the sole of the foot caused by a rusty nail), particularly virulent organisms are inoculated deep into the wound, causing a significant infection. A puncture in the heel that penetrates the calcaneus would be classified as a type I wound; however, this type of puncture wound is notorious for becoming infected, in part because the initial treatment was inadequate. In addition, these puncture wounds are often contaminated by gram-negative organisms, such as *Pseudomonas*, which can cause a chronic infection that is very difficult to cure.

Puncture wounds resulting from human bites are also serious and are often initially overlooked by the patient. In a fist fight, for example, a metacarpophalangeal joint may be punctured by a tooth and contaminated by anaerobic or microaerophilic bacteria contained in the mouth. These organisms can cause especially aggressive and destructive infections in the hand (see Section II, Plate 1).

Even a closed fracture may become infected during open reduction and internal fixation. Although the incidence of infection in these cases is less than 1%, the risk of converting a closed fracture into an open one must be considered in choosing surgical treatment for a fracture.

Failure to remove contaminating organisms from an open fracture site may result in severe complications. Acute infections with *Clostridium* species, as well as with streptococci and other bacteria, can lead to cellulitis, sepsis, and even death. Even if acute infections do not develop, osteomyelitis, a low-grade chronic infection of bone, may result (see Section II, Plates 11–18). This condition is distinguished from soft tissue infections by its persistence and severity. Once established, osteomyelitis is very difficult, if not impossible, to eradicate. Although soft tissue infections are usually cured by incision and drainage, bacteria can become sequestered in bone, where perfusion is inadequate and bactericidal antibiotic levels cannot be achieved. Chronic osteomyelitis may not respond to surgical debridement and intravenous antibiotics, and purulent drainage often persists.

Surgical Management of Open Fractures

All open fractures should undergo immediate and thorough surgical debridement to remove all

Surgical Management of Open Fractures

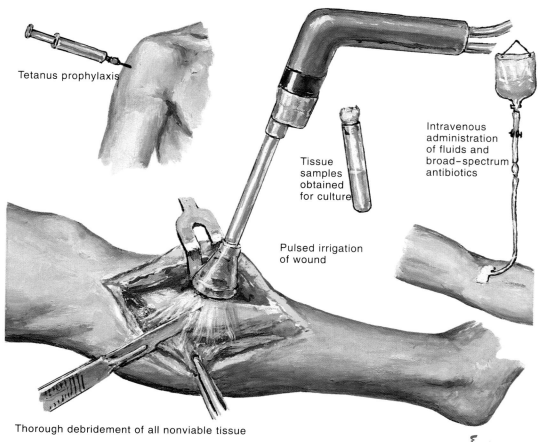

Tetanus prophylaxis

Tissue samples obtained for culture

Pulsed irrigation of wound

Intravenous administration of fluids and broad-spectrum antibiotics

Thorough debridement of all nonviable tissue

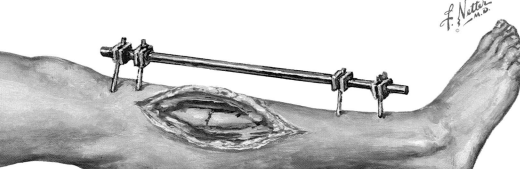

Wound left open. External fixation device allows access to wound for dressing. Delayed primary closure after 3 – 5 days, if wound remains clean

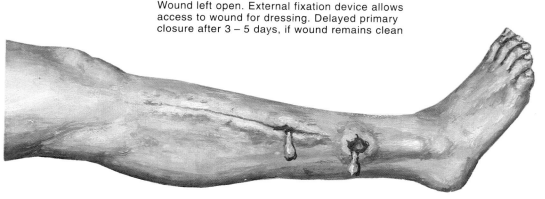

Despite good care, chronic osteomyelitis may develop with sequestra and drainage

contaminating material (Plate 143). Debridement should be done as soon as possible after the injury (always within 6–8 hours). Tissue samples are taken from deep in the wound and broad-spectrum antibiotics administered intravenously for at least 48 hours thereafter. To avoid sealing contaminants inside the wound, all wounds are left open following debridement. Delayed primary closure of

the wound can be considered 3 to 5 days after the injury if the wound remains clean. For all patients with an open fracture, the immunization record is checked and adequate tetanus prophylaxis provided, if needed.

If the fracture is accompanied by severe soft tissue injury, stabilization of the fracture with an external fixation device facilitates wound care.

Gas Gangrene

Complications of Fracture

(Continued)

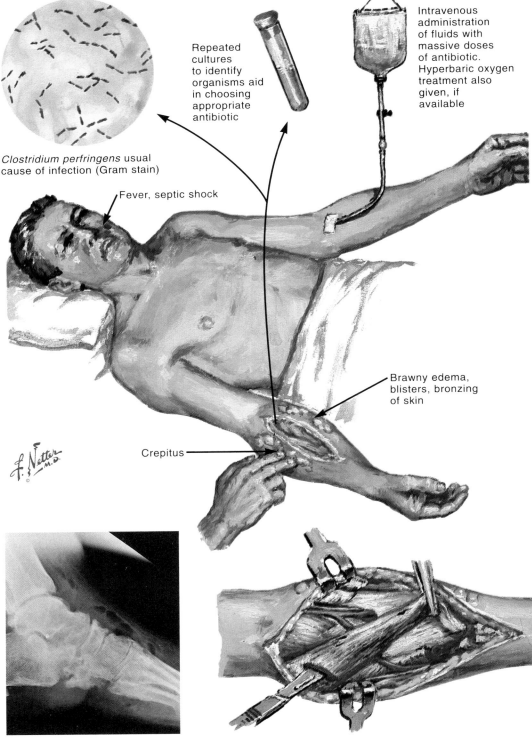

Repeated cultures to identify organisms aid in choosing appropriate antibiotic

Intravenous administration of fluids with massive doses of antibiotic. Hyperbaric oxygen treatment also given, if available

Clostridium perfringens usual cause of infection (Gram stain)

Fever, septic shock

Brawny edema, blisters, bronzing of skin

Crepitus

Radiograph of foot may reveal gas spaces between tissue layers

All nonviable tissue, especially muscle, debrided. Vessels and nerves sometimes spared

Gas Gangrene

The most serious acute infection that can result from a contaminated open fracture is gas gangrene (Plate 144). Although this complication is rare, the causative organism, *Clostridium perfringens*, is found virtually everywhere and should be considered a possible contaminant in every open wound. The reduced oxygen tension in the wound provides an excellent environment for the growth of clostridia.

Gas gangrene develops when a contaminated open fracture is inadequately debrided. The infection tends to involve the subcutaneous tissue and muscles, sometimes sparing blood vessels, nerves, and bone. Once established, the infection may produce a localized cellulitis or extensive and aggressive myonecrosis. The onset of infection usually occurs within 72 hours after injury. Characteristic manifestations are localized pain, swelling, brawny edema, blister formation, and bronzing of the skin. Pockets of subcutaneous gas produce crepitus on palpation, and the wound often drains a thin, brownish, watery material. Severe systemic symptoms of fever, tachycardia, and lethargy may progress rapidly to septic shock and coma.

As with other wound infections, prevention is the keystone in the management of infections caused by *Clostridium*. The contaminated hematoma and all necrotic tissue should be debrided promptly after any open fracture. Antibiotics are administered to prevent infection, and the wound is left open. Primary closure is delayed until the wound is clean and there is no evidence of infection.

Gas gangrene is a true surgical emergency that demands immediate attention to preserve life and limb. Once gas gangrene, cellulitis, or myonecrosis develops, treatment must be swift and aggressive. Intravenous administration of fluid and blood is carried out as necessary to treat the systemic complications. Large doses of the appropriate antibiotic are also administered intravenously. It is essential to open the infected wound as soon as possible and perform a radical debridement of all necrotic and infected tissue. This precaution means that frequently the surgical procedures must be repeated every few hours because of the rapid and aggressive nature of the infection. Hyperbaric oxygen treatment should be considered if such a facility is available.

Complications of Fracture
(Continued)

Implant Failure

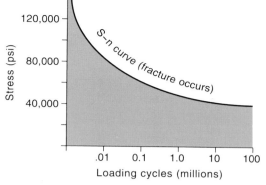

In above test, implant material will fracture with single stress of 140,000 psi. Material fatigues with repeated loading cycles, fracturing at 40,000 psi at 10 million cycles. In walking, estimated average of loading cycles on femur is 1 million/year

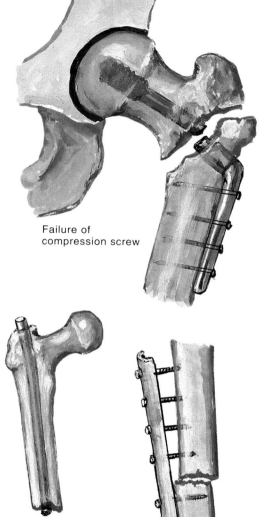

Failure of compression screw

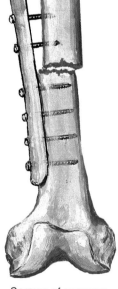

Crutches, brace, or cast provides external support to lessen stress on internal fixation implants during healing of bone

Failure of intramedullary rod

Screws of compression plate pulled loose from osteoporotic femur

Implant Failure

Implant devices used in the internal fixation of fractures may fail with normal use, either by breaking or by loosening (Plate 145). After implantation of an internal fixation device, a race begins between the normal healing process and failure of the device due to metal fatigue. Normal, healthy bone has the ability to remodel, repair, and reinforce itself when subjected to repetitive loading forces, as in walking. However, metal fixation devices subjected to repetitive bending loads weaken and eventually fail, much as paper clips break with repeated bending. Metal fatigue occurs only after many loading cycles, and the fracture usually heals before the device fails. If the fracture repair process is slow or inadequate, the body continues to depend on the implant to withstand stresses on the limb. All implants have a finite life span, and if the fracture fails to heal in the normal time frame, fatigue failure of the implant becomes more and more likely.

Bone mass deficiency may also contribute to implant failure, because stabilization of a fracture with plates and screws depends on the secure fixation of screws in the bone fragments. In bone weakened by osteoporosis or other metabolic bone diseases, the screws pull out, resulting in loss of fracture fixation and loss of reduction. When loads are applied to the fractured limb, the screw fixation is often not secure.

The risk of implant failure can be minimized by protecting the bone from excessive and repetitive stresses until full fracture healing has occurred. If the fixation is not secure, all loads must be avoided until radiographs clearly show evidence of fracture healing. For this reason, patients with osteoporosis who are treated with plate and screw fixation for an intertrochanteric fracture should avoid weight bearing, remaining first in a bed and then in a chair, for 3 months after the injury. Patients can begin protected weight bearing using crutches when fracture healing has been demonstrated. When delayed healing increases the risk of fatigue failure in a metal fixation device, the stresses of weight bearing should be minimized by external support of the fracture through the use of crutches, casts, or braces until adequate healing is documented on radiographs.

If the implant fails, it is usually removed and replaced with another fixation device. Bone autografts are usually incorporated in the revision surgery to expedite the healing process and minimize the risk of repeat implant failure.

Complications of Fracture
(*Continued*)

Malunion of Fracture

A malunion is a functional or cosmetic deformity that persists after fracture healing (Plate 146). The deformity may be angular or rotational or may consist of a discrepancy in length (usually shortening).

Angular Malunion. Supracondylar fractures of the humerus are quite unstable, and reduction is difficult to maintain. Even an acceptable reduction may be lost, and the bone heals with a varus deformity (called gunstock deformity, if severe). The normal carrying angle of the elbow (5°–20°) is decreased or reversed. Despite the abnormal appearance of the elbow, function is not compromised, even with a severe gunstock deformity. Closed reduction and percutaneous pinning, or even open reduction and pinning, of these unstable fractures are used to prevent gunstock deformity. Angular malunions that result in a significant loss of function or cosmetic deformity are best treated with a corrective osteotomy at the site of the original fracture. The alignment of the corrective osteotomy is maintained with a plate and screws or an intramedullary nail. The osteotomy is often supplemented with cancellous bone grafts to ensure healing.

Rotational Malunion. This complication can occur with fracture of any long bone and is very difficult to recognize on standard radiographs. After every fracture reduction, a clinical examination is essential to ascertain that there is no residual rotational malalignment. This is most easily accomplished by comparing the rotational alignment in the injured limb to that of the uninjured limb. Rotational malunions are common in spiral fractures of the second, third, or fourth metacarpal. Residual malalignment is frequently missed because the deformity can be detected only when the fingers are flexed. On flexion of the metacarpophalangeal joints, all four digits should point toward the scaphoid on the medial aspect of the wrist.

Change in Limb Length. Shortening of the limb is a particularly common complication of fractures of long bones, especially if the fracture is significantly displaced or comminuted. Loss of structural support of the skeleton allows the muscles to contract, causing the bone to overlap and the limb to shorten. Moderate shortening of the upper limb does not significantly limit function, and mild shortening in the lower limb is usually well tolerated. A leg length discrepancy greater than ½ inch, however, often results in a limp. Simple shoe lifts compensate for leg length discrepancies between ½ inch and 1 inch, but discrepancies greater than 1 inch usually necessitate surgical treatment.

Malunion of Fracture

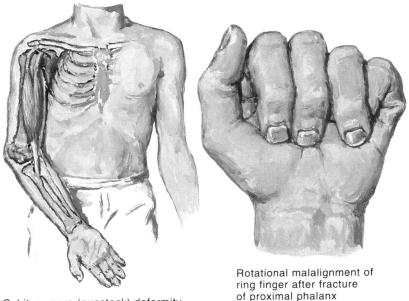

Cubitus varus (gunstock) deformity due to malunion of supracondylar fracture of humerus

Rotational malalignment of ring finger after fracture of proximal phalanx

Fracture of shaft of femur with malunion (shortening)

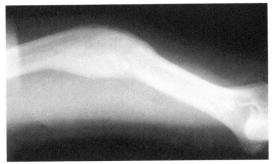

Malunion of shaft of humerus after fracture

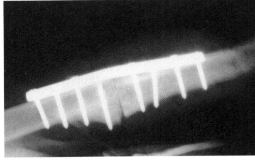

Correction of malunion of humerus with osteotomy and cancellous bone grafts from ilium and fixation with compression plate

For shortened limb in adults, opposite limb may be compensatorily shortened with osteotomy and intramedullary nailing. A. Magnified tip of saw. B. After reaming of medullary canal, saw introduced and two rotary cuts made, demarcating segment of bone to be removed. C. Hook chisel used to split bone segment into several parts and push them out of the way. D. Osteotomy gap closed and intramedullary nail inserted

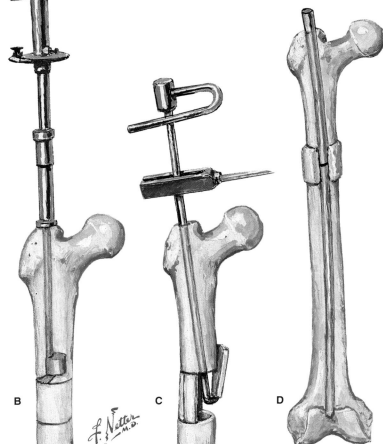

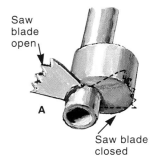

Saw blade open

Saw blade closed

A   B   C   D

Growth Deformity After Fracture

Complications of Fracture
(Continued)

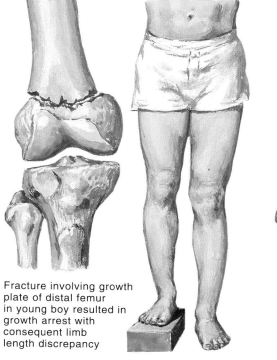

Fracture involving growth plate of distal femur in young boy resulted in growth arrest with consequent limb length discrepancy

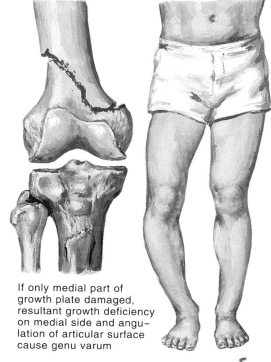

If only medial part of growth plate damaged, resultant growth deficiency on medial side and angulation of articular surface cause genu varum

If limb shortening occurs in a growing child, growth of the longer limb should be arrested with fusion of the growth plate (epiphysiodesis) at the appropriate time, as determined with standardized growth charts (see CIBA COLLECTION, Volume 8/II, page 89). In a young child, a leg length discrepancy of up to 1 inch can be corrected with epiphyseal arrest. In adults, the longer femur is usually shortened with osteotomy. An appropriately sized segment of the femoral shaft is morselized with an intramedullary saw, and the two major fragments of the femoral shaft are reduced and held in anatomic alignment over an intramedullary nail. (See pages 154–157 for other problems of fracture healing.)

Growth Deformity

In children, fractures that involve the growth plate (physis) may require special treatment to prevent a deformity that develops with growth (Plate 147). One of the most common causes of growth deformity is damage to the growth plate, which is responsible for the longitudinal growth of a limb. Particularly in younger children, damage to the growth plate (even though the fracture heals) will arrest limb growth, producing a shortened limb or an angular deformity.

Limb Shortening. Although limb shortening is a risk in virtually any growth plate fracture, it is particularly common in Salter-Harris type V injuries, in which the growth plate is crushed and destroyed (Plate 128). Children with growth plate injuries require periodic reexamination to ascertain that normal bone growth is occurring. Radiographs taken 6 to 9 months after fracture should show an open growth plate and continued longitudinal growth. The physical examination must document that the limb lengths are remaining equal. This determination is most important

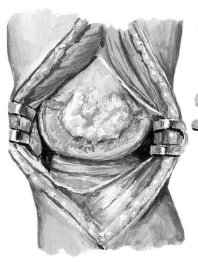

Medial exposure of knee after injury reveals development of bone bridge across one side of growth plate, limiting growth

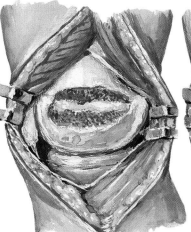

Bone bridge removed with dental burr, revealing normal growth plate underneath

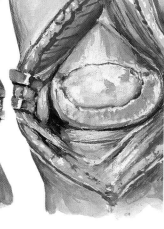

Defect filled with Silastic or autogenous fat to prevent reformation of bone bridge

because modest limb length discrepancies are best treated by stopping the growth of the uninjured limb with epiphysiodesis as soon as complete growth arrest is demonstrated in the injured limb.

Angular Deformity. Partial damage to the growth plate may produce a partial growth arrest. When a portion of the growth plate ceases to grow, an angular deformity results. This particular deformity is frequently seen in the distal femur after a Salter-Harris type II fracture in which the medial portion of the growth plate is damaged (Plate 128). The medial portion of the physis stops growing while the lateral portion continues to grow, producing a varus deformity of the limb. A similar angular deformity can occur in the forearm or the leg when the growth plate of one bone is injured and fuses prematurely, while the remaining bone continues to grow. For example, when a fracture

of the tibia damages the entire proximal or distal growth plate, continued longitudinal growth of the fibula forces the limb into a varus position.

After some growth plate injuries, a bone bridge forms across a portion of the growth plate, arresting growth and creating a significant deformity. To prevent these complications, the bone bridge must be completely removed. Extensive preoperative planning is necessary to identify the extent of the bone bridge. After resection of the bone bridge, Silastic or autogenous fat is packed into the defect to prevent the bridge from reforming. If this surgical procedure is effective in maintaining an open growth plate, longitudinal growth resumes, reducing the risk of further angular deformity. Alternatively, an osteotomy can be performed to correct a residual deformity when the child reaches skeletal maturity.

Posttraumatic Osteoarthritis

Complications of Fracture
(Continued)

Posttraumatic Osteoarthritis

Posttraumatic osteoarthritis is a common consequence of some fracture malunions and also frequently results from intraarticular fractures (Plate 148). A malunion, especially in a lower limb, may create an angular deformity that produces excessive loading stresses on the adjacent joints. A varus deformity of the tibia, for example, puts excessive loads on both the ankle joint and the knee joint. The biomechanical imbalance concentrates the forces on one small area of the articular cartilage, increasing stress and wear on this area. With continued use of the limb, a degenerative process occurs in the articular cartilage and subchondral bone.

Intraarticular fractures are particularly likely to lead to posttraumatic osteoarthritis. Whenever a fracture line extends across the articular surface, the articular cartilage is permanently damaged. The amount of injury can be minimized by anatomic reduction of the articular surfaces. Therefore, virtually all displaced intraarticular fractures require open reduction and rigid internal fixation of the articular fragments to restore joint congruity. However, even if joint congruity is reestablished, the cartilage injury does not fully heal. The smooth hyaline cartilage of the articular surface cannot regenerate, and a fracture through the hyaline articular cartilage is repaired with fibrocartilage. Fibrocartilage does not have the mechanical strength or durability of hyaline cartilage. When this reparative fibrocartilage is subjected to repeated stresses, it wears out, also leading to posttraumatic osteoarthritis. The arthritis may develop in the first few months after fracture healing, or it may develop insidiously with time as the articular surface gradually wears away. Arthritic symptoms may appear 15 to 20 years after the injury.

Conservative management is adequate for mild posttraumatic osteoarthritis. These measures include limitation of activity, avoidance of stress, use of braces and other support devices for walking, and administration of nonsteroidal antiinflammatory drugs (NSAIDs). Severe, disabling osteoarthritis of the hip, knee, or shoulder is best treated with total joint replacement. Total joint replacement restores joint motion and relieves pain by replacing the articular surfaces with plastic and metal prostheses. Arthrodesis (fusion) of the joint is the preferred treatment of degeneration in other joints, particularly the ankle joint and the small joints of the foot and hand. However, although a successful arthrodesis eliminates pain in the arthritic joint, it also sacrifices joint motion.

Osteonecrosis

Osteonecrosis, also called avascular necrosis, is an occasional but severe complication of certain fractures (Plate 149). In healthy bone, a rich blood

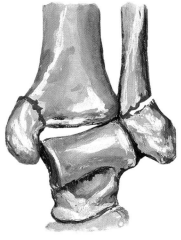
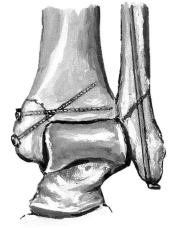
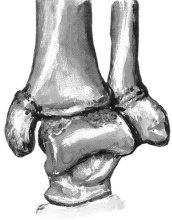

Intraarticular fracture of both malleoli with lateral displacement of talus

Open reduction to restore congruity of articular surfaces and fixation with screws and intramedullary rod essential to avoid posttraumatic osteoarthritis

Posttraumatic osteoarthritis following inadequate reduction of bimalleolar fracture with loss of joint congruity

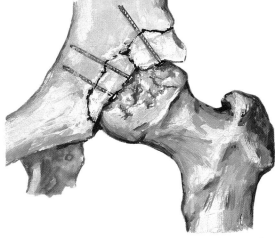
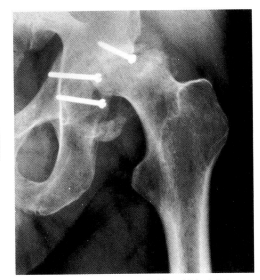

Fracture of acetabulum healed with loss of congruity of articular surface, leading to painful posttraumatic osteoarthritis of hip joint

Posttraumatic osteoarthritis of hip joint after repair of acetabulum fracture. Total hip joint replacement may be indicated for pain relief

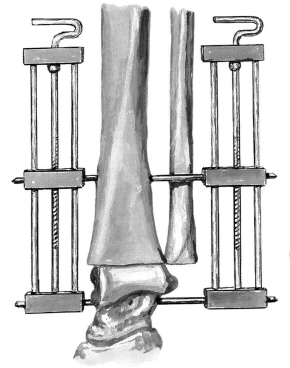
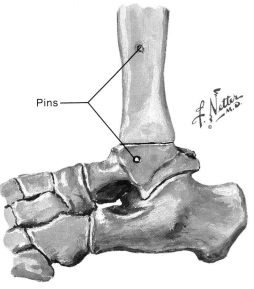

Pins

Ankle arthrodesis with use of compression clamp performed after horizontal resection of articular surfaces of tibia and fibula and proximal portion of articular surface of talus

Lateral view of ankle with compression arthrodesis. Padded cast from below knee to toes applied over compression clamp and worn for 6 weeks, then removed together with clamps and pins. Procedure effectively relieves pain

Complications of Fracture
(Continued)

Osteonecrosis After Fracture

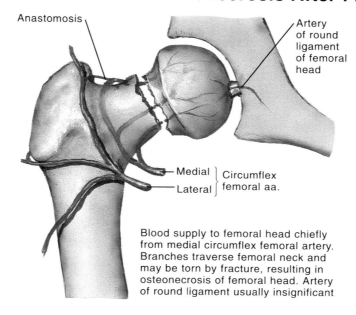

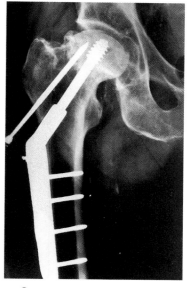

Blood supply to femoral head chiefly from medial circumflex femoral artery. Branches traverse femoral neck and may be torn by fracture, resulting in osteonecrosis of femoral head. Artery of round ligament usually insignificant

Osteonecrosis with collapse of femoral head. Total hip replacement indicated

supply normally provides nourishment and enables the bone both to repair itself following fracture and to remodel when new stresses are applied to it. Osteonecrosis occurs when the blood supply to a segment of a bone is destroyed and the bone cells die. Extensive stripping of soft tissue away from bone, particularly in a high-velocity injury, may render any bone fragment avascular. When a large fragment at a fracture site loses its blood supply, it cannot participate in the normal reparative processes, and delayed union or nonunion may result.

The blood supply to particular segments of certain bones is unique and one directional. Consequently, some specific fracture patterns are especially likely to create an avascular segment of bone. For example, the femoral head is particularly susceptible to osteonecrosis because virtually all the blood vessels to the femoral head traverse the femoral neck. A fracture of the femoral neck disrupts these blood vessels, leaving the head with no blood supply. Similarly, the body of the talus has very few soft tissue attachments and derives virtually all its blood supply from vessels that pass up through the talar neck in a retrograde fashion. A fracture of the neck disrupts these blood vessels and impairs the circulation. Another vulnerable area is the proximal pole of the scaphoid, because its circulation is supplied by blood vessels that enter the distal pole and waist of the bone. A fracture of the waist of the scaphoid, therefore, leaves the proximal pole with inadequate circulation or none at all (Plate 60).

Although the loss of circulation to a major bone segment impairs healing, healing does proceed, because the segment that retains its blood supply often generates sufficient callus to incorporate the avascular segment. Once healing occurs, the body removes the necrotic bone by a process called creeping substitution. In this process, osteoclasts proliferate from the vascularized bone into the necrotic segment and remove the dead bone trabeculae. While this is happening, the necrotic segment is weakened and becomes susceptible to collapse. The process of creeping substitution is slow, taking as long as 3 years for the necrotic bone to be removed and replaced with new osteons. Stress applied to the weakened bone during this time causes it to collapse. This phenomenon, called late segmental collapse, removes the normal underlying support for the articular cartilage of the segment, disturbing the congruity of the adjacent joint surfaces and predisposing to osteoarthritis. If excessive stresses are avoided during the process of creeping substitution, the necrotic segment is eventually replaced with strong viable bone, late segmental collapse does not occur, and the risk of osteoarthritis is minimized.

In the early stage of osteonecrosis, when the dead bone is present and not yet replaced with

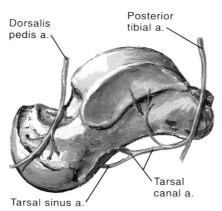

Most nutrient arteries to talus enter neck. Rupture of arteries by fracture may result in osteonecrosis of talar body

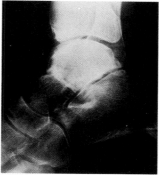

Osteonecrosis of talar body (dead bone appears dense on radiographs)

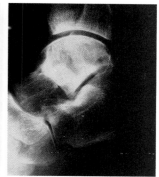

Revascularization (creeping substitution) in progress 1 year later

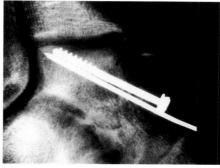

Hawkins sign. Resorption of subchondral bone indicates vascularity of talar body

In some persons, nutrient arteries enter only distal half of scaphoid. Fracture of scaphoid waist results in osteonecrosis of proximal fragment

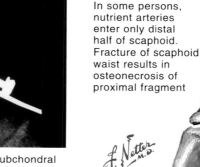

new bone, the avascular segment is characterized by a very dense appearance on radiographs. This apparent increase in density is only relative because the surrounding bone, which is still alive, is undergoing disuse osteoporosis, a normal phenomenon seen in the early stages of fracture healing. Without an adequate blood supply, the necrotic fragment does not become osteoporotic and thus appears relatively dense.

The absence of osteonecrosis can be inferred when Hawkins sign is seen on the radiograph. Hawkins sign is evidence of the resorption of subchondral bone as a consequence of disuse osteoporosis and suggests that the bone segment has adequate

circulation, that normal bone healing is occurring, and that osteonecrosis has not occurred.

Usually, osteonecrosis is a consequence of the pattern of injury, and little can be done to prevent it besides stable anatomic fixation of the fracture. When osteonecrosis is detected, the bone must be protected from excessive stresses until it is fully reconstituted, a process that may take as long as 3 years. During this time, patients should wear a brace or use crutches until radiographs show evidence that the avascular segment has been replaced with new bone. These simple measures reduce the risk of late segmental collapse and the development of osteoarthritis.

Complications of Fracture
(Continued)

Joint Stiffness After Fracture

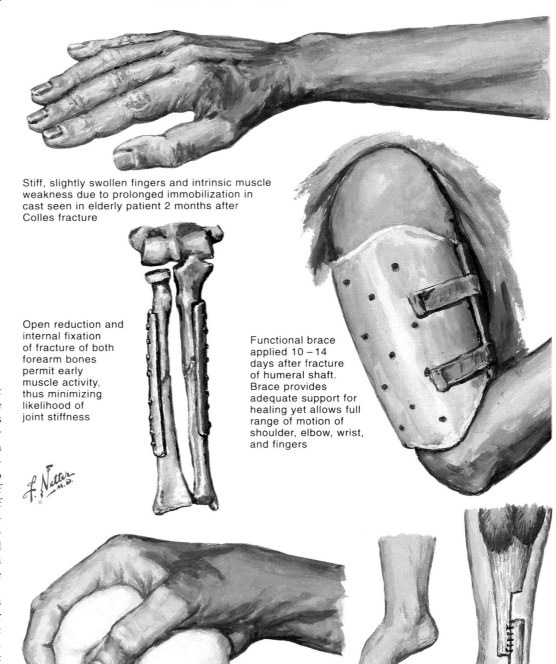

Stiff, slightly swollen fingers and intrinsic muscle weakness due to prolonged immobilization in cast seen in elderly patient 2 months after Colles fracture

Open reduction and internal fixation of fracture of both forearm bones permit early muscle activity, thus minimizing likelihood of joint stiffness

Functional brace applied 10 – 14 days after fracture of humeral shaft. Brace provides adequate support for healing yet allows full range of motion of shoulder, elbow, wrist, and fingers

When stiffness develops or threatens, patient begins gentle passive and active range–of–motion exercises, plus exercises to strengthen atrophic muscles (such as squeezing ball or lump of putty)

Lengthening of Achilles tendon with Z–plasty plus posterior capsulotomy may be needed to correct severe equinus contracture in some patients

Joint Stiffness

Effective immobilization of a fracture in a cast usually includes immobilization of the joints above and below the site of injury (Plate 150). This extensive, prolonged immobilization frequently leads to joint stiffness, which may prove to be a bigger problem than the fracture itself. Immobilization lasting more than a few weeks leads to scarring of the joint capsule and contracture of the muscles, and it also impairs the nutrition of the articular surfaces. With prolonged immobilization, adhesions develop across the articular surfaces, even in joints that had not been injured directly. In addition, prolonged immobilization in a plaster cast results in marked atrophy of the muscles in and around the site of injury.

One of the best examples of this problem is Colles fracture of the distal radius in the older patient (Plate 52). Although this fracture almost always heals, adequate healing takes 8 to 10 weeks. If the limb is immobilized in a cast for this amount of time, severe stiffness of the elbow and wrist may occur, and even the shoulder and finger joints may become stiff. Therefore, again, although the fracture heals, the resulting joint stiffness and muscle atrophy render the arm useless. Rehabilitation of the joints and muscles is a long and difficult process that rarely restores full limb function.

Methods have been developed to ensure adequate fixation of the fracture fragments yet maintain joint motion and muscular activity to prevent the stiffness and atrophy that result from cast immobilization. If joint stiffness appears likely, the fracture is treated with early open reduction and internal fixation. A few days after surgery, the patient resumes gentle active range-of-motion exercises of the adjacent joints. Surgical stabilization and early rehabilitation are most effective in fractures of the shafts of both forearm bones in adults. Open reduction and internal fixation can restore a stable anatomic configuration of the bone architecture, which allows early restoration of motion in the elbow, wrist, and hand.

With certain fractures, such as a fracture of the shaft of the humerus, use of a functional brace

accomplishes the same objectives. Traditional cast immobilization for a fracture of the humeral shaft requires immobilization of the shoulder and elbow joints in a shoulder spica cast. Such immobilization of both joints for 8 to 10 weeks would lead to a significant loss of function. Conversely, a functional brace allows active range of motion in the shoulder and elbow joints yet provides adequate support of the healing fracture. A functional brace is applied 10 to 14 days after injury, once the initial swelling has subsided. The brace is adjustable and can be tightened to provide firm support about the arm and maintain acceptable alignment of the fracture.

When joint stiffness develops, restoring motion requires a long-term rehabilitation program, usually lasting more than 1 year. After the patient regains joint motion with gentle passive range-of-motion exercises, active exercises are begun to strengthen the atrophied muscles. When fixed muscle contractures fail to respond to aggressive and prolonged rehabilitation, surgical release of soft tissue may be necessary as a last resort. One of the most effective soft tissue releases is a Z-plasty lengthening of the Achilles tendon for persistent equinus contracture following injury to the ankle. A posterior capsulotomy may also be needed to restore full mobility of the ankle joint.

Complications of Fracture
(Continued)

Reflex Sympathetic Dystrophy

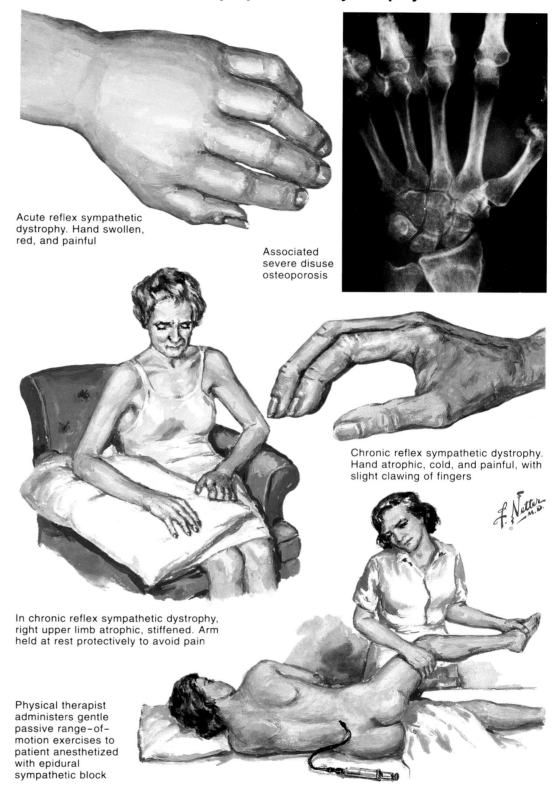

Acute reflex sympathetic dystrophy. Hand swollen, red, and painful

Associated severe disuse osteoporosis

Chronic reflex sympathetic dystrophy. Hand atrophic, cold, and painful, with slight clawing of fingers

In chronic reflex sympathetic dystrophy, right upper limb atrophic, stiffened. Arm held at rest protectively to avoid pain

Physical therapist administers gentle passive range-of-motion exercises to patient anesthetized with epidural sympathetic block

Reflex Sympathetic Dystrophy

In 2% to 3% of patients with limb injuries, a persistent and severe pain develops shortly after the fracture or joint injury has healed (Plate 151). The pain is out of proportion to the severity of the initial injury and often involves the entire limb, not just the injured area. The precise pathophysiology of this disorder is not yet understood. The first clinical manifestations are redness, swelling, and hyperesthesia of the limb at the injury site as well as proximally and distally. Frequently, severe disuse osteoporosis is evident on radiographs. The initial phase of acute pain and hypersensitivity is eventually followed by limb stiffness, loss of function, and severe muscle atrophy. In many patients, the entire limb becomes cold, pale, and useless.

Diagnosis of reflex sympathetic dystrophy is based on clinical and radiographic manifestations, but other procedures may help confirm the diagnosis. Thermography shows asymmetry of skin temperature in a stocking or glove distribution, and skin temperature in the affected limb is often at least 1°F lower than in the opposite limb. In 40% to 60% of patients, technetium 99m bone scans show a generalized increase of radioisotope uptake.

The most effective management of this potential complication is aggressive prevention. Since prolonged immobilization appears to be the most common cause, the patient should be encouraged to begin active range-of-motion exercises as soon as possible after the injury. After immobilization, the patient should gradually resume normal activities, progressively increasing them as the injury heals. A very structured physical or occupational therapy program should be instituted.

Pain must be controlled with the administration of transcutaneous electric stimulation (TENS), mild analgesics, or NSAIDs. Tricyclic antidepressants help decrease anxiety and apprehension. Some patients respond promptly to sympathetic blockade, and a series of sympathetic blocks provides at least temporary relief from pain, allowing the patient to begin a vigorous rehabilitation program. Restoring the limb to pain-free function takes a long time, and patients may need substantial psychologic support during the long rehabilitation period.

Nonunion of Fracture

Test for nonunion

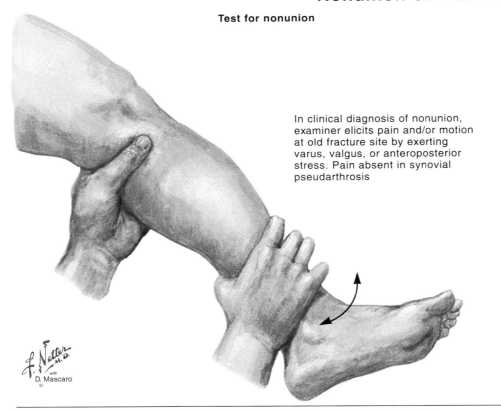

In clinical diagnosis of nonunion, examiner elicits pain and/or motion at old fracture site by exerting varus, valgus, or anteroposterior stress. Pain absent in synovial pseudarthrosis

Synovial pseudarthrosis

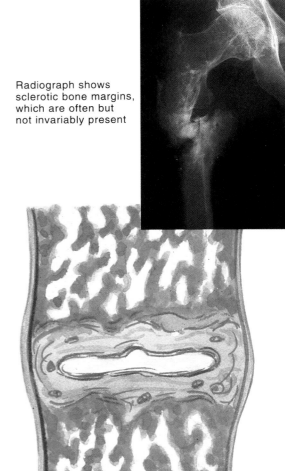

Radiograph shows sclerotic bone margins, which are often but not invariably present

Histologic section shows false joint lined with synovial membrane and filled with fluid

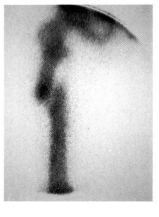

Bone scan shows characteristic increase in radioisotope uptake at both margins of synovial pseudarthrosis with intervening cold area

Fibrous nonunion

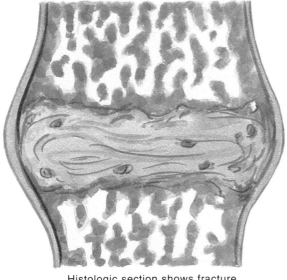

Histologic section shows fracture gap filled with nonossified fibrous cartilage

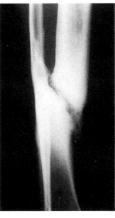

Radiograph shows persistent fracture gap in nonunion of tibia 3 months after injury. Note sclerosis of bone ends

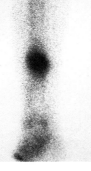

Bone scan demonstrates fibrous nonunion

SECTION I PLATE 152   Slide 4928

Complications of Fracture
(Continued)

Nonunion of Fracture

Normally, when a bone breaks, the fracture heals uneventfully to a solid bony union within a few months. In a typical long bone, such as the tibia, union usually takes about 3 months. Smaller bones heal faster. About 3% to 5% of fractures do not heal, however; these are called nonunions.

In a nonunion, all of the reparative processes in the fractured bone have ceased, but bone continuity has not been restored.

The diagnosis of nonunion is made both clinically and radiographically (Plate 152). On clinical examination of a nonunion, the fracture fragments are still mobile after the appropriate healing time. Radiographs show no bony trabeculae spanning the fracture gap in the anteroposterior, lateral, or both oblique views. If the fracture was treated with an internal fixation device, diagnosis is based entirely on the radiographic evidence.

The causes of nonunion include inadequate reduction or immobilization of the fracture, interposition of soft tissue in the fracture gap, significant soft tissue loss or vascular damage at the

time of the original injury, and osteomyelitis at the fracture site. In some cases, the cause remains unknown.

In most cases of nonunion, histologic examination shows a gap between the fracture fragments that is filled with a combination of fibrous, cartilaginous, and bony tissue. Because the fibrous tissue usually dominates, this type of nonunion is called a fibrous nonunion. In about 12% of nonunions, however, the histologic composition of the fracture gap is quite different. The nonunion site is a cleft filled with fluid and lined with a synoviallike membrane. This type of nonunion, called synovial pseudarthrosis, is usually caused by excessive movement of the fracture fragments during the healing process.

Surgical Management of Nonunion

Complications of Fracture
(Continued)

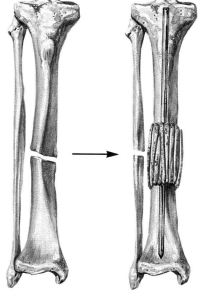

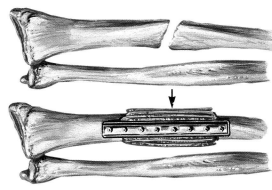

Nonunion of tibia. Fixation with intramedullary device plus matchstick bone autografts from ilium. Short segment of fibula excised to permit growth-stimulating compression of tibia

Nonunion of radius. Firm fixation with compression plate plus matchstick bone autografts

The diagnosis of synovial pseudarthrosis is based on two factors: (1) manipulation of the nonunion site produces excessive motion but no pain, and (2) the nonunion has been present for a considerable time, usually more than 1 year. On routine radiographic examination, the ends of the bone fragments appear rounded and sclerotic, producing a mortar-and-pestle appearance. The diagnosis is frequently confirmed with a technetium 99m bone scan. As in all nonunions, the bone fragments show an intense uptake of the radioisotope, but in synovial pseudarthrosis, a cold cleft is visible between the bone fragments on at least one of the radiographic views (anteroposterior, lateral, and both obliques).

Surgical Management of Nonunion

Bone graft surgery is the gold standard in the treatment of nonunion (Plate 153). In the surgical management of fibrous nonunion, only enough soft tissue is reflected back from the bone fragments to adequately expose the nonunion site. The material between the fractured bone ends (which usually consists of fibrous, cartilaginous, and bony tissue) is not excised. Fresh iliac bone autograft, cut in matchstick strips, is laid in and around the nonunion site, completely surrounding the bone. The bone graft is usually supplemented with some form of internal fixation—either an intramedullary rod (for nonunion of the femur) or a plate and multiple screws.

In the treatment of synovial pseudarthrosis, an entirely different procedure is performed. All of the synoviallike tissue is removed from between and around the nonunion fragments. If this tissue is not thoroughly removed, the synovial pseudarthrosis may recur. After complete excision of this material, bone autograft is packed in and around the nonunion fragments. Internal fixation is invariably required to secure a synovial pseudarthrosis because the fracture fragments are excessively mobile (which caused the synovial pseudarthrosis to form in the first place).

In nonunion of the tibia, some surgeons excise a short segment of the intact fibula to permit compression of the tibial fragments. The compression, which stimulates bone formation, results in slight shortening of the limb. However, once the nonunion has healed, a heel lift in the shoe easily compensates for the slight leg length discrepancy.

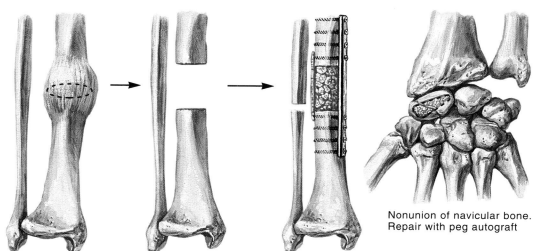

Nonunion of navicular bone. Repair with peg autograft

Synovial pseudarthrosis of tibia. Bone margins, synoviallike tissue, and false joint cavity between bone ends excised. Gap filled with cancellous and cortical bone autografts. Fracture site rigidly secured with compression plate. Fibula osteotomized to allow compression of tibia

Free vascularized bone graft in large bone defects

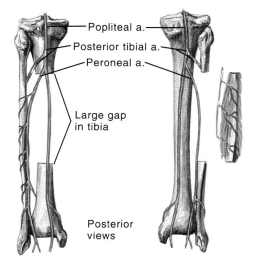

Popliteal a.
Posterior tibial a.
Peroneal a.

Large gap in tibia

Posterior views

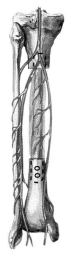

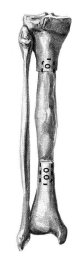

Large gap in tibia to be filled with free vascularized bone autograft from fibula. Rib or iliac crest alternate donor site

Appropriate segment of contralateral fibula excised with cuff of muscle and vascular pedicles containing nutrient artery

Vascularized fibular segment secured in tibial defect. Vessels anastomosed with microsurgical technique

With time, implanted segment of fibula grows in diameter, eventually matching tibia in strength

Experimental Electric Stimulation of Bone Growth

Complications of Fracture

(Continued)

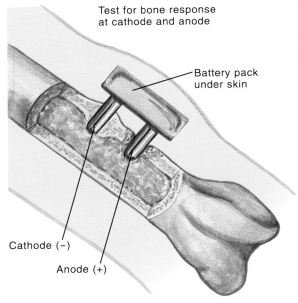

Test for bone response
at cathode and anode

Battery pack
under skin

Cathode (−)

Anode (+)

Cathode and anode electrodes inserted in drill
holes in femur of rabbit, with battery pack under
skin. Constant direct current applied for 18 days.
At currents between 5 μA and 20 μA, new bone
formed around cathode but only necrosis occurred
around anode. Current under 5 μA produced
no effect, and current over 20 μA caused
necrosis around both cathode and anode

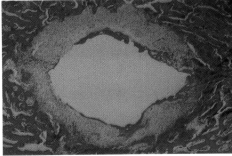

Section of bone at site of cathode. Small area
of pink debris around cathode hole, then area
of cartilage, surrounded by large zone of new
bone formation

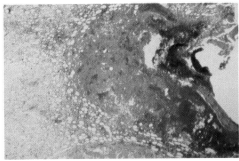

Section at anode site shows only necrosis

Experiment for best location of cathode

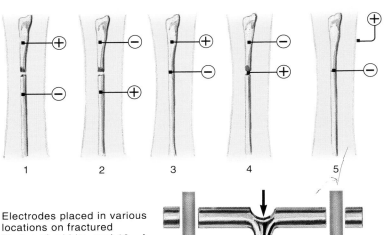

1   2   3   4   5

Electrodes placed in various
locations on fractured
fibulas of rabbits, and 10 μA
current applied for 18 days.
Significantly greater healing
occurred when cathode
placed directly in fracture
site (fibulas 3 and 5).
Degree of healing evaluated
by measuring resistance to
bending with apparatus
at right

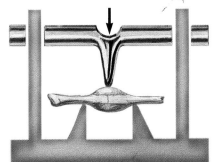

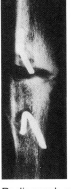

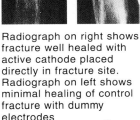

Radiograph on right shows
fracture well healed with
active cathode placed
directly in fracture site.
Radiograph on left shows
minimal healing of control
fracture with dummy
electrodes

f. Netter
with
D. Mascaro

The incidence of nonunion after fracture is higher in the navicular than in most other bones. The nonunion is usually treated surgically with a peg of autograft bone inserted in the medullary cavity of both fragments.

Severe injuries or open fractures in which large segments of bone are lost may create a large bone defect at the nonunion site. The routine method of bone grafting with autogenous bone may not be successful for large defects. A free vascularized bone graft is frequently used to heal this type of nonunion. The midshaft of the fibula with the accompanying arterial supply is typically used as the free vascularized graft, although a rib or iliac crest is an alternative donor site. An appropriate segment of the contralateral fibula is excised along with a cuff of muscle and vascular pedicle containing a nutrient artery. The vascularized fibular segment is secured between the nonunion fracture fragments, and the vessels are anastomosed using microsurgical technique. The nonunion containing the vascularized fibular graft must be protected with a cast or brace until a solid bony union develops between the host bone and both ends of the vascularized graft. The diameter of the free vascularized graft from the fibula is obviously smaller than that of the host tibia or femur. However, with time and use, the fibular graft tends to hypertrophy, and its diameter may eventually approach that of the host tibia or femur. During this period of bone remodeling, however, the limb must be protected with a brace.

Experimental Electric Stimulation of Bone Growth

The unique electric properties of bone were discovered in the 1950s. When bone is mechanically deformed, the side of bone under compression becomes electronegative and the side of bone under

tension becomes electropositive. In the 1960s, researchers discovered that active areas of bone growth and repair were electronegative in relation to less active areas. These findings led to a series of experiments by different investigators (Plate 154). In studies on laboratory animals, electrodes were inserted through drill holes in the cortex of a long bone, with the free ends of the electrodes extending into the medullary canal. Using constant direct current of various intensities, the researchers explored the relationship between the application of electric current and new bone formation. When the current levels were between 5 and 20 microamperes (μA), new bone formed around the cathode

(negative electrode) in the medullary canal. When the current was less than 5 μA, no bone formed around the cathode, and current of more than 20 μA led to necrosis around both the cathode and the anode (positive electrode).

Another series of experiments was performed to determine if electricity could augment fracture repair in laboratory animals. The anode and cathode were placed in various configurations in relation to the fracture site in the fibula of a rabbit. Results showed that fracture healing increased only when the cathode was positioned directly in the fracture site. The augmentation of fracture healing by electricity was determined by testing

Complications of Fracture
(Continued)

Pulsed Inductive Coupling Method of Electric Stimulation of Bone Growth (method of Bassett et al)

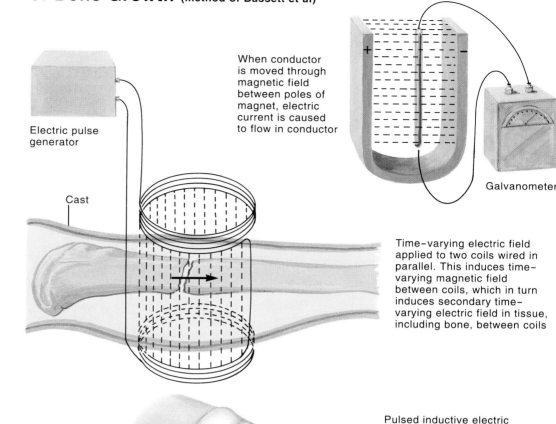

Electric pulse generator

Cast

When conductor is moved through magnetic field between poles of magnet, electric current is caused to flow in conductor

Galvanometer

Time–varying electric field applied to two coils wired in parallel. This induces time-varying magnetic field between coils, which in turn induces secondary time-varying electric field in tissue, including bone, between coils

Pulsed inductive electric stimulation system. Coil units applied by patient at home for 8–10 hours a day. Placement of coils critical and centered over site of nonunion. Placement predetermined radiographically. When healing has progressed (usually after 12 weeks or more), electric treatment stopped and axial compression exercises begun. Treatments may be repeated, if necessary

F. Netter M.D.
with D. Mascaro ©

the mechanical integrity of the fracture callus. Although the location of the cathode was critical for the stimulation of fracture healing, the location of the anode was not important; that is, as long as the anode made electric contact and completed the circuit, it made no difference whether it was placed in the bone, on the surface of the skin, or anywhere in between.

Based on these findings, clinical trials were performed in which cathodes delivering 20 μA each were inserted into the nonunion site by two different methods: (1) percutaneous insertion under radiographic control or (2) surgical implantation, using an open procedure. In the percutaneous technique, a battery pack was connected to the portion of the cathodes that protruded externally through the skin. In the invasive method, a very small implantable battery pack was connected to the cathodes and placed into the subcutaneous tissue under the skin. The clinical trials demonstrated that direct current could heal a nonunion in about the same time and with the same rate of success as bone graft surgery. These methods were soon approved by the Food and Drug Administration for use in treating nonunion.

Noninvasive Coupling Methods of Electric Stimulation of Bone

Two entirely noninvasive techniques can be used to apply electricity to bone (Plate 155). The first, the inductive coupling method, takes advantage of the fact that an electric current is caused to flow in a conductor when the conductor is moved through a magnetic field between the poles of a magnet. When a time-varying electric field is applied to two coils placed on either side of a limb, a time-varied magnetic field is produced between the coils, which in turn induces a sec-

ondary time-varying electric field in the tissues, including bone, between the coils.

Pulsed Inductive Coupling Method. In the treatment of nonunion, coils are placed around the cast on the limb and, with radiographic guidance, are centered directly over the nonunion site. An asymmetric pulse signal is applied for 8 to 10 hours daily. The inductive coupling method heals a nonunion in about the same amount of time as do direct current and bone graft surgery, and the rate of successful healing is also about the same for the three techniques.

Capacitive Coupling Method. In this second noninvasive method of applying electricity to a

nonunion, capacitor plates or electrodes are placed on the surface of the skin on either side of the underlying nonunion. A time-varying electric field is applied to the electrodes, which induces a secondary time-varying electric field in the tissues, including bone, between the electrodes. This noninvasive treatment also takes approximately the same amount of time as the other electric treatments and bone graft surgery and has approximately the same degree of success.

The pulsed inductive coupling and capacitive coupling methods have both been approved by the Food and Drug Administration for use in the treatment of nonunion. □

Section II
Infection

Frank H. Netter, M.D.

in collaboration with

James D. Heckman, M.D. *Plates 6 – 18*
Ronald L. Linscheid, M.D. *Plates 1 – 5*

Infections of Hand

Infected Wounds of Hand and Fingers

(Note: a thorough knowledge of the anatomy of the hand is essential for the proper treatment of hand infections. Please refer to CIBA COLLECTION, Volume 8/I, pages 55–73.)

Before the introduction of antibiotics, infections of the hand often led to prolonged morbidity, severe deformity, amputation, and even death. Kanavel's classic studies on the pathways of purulent infection within the anatomic compartments of the hand opened the modern era of treatment for these problems. Although injuries in the industrial workplace are less prevalent than in Kanavel's time, wounds of the hand still account for a large percentage of hand infections. A high incidence of hand infections is also associated with societal problems, such as intravenous injection of drugs with contaminated needles, wounds inflicted with various weapons in gang-related incidents, and complications of treatment with immunosuppressive agents. Human and animal bites may also have severe consequences.

The evaluation of a hand wound must include the duration of time since the injury, the contamination likely at the site of injury, and the severity of the wound (Plate 1). After the initial evaluation of the patient's neurovascular and musculoskeletal status, the examiner must make a decision about further evaluation and treatment. It is generally better to err on the side of caution and thoroughly inspect the wound under surgical control in the operating room. Regional, intravenous, or general anesthesia is induced. In a fresh wound, exsanguination is performed with an elastic bandage; if the wound is already infected, elevating the limb for 2 minutes reduces the risk of forcing the inflammation deeper into normal tissue. Hemostasis is obtained with an axillary pneumatic or an Esmarch forearm tourniquet.

Foreign material and devitalized tissue are debrided, and the wound is thoroughly irrigated. Pulsed lavage with 3 liters or more of saline solution significantly reduces bacterial contamination. Reducing the bacterial population below 1 million organisms/mm^3 allows the normal immune defenses to control contaminants. After debridement, exposed tendons, vessels, nerves, and joints should be protected, but wound closure should be delayed. Fine-meshed gauze soaked with dilute iodine solution provides moisture and protection to the exposed tissues. The hand is mobilized in a sterile setting before closure. This open treatment followed by repeat debridement at 3 to 5 days and delayed primary closure produces excellent results.

The same approach to postoperative care is appropriate following incision and drainage of abscesses. In the immediate postoperative period, the wrist is generally immobilized in dorsiflexion, the metacarpophalangeal joints in 30° to 40° flexion, and the proximal interphalangeal joints in relative extension. A bulky dressing provides pressure to reduce edema and capillary drainage to extract exudate. These measures minimize the likelihood of joint contractures due to immobility.

Infected Wounds of Hand and Fingers

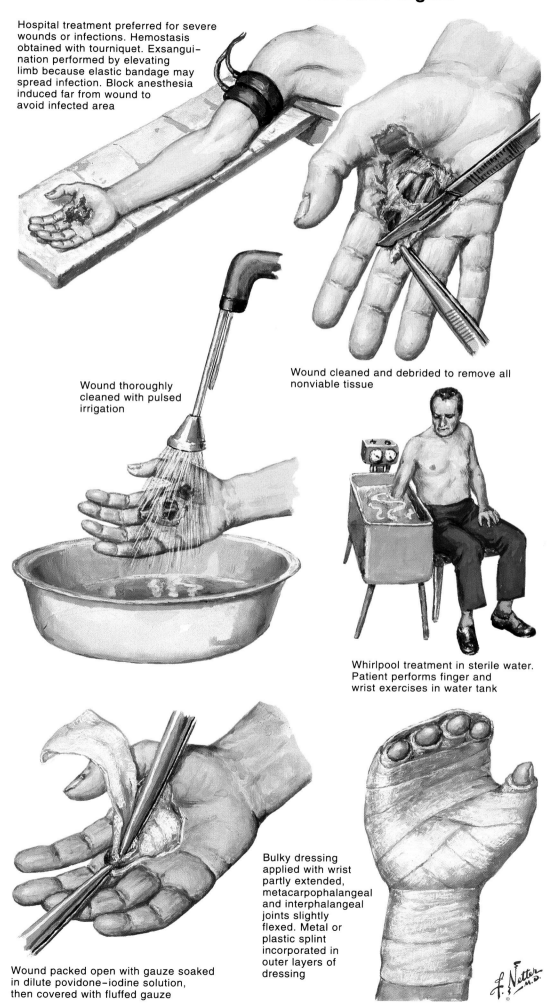

Hospital treatment preferred for severe wounds or infections. Hemostasis obtained with tourniquet. Exsanguination performed by elevating limb because elastic bandage may spread infection. Block anesthesia induced far from wound to avoid infected area

Wound cleaned and debrided to remove all nonviable tissue

Wound thoroughly cleaned with pulsed irrigation

Whirlpool treatment in sterile water. Patient performs finger and wrist exercises in water tank

Wound packed open with gauze soaked in dilute povidone–iodine solution, then covered with fluffed gauze

Bulky dressing applied with wrist partly extended, metacarpophalangeal and interphalangeal joints slightly flexed. Metal or plastic splint incorporated in outer layers of dressing

Infections of Hand
(Continued)

Cellulitis and Epidermal Abscess

If possible, cultures should be obtained before beginning antibiotic therapy for any hand infection. Gram-positive cocci are responsible for most abscesses, particularly those resulting from infections incurred around the home or in the industrial workplace. Wounds due to agricultural or garden accidents are more likely to be contaminated with gram-negative or mixed organisms (Plate 2).

Felon. A felon, or whitlow, may begin as a subepidermal abscess that penetrates a pulp space of the finger. Further extension into adjacent fibrofatty spaces causes distention with severe pain and throbbing. If the spread continues, osteomyelitis of the distal phalanx may result in loss of the tuft, septic arthritis of the distal interphalangeal joint, or tenosynovitis of the flexor tendon sheath.

In the earliest phase, release of the subepidermal abscess and antibiotic treatment may abort the infection. However, when the felon is well established, incision and drainage are imperative. A longitudinal incision is made directly over the site of drainage or necrosis to minimize the chance of injuring a digital nerve. A fish-mouth incision or through-and-through incision is seldom necessary. A wick of gauze is left in the wound for 1 or 2 days, after which irrigation or soaks may be started.

Paronychia. Paronychia usually originates with an undetected break in the eponychium (cuticle) or with a hangnail. Dryness of the skin may be a factor, and the infectious organisms are often supplied from the patient's nasopharynx. The early signs are redness and burning that spread along the nail fold. Pain is often inordinate for the apparent degree of inflammation. At this early stage, gently lifting the eponychium with a No. 11 Bard Parker blade evacuates the pus, allowing the inflammation to resolve without further treatment. A partial finger block suffices for anesthesia.

If untreated, the infection may progress beneath the nail, causing it to loosen. At this stage, excision of the proximal nail produces satisfactory decompression, but the excision often requires a radial incision in the nail fold. Rarely, a mucous cyst simulates a paronychia or actually becomes infected. The infection may progress up the stalk of the cyst to the joint cavity, resulting in a septic distal interphalangeal joint.

Subcutaneous Abscess. Subcutaneous abscesses may occur anywhere in the fingers or hand and usually result from minute breaks in the skin that become infected. They announce their presence with pain, swelling, redness, and turgor. On the dorsum of the hand, abscesses are likely to originate in a hair follicle, or there may be several drainage sinuses that coalesce into a carbuncle.

Subcutaneous abscesses often have a purulent center, which aids identification. Incision and drainage are performed, with suitable regional anesthesia induced proximal to any obvious inflammation and avoiding areas of lymphangitis. The

Cellulitis and Epidermal Abscess

Felon. Line of incision indicated

Purulent drainage

Cross section shows division of septa in finger pulp

Paronychia

Eponychium elevated from nail surface

If subungual space involved, nail flap pulled down and nail root excised

Small gauze wick inserted

Subcutaneous abscess. V–shaped line of incision indicated

Carbuncle treated with incision and drainage

Pyoderma (subepidermal cellulitis) treated with oral antibiotics, not incision

Herpes simplex cellulitis. Usually heals well in 10–14 days if often washed gently and kept covered; not incised

incision is centered over the fluctuant area, placed in skin creases, or angled at them obliquely. The incision should avoid underlying structures, particularly cutaneous nerves.

Pyoderma. Also called subepidermal or vesicular cellulitis, pyoderma is most often seen in children and usually involves the dorsal aspect of the two distal segments of a finger. This infection is often due to *Streptococcus* from the nasopharynx, although both *Staphylococcus* and *Pseudomonas* species may also be present. The blebs may be aspirated and the fluid cultured to obtain definitive diagnosis, but the lesions invariably respond to antibiotics and protection from contact with the mouth.

Pyoderma is highly contagious, and precautions should be taken to avoid spreading it to family members or schoolmates.

Herpes Simplex Cellulitis. A vesicular cellulitis of the hand or fingers due to infection with herpes simplex virus occurs most often in dentists and health care workers. Although the infection is contagious and often quite uncomfortable, it tends to run a benign course: several crops of vesicles develop slowly and heal over 2 to 3 weeks. The vesicles may be punctured under sterile conditions. Involved hands must be kept clean and dry, and the patient must be very careful to avoid further self-contamination or cross-contamination.

Infections of Hand
(Continued)

Tenosynovitis and Infection of Fascial Space

Tenosynovitis. Purulent tenosynovitis can be a devastating infection because it produces adhesions within the tenosynovial canal that markedly limit finger motion. If the infection affects one of the ulnar three fingers, the quadrigia effect may limit motion of the adjacent fingers as well. Once a granulation response has begun, the ability to restore full function is compromised. If treatment is delayed or the antibiotics used are insufficient or ineffective, the infection may convert to a subacute state that produces progressive destruction (Plate 3).

The infection is usually secondary to a puncture wound, and initial onset is insidious. Infection with a virulent organism such as *Staphylococcus*, however, can produce severe pain within a few hours. The four cardinal signs of tendon sheath infection (described by Kanavel) are uniform swelling, fixed flexion, pain on attempted passive extension of the finger, and tenderness along the course of the tendon sheath into the distal palm.

In the thumb and little finger, the tendon sheath usually extends into the radial and ulnar bursae, respectively, allowing infection to spread well into the distal forearm. A communication between the two bursae allows the establishment of a horseshoe abscess that affects both the thumb and the little finger, although effective treatment with antibiotics has made this complication rare. By the time the horseshoe abscess occurs, irrevocable damage to the delicate gliding tissues of the tenosynovial sheath may have occurred. Avascular necrosis of the tendons follows quickly from vincular occlusion and intracompartmental pressure. Less virulent organisms cause a less acute infection, but if they are unrecognized and untreated, the residual effect may be no less detrimental.

A subcutaneous abscess directly over the tendon sheath may be confused with true purulent tenosynovitis. Therefore, if the diagnosis is not clear, incision and drainage should be performed. The initial incision is made over the site of maximum tenderness. If a subcutaneous abscess is found and the underlying sheath appears transparent and free of effusion, further dissection is not necessary. However, if there is effusion, purulence, distention, or thickening and opacity of the sheath, the incision should be extended as a Brunner zigzag incision.

To ensure adequate drainage and perfusion of the sheath, one or more flaps are raised at the sites of the cruciate pulleys. Any fluid should be aspirated and cultured immediately. If the tenosynovial sheath is inflamed, tissue samples should be sent for culture, Gram stain, and histologic examination. Determining the causative organism is essential because a number of unusual organisms, including *Brucella*, *Pasteurella multocida*, and various *Mycobacterium* species, may also induce tenosynovitis.

Tenosynovitis and Infection of Fascial Space

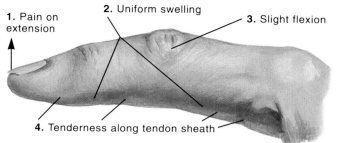

1. Pain on extension
2. Uniform swelling
3. Slight flexion
4. Tenderness along tendon sheath

Tenosynovitis. Four cardinal signs of Kanavel

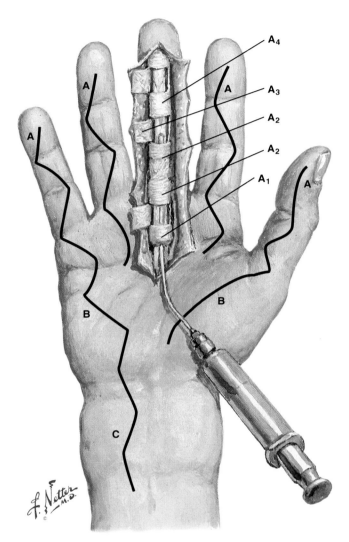

A₄ A A₃ A₂ A₂ A₁ A B B C

Tenosynovitis of middle finger. Treated with zigzag volar incision. Tendon sheath opened by reflecting cruciate pulleys. Fine plastic catheter inserted for irrigation. Lines of incision indicated for tendon sheaths of other fingers (A); radial and ulnar bursae (B); and Parona subtendinous space (C)

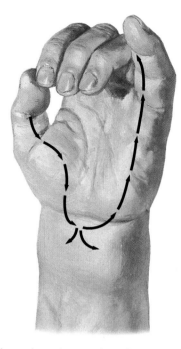

Horseshoe abscess from focus in thumb spreads through radial and ulnar bursae and tendon sheath of little finger, with rupture into Parona subtendinous space

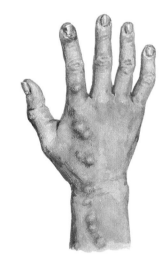

Sporotrichosis. Begins as small nodule and spreads to hand, wrist, forearm (even systemically). This and other mycotic infections (nocardiosis, brucellosis, coccidioido-mycosis, tuberculosis) diagnosed with biopsy and culture

The tendon sheath can be milked by passive movements of the fingers. The sheath may also be irrigated through a small catheter, which is left in place for 1 or 2 days, and the effusion allowed to drain. The skin may be closed loosely to protect the underlying tendon. Active movement of the finger should be started immediately after surgery and continued under supervision. If the ulnar or radial bursa is involved, separate incisions are made at the wrist or the digital incisions extended, with care to preserve the transverse carpal ligament.

Sporotrichosis. Sporotrichum schenckii, a fungus frequently found in soil or on garden plants, produces cutaneous and subcutaneous lesions and inflammation of the lymph vessels (lymphangitis). This indolent infection is characterized by a pilot lesion at the site of inoculation, followed by the appearance of a succession of satellite lesions, which progress proximally along a lymphatic chain. The lesions are raised, red, swollen, and usually about 1 cm in diameter; the center may ulcerate and drain. Pain is minimal. Diagnosis requires isolating the organism from the ulcerations.

The treatment of choice is topical application of potassium iodide, which is effective in the benign form of the disease. Lesions heal in 2 to 3 weeks. Sporotrichosis may remain localized or spread systemically to involve other organ systems.

Infections of Hand

(Continued)

Infection of Deep Compartments

The deep compartments of the hand may become infected by direct inoculation via penetrating wounds or by extension of infection in adjacent areas (Plate 4). Such infections are relatively infrequent, but when present they cause rapid deleterious changes and are prone to spreading. Unless treated with incision and drainage, deep infection may cause permanent deformity.

Infection of Midpalmar Space. The midpalmar space lies under the flexor tendons of the ulnar three fingers and over the deep fascia covering the intrinsic muscles. Ulnarly the hypothenar muscles and radially the adductor pollicis muscle define the space, which is partially separated by fibrous septa that attach the palmar floor to the central ridges of the metacarpal shafts. Purulence may enter or extend through the lumbrical canals or break through into the carpal canal or thenar space.

Symptoms such as pain on movement, swelling, and marked tenderness may rapidly increase in severity. The dorsum of the hand swells as the lymphatic drainage becomes involved. Tenosynovitis may also develop. The diagnosis is suggested by exquisite tenderness over the palm.

Treatment is by incision, which follows skin creases and is centered to allow access to the midpalmar space and retraction of the flexor tendons. The neurovascular bundles must be carefully identified and retracted. Usually, the purulence is under pressure when the midpalmar space is opened, and can be aspirated and the space irrigated. Extensions into adjacent spaces can be identified by massaging the palm, starting at the perimeter. Drains are inserted and kept in place for 1 or 2 days.

Infection of Thenar Space. The thenar space lies under the flexor tendons of the index finger and over the adductor pollicis muscle. The septum to the third metacarpal defines the ulnar border, and the thenar muscles define the radial border. The infection may extend into the lumbrical canal of the index finger and over the distal aspect of the adductor pollicis muscle. A dorsal thenar space infection on the dorsal aspect of the adductor pollicis muscle may dissect under the first dorsal interosseous muscle. An incision along the thenar space must avoid the recurrent motor branch of the median nerve. The nerve is identified by surface anatomic landmarks, using Kaplan's cardinal line intersection with the thenar crease. The incision can be extended distally as a Z-plasty over the first web space.

Collar Button Abscess. These types of abscesses derive their name from the dumbbell contour of the abscess around the margin of the superficial transverse metacarpal ligament in one of the web spaces. Thus, they may present on both dorsal and volar aspects of the hand. Drainage is through a zigzag incision over the distal web space.

Infection of Parona Space. The Parona space lies deep to the flexor tendon sheaths in the distal

Infection of Deep Compartments of Hand

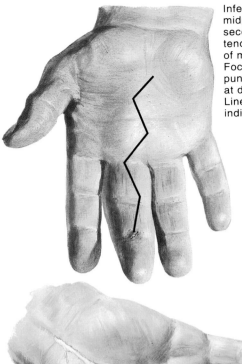

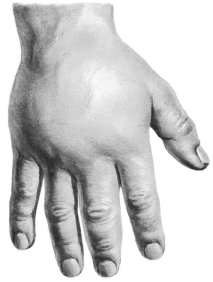

Infection of midpalmar space secondary to tenosynovitis of middle finger. Focus is infected puncture wound at distal crease. Line of incision indicated

Dorsal edema characteristic of palmar infections. Should not be incised unless fluctuant or pointing

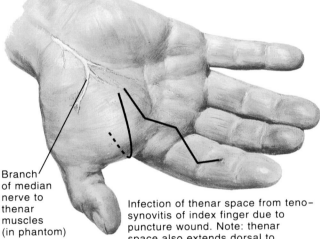

Branch of median nerve to thenar muscles (in phantom)

Infection of thenar space from tenosynovitis of index finger due to puncture wound. Note: thenar space also extends dorsal to adductor pollicis muscle. Line of incision indicated

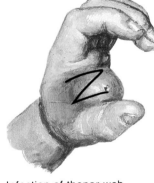

Infection of thenar web space in infant. Incision line for Z-plasty indicated

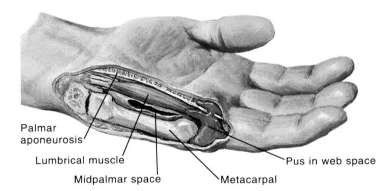

Palmar aponeurosis

Lumbrical muscle

Midpalmar space

Metacarpal

Pus in web space

Sagittal section shows infection of web space (collar button abscess)

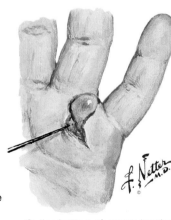

Collar button abscess treated with incision and drainage

forearm and volar to the pronator quadratus muscle. Infections are usually due to direct inoculation or extension from an infection of the tendon sheaths. An abscess may be drained through a direct palmar incision if the radial and ulnar bursae are involved. The median nerve must be identified and protected. If the tendon sheaths are not involved, an incision between the flexor tendons and ulnar neurovascular bundle allows access to the Parona space, as does a direct ulnar incision sliding along the pronator quadratus muscle.

Infections From Human and Animal Bites. Teeth carry a variety of virulent organisms, and a bite may inoculate these organisms deeply into tissues of the hand. Most dogs and cats are carriers of *Pasteurella multocida*, an organism that produces a rapidly spreading inflammation that may penetrate subcutaneous and subfascial spaces as well as tendon sheaths and deep compartments. Human bites carry streptococcal, staphylococcal, spirochetal, and gram-negative organisms. *Eikenella corrodens* is an especially invasive organism that is difficult to eradicate. Penetration of the metacarpophalangeal joint by an incisor may lead to a destructive septic arthritis and dissemination of infection into the adjacent spaces. Treatment of this type of infection requires early recognition, adequate incision and irrigation.

Infections of Hand
(Continued)

Lymphangitis

Lymphangitis often originates from an insignificant break in the skin or a small wound in the hand (Plate 5). Pain and a burning erythema develop at the site of inoculation. Lymphangitic erythematous streaks begin to form over the dorsum of the hand, progressing in just a few hours into the forearm and then into the arm. Pain intensifies and fever and chills develop. The axilla and epitrochlear areas become tender and swollen.

On examination, the patient appears anxious, protects the involved arm, and may shiver with chills. The wound and the lymphangitic streaks are tender to the touch, as are the soft, swollen epitrochlear and axillary nodes. There may be a small serous drainage at the wound site, which should be cultured and Gram stained. Because streptococci are the usual causative organisms, treatment with penicillin or cephalosporin is started immediately. The perimeter of the erythema at the wound site and the lymphangitic streaks can be marked with a pen for later reference, and the size of the nodes is noted. If the infection does not respond to treatment with antibiotics or if the signs worsen in 12 to 24 hours, a culture sample should be obtained by aspiration or incision, or the antibiotic regimen should be changed.

Necrotizing Fasciitis. Also called Meleney ulcer, necrotizing fasciitis is a severe manifestation of lymphangitis that progresses in a frightening manner within a few hours. Anaerobic or microaerophilic streptococci are believed to be the usual cause, but these microorganisms are difficult to culture. Tissue necrosis develops rapidly behind an advancing wall of inflammation that limits penetration by antibiotics. Desquamation followed by gangrene may be relentless. The clinical signs of pain, hyperpyrexia, and chills are severe.

The skin lesions are incised and drained or aspirated to obtain fluid for culture. Intravenous infusion of aqueous penicillin must be instituted immediately; additional antibiotics may be recommended by an infectious disease specialist. The

Lymphangitis

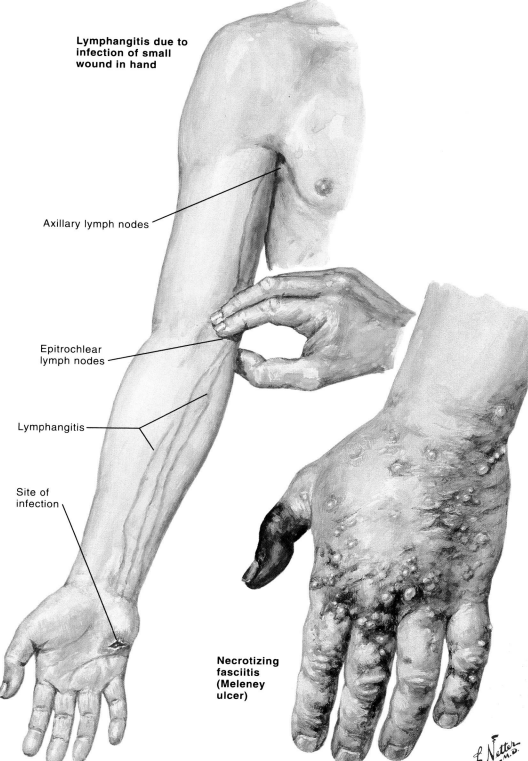

Lymphangitis due to infection of small wound in hand

Axillary lymph nodes

Epitrochlear lymph nodes

Lymphangitis

Site of infection

Necrotizing fasciitis (Meleney ulcer)

f. Netter M.D.

progress of the inflammation and necrosis must be carefully monitored. Even when the necrotizing lymphangitis is controlled early, however, autoamputation may be a sequela, and death is an occasional outcome.

Other Hand Infections. The preceding discussion is merely an introduction to the greater scope of infections of the hand. Mycobacterial tenosynovitis and arthritis still occur. *Mycobacterium marinum* is an organism frequently associated with injuries due to marine activities. Gonococcal septic arthritis rapidly destroys involved joints. Rare invaders of the musculoskeletal system are fungal infections, including coccidioidomycosis and

blastomycosis. *Clostridium perfringens* may colonize crushed muscle in the hand, producing gas gangrene (see Section I, Plate 144). Rare viral infections transmitted from domestic animals occasionally produce lesions on the hand, and inflammation that mimics infection (eg, calcium pyrophosphate dihydrate disease) should also be considered in the diagnosis.

The introduction of antibiotics has dramatically improved the prognosis for infections of the hand. For optimal treatment, however, the correct diagnosis must be established, the organism identified, the purulence drained, and an appropriate rehabilitation program instituted. □

Common Infections of Foot

Infections of Foot

Ingrown Toenail

Ingrown toenail is one of the most common foot problems (Plate 6). Usually affecting the great toe, ingrown toenail may involve the medial or the lateral skin fold. First, the toenail grows underneath the skin fold. Continual longitudinal growth of the toenail puts pressure on the undersurface of the skin fold, creating an area of inflammation and swelling that becomes infected secondarily. Wearing tight shoes that pinch the lateral skin fold between the shoe and the underlying toenail often precipitates or aggravates the problem.

Ingrown toenail is best prevented with proper toenail-trimming techniques. The toenail should be allowed to grow beyond the lateral skin fold and should be cut straight across, not rounded at the corners. The risk of ingrown toenail is minimized by making sure that the square edge of the nail extends beyond the skin fold and by wearing well-fitting shoes.

An inflamed, ingrown nail is treated initially with removal of all compressive shoes and stockings, soaking of the foot in warm water, and oral administration of antibiotics if seropurulent drainage or extensive cellulitis is evident about the nail. If the inflammation or infection fails to resolve with these measures, surgical excision may be required. Longitudinal incisions are made at the base of the hypertrophic skin fold and at a point approximately one quarter of the width of the toenail; the hypertrophic skin fold and underlying granulation tissue are excised en bloc. The entire length of this portion of the toenail is removed, with special attention given to complete excision of the nail matrix.

The nail matrix is a dense white structure lying at the most proximal margin of the toenail. Failure to fully excise the nail matrix leads to regrowth of the toenail and creates the potential for the recurrence of an ingrown toenail. After partial excision of the toenail and the surrounding granulation tissue, the patient is given broad-spectrum oral antibiotics and encouraged to soak the toe twice a day in warm water. The excised area heals by secondary intention.

Fungal Infection of Toenail

Chronic fungal infections of the skin, particularly athlete's foot, may eventually lead to infection of the nail bed and a condition called onychomycosis. The fungal infection causes the toenail to become hypertrophic, deformed, yellow, and friable (Plate 6). Once established, a fungal infection is virtually impossible to eradicate.

Conservative treatment includes simple trimming of the toenail to maintain an approximation of the normal shape and appearance. When the toenail becomes severely deformed and thickened, it may cause painful pressure on the adjacent skin. Occasionally, pressure from large, deformed nails creates a secondary, low-grade cellulitis around the periphery of the nail. Removal of the toenail may be necessary to decrease the pain and inflammation.

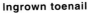

Ingrown toenail

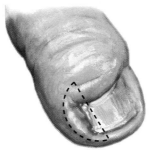

Broken lines show lines of incision for excision of lateral ¼ of toenail, nail bed, and matrix

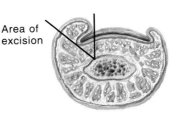

Area of excision

En bloc excision includes nail matrix

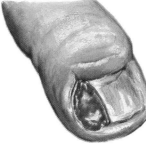

After excision, wound allowed to granulate

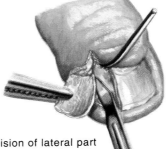

En bloc excision of lateral part of toenail, nail bed, and matrix

JOHN A. CRAIG —AD
& D. Mascaro

Fungal infection of toenail

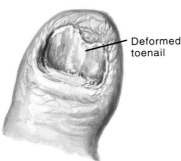

Deformed toenail

Toenail deformity caused by chronic fungal infection

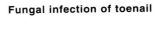
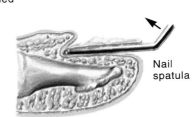

Nail spatula

Toenail plate freed from nail bed and proximal nail fold

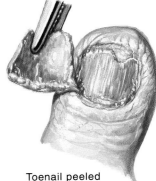

Toenail peeled away from nail bed, using clamp

Puncture wound

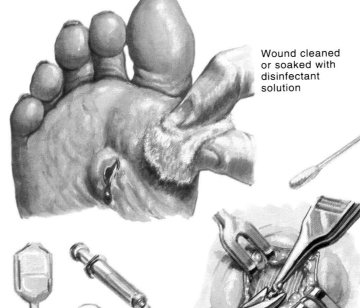

Wound cleaned or soaked with disinfectant solution

Specimens obtained for culture of aerobic and anaerobic bacteria

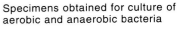

Wound debrided

Tetanus prophylaxis and intravenous administration of antibiotics

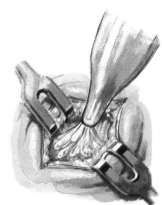

Wound copiously irrigated

Infections of Foot

(Continued)

Deep Infections of Foot

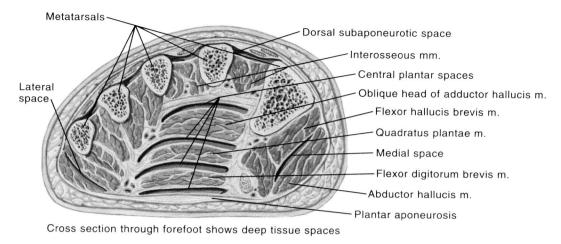

Cross section through forefoot shows deep tissue spaces

Metatarsals

Lateral space

Dorsal subaponeurotic space
Interosseous mm.
Central plantar spaces
Oblique head of adductor hallucis m.
Flexor hallucis brevis m.
Quadratus plantae m.
Medial space
Flexor digitorum brevis m.
Abductor hallucis m.
Plantar aponeurosis

After administration of local anesthesia, the surgeon may elevate the toenail from its bed and remove it entirely. Avulsion of the toenail in this manner provides temporary relief; however, as the toenail regrows, the fungal infection persists and the toenail deformity recurs. The only way to eliminate the problem completely is by surgical excision of the entire toenail and its matrix.

Puncture Wound

Puncture wound of the foot remains one of the most common presenting injuries seen in hospital emergency departments (Plate 6). The sole of the foot is highly vulnerable to puncture by sharp objects hidden from sight. Although shoes provide some protection from injury, large, sharp objects such as nails can pierce the sole of the shoe and penetrate the foot. Most patients come to the emergency department for tetanus prophylaxis. Although tetanus, which is caused by *Clostridium tetani*, is a theoretical complication of a puncture wound, such an infection is exceedingly rare because of widespread effective immunization. On the other hand, penetration of the sole of the foot by contaminated, sharp objects may seed the foot with other aggressive bacteria that can produce extensive local infection. Gram-positive cocci (*Staphylococcus* and *Streptococcus*) remain common causes of foot infection after puncture wounds, but a surprisingly large number of infections are due to gram-negative organisms, particularly *Pseudomonas aeruginosa*. It has been postulated that this pathogen resides in the sole of the shoe and is carried into the foot when the puncturing object penetrates both the shoe and the foot. Gram-negative infections can be quite aggressive, particularly if the puncture wound extends to bone, causing osteomyelitis.

To avoid the development of significant infection after a puncture wound, adequate tetanus prophylaxis is administered and the wound is soaked. The skin edges of the puncture wound should be sharply excised, and the depths of the wound debrided of all necrotic tissue and foreign bodies left in the foot. After debridement, the wound is thoroughly irrigated and left open. Some surgeons recommend administration of a short course of intravenous antibiotics to help prevent infection.

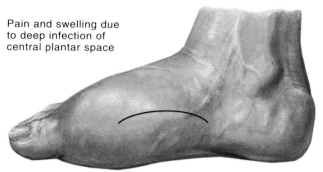

Pain and swelling due to deep infection of central plantar space

Incision site for drainage of central plantar spaces

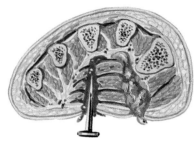

Puncture wound or perforating ulcer may penetrate deep central plantar spaces, leading to abscess

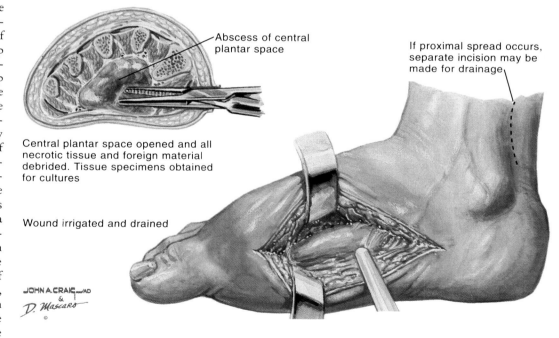

Abscess of central plantar space

Central plantar space opened and all necrotic tissue and foreign material debrided. Tissue specimens obtained for cultures

Wound irrigated and drained

If proximal spread occurs, separate incision may be made for drainage

JOHN A. CRAIG—AD
& D. Mascaro

Deep Infection

A neglected puncture wound of the foot may lead to an extensive deep infection in the foot, causing fever, pain, diffuse swelling, and redness of the foot within a few days of injury. The sole of the foot has five separate fascial compartments in which infection may be localized (Plate 7). The central plantar space is particularly susceptible to the accumulation of a large abscess.

A well-established abscess in one of the closed spaces of the foot must be treated with surgical incision and drainage. The central space of the plantar aspect of the foot is best approached

through a medial foot incision, which reflects the abductor hallucis muscle plantarly and allows both access to the central space and visualization of the critical neurovascular structures coursing to the toes. All necrotic and infected tissue is debrided and the wound thoroughly irrigated and left open. Either repeated wet-to-dry dressings applied to the wound or repeated debridement in the operating room may be needed to eradicate the infection.

Tissue specimens are obtained for culture and broad-spectrum antibiotics administered. Appropriate antibiotics are administered when cultures identify the infective organism.

Infections of Foot

(Continued)

Lesions in Diabetic Foot

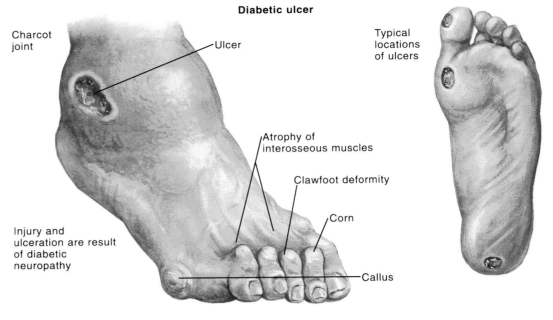

Diabetic ulcer

Charcot joint

Ulcer

Typical locations of ulcers

Atrophy of interosseous muscles

Clawfoot deformity

Corn

Injury and ulceration are result of diabetic neuropathy

Callus

Infection

Cross section through forefoot shows abscess in central plantar space. Infection due to impaired immune response, skin defects, and poor perfusion

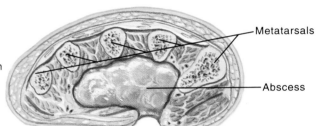

Metatarsals

Abscess

Gangrene

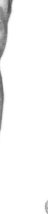

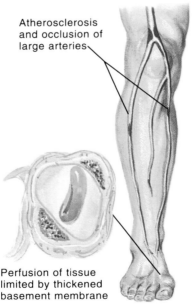

Atherosclerosis and occlusion of large arteries

Perfusion of tissue limited by thickened basement membrane

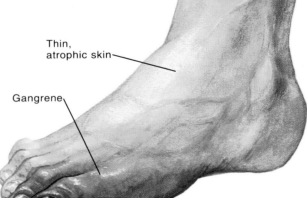

Hair loss

Thin, atrophic skin

Gangrene

JOHN A. CRAIG—AD
& D. Mascaro

Lesions in Diabetic Foot

Infections of the foot are extremely common in patients with diabetes mellitus (Plate 8). Several factors combine to increase the risk of foot infections in the diabetic patient. Diabetes produces a typical pattern of sensory neuropathy that results in loss of protective sensation in the feet and hands in a stocking or glove distribution. Consequently, the foot is more susceptible to injury; in particular, the skin may be blistered, cut, or otherwise injured without the patient's awareness. Once an open wound develops, it is likely to become infected, because the patient with diabetes mellitus has an impaired immune response and cannot fight infection effectively. In addition, the patient frequently has impaired circulation, particularly to the skin and soft tissues of the foot, because of arteriosclerotic vascular disease and because of a specific thickening of the capillary basement membrane. Such abnormalities combine to impair vascular inflow and perfusion of oxygen to the local tissues of the foot, further impeding the normal healing process.

These factors make the patient with diabetes mellitus particularly susceptible to the development of ulcerations over bony prominences on the toes and under the metatarsal heads. The ulcerations may become infected with aggressive and virulent bacteria, creating extensive deep abscesses in the foot or actual gangrene of all or part of the foot. Gangrene usually results from significant impairment of vascular perfusion to the foot. Occasionally, a local infection in the foot spreads rapidly, ascending the leg and causing necrotizing fasciitis and life-threatening septicemia.

Clinical Evaluation of Patient

Because of the severity of these infections, foot lesions in all diabetic patients must be evaluated carefully (Plate 9). The patient with a foot infection must be examined for signs and symptoms of sepsis (fever, elevated leukocyte count, and excessively elevated blood glucose levels). In addition, the level of serum albumin and the total lymphocyte count in the circulating blood can be used as guides to the patient's immune system and nutritional status. A serum albumin level greater than 3.0 g/dl and a serum total lymphocyte count greater than 1,500 cells/mm³, are indirect

indications of a healthy immune system and an adequate nutritional status.

The patient's vascular status must be evaluated as well. A clinical examination should be carried out to palpate the peripheral pulse and assess capillary refill in the toes. Skin temperature and turgor are also assessed. The amount of oxygen available to the tissues to fight infection and heal the wound can be estimated by measuring the transcutaneous oxygen tension. When oxygen tension is extremely low (<30 mmHg), the wound will probably not heal and any infection present will progress. The adequacy of perfusion of the tissues is judged by calculating the ankle/arm

Infections of Foot
(Continued)

index. The ankle/arm index is a ratio of the systolic blood pressure in the lower limb to that in the upper limb. A ratio below 0.45 indicates that perfusion of the tissues is inadequate, increasing the likelihood of gangrene and the failure of wound healing in the ankle and foot.

Wagner categorized diabetic foot ulcerations into five grades based on the natural history of the lesions: grade I, noninfected ulcer; grade II, noninfected deep ulcer; grade III, deep infection of the soft tissues and bone; and grades IV and V, ulcerations with gangrene of some (grade IV) or most (grade V) of the tissues of the foot. The process is potentially reversible for all grades, except grades IV and V. This classification system is useful in monitoring the progression of diabetic foot ulcers and devising treatment. Therefore, all ulcerations should be graded at the beginning of treatment.

Successful treatment of diabetic foot ulcers depends on several factors. The patient's nutritional and immune status should be maximized, and the diabetes must be well controlled to prevent ketoacidosis. The infected area must have adequate vascular perfusion. If the blood supply is impaired, operative intervention may be necessary to improve large-vessel perfusion of the ischemic limb. The local area of infection must be promptly surgically debrided of all necrotic or infected tissue. Repeated debridement, combined with open drainage and frequent dressing changes, is often necessary to control these very aggressive infections. Broad-spectrum antibiotics are administered immediately, followed by specific antibiotics as soon as the infective organism is identified with tissue cultures.

In some patients, extensive infection or gangrene develops despite aggressive and thorough treatment, and the infected limb cannot be saved. In diabetic patients, what begins as a simple infection may result in amputation of the limb. □

Clinical Evaluation of Patient With Diabetic Foot Lesion

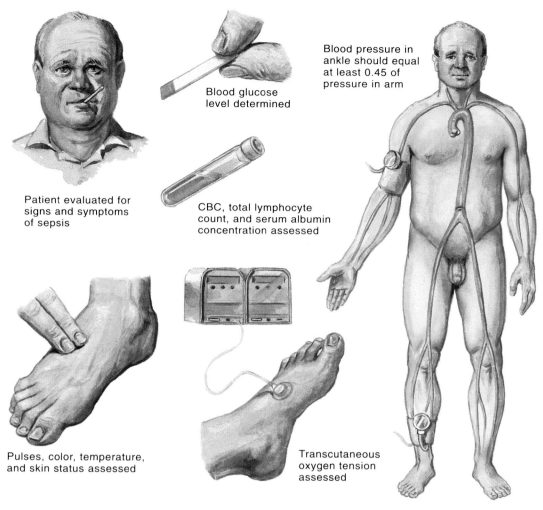

Patient evaluated for signs and symptoms of sepsis

Blood glucose level determined

CBC, total lymphocyte count, and serum albumin concentration assessed

Blood pressure in ankle should equal at least 0.45 of pressure in arm

Pulses, color, temperature, and skin status assessed

Transcutaneous oxygen tension assessed

Wagner classification of diabetic foot lesions

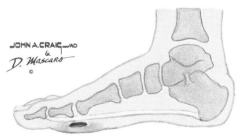

Grade 0. No open lesion

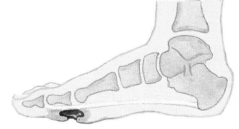

Grade I. Noninfected superficial lesion

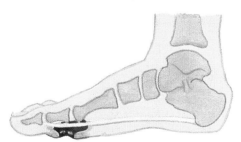

Grade II. Noninfected deep lesion

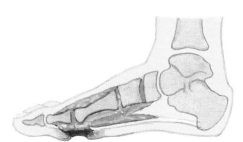

Grade III. Abscess and osteitis

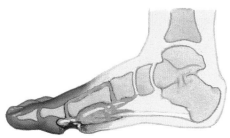

Grade IV. Gangrene of forefoot

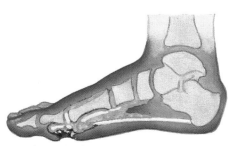

Grade V. Gangrene of entire foot

Septic Joint

Septic Bursitis

The human body contains more than 150 bursae, which are sacs or potential spaces lined with a synovial membrane and containing synovial fluid. Bursae, located in the subcutaneous tissue over bony prominences, permit virtually friction-free movement of the skin over these prominences, minimizing irritation. With excessive irritation or use of a joint, a bursa can become swollen as more synovial fluid is produced to lubricate the movement of adjacent tissues (Plate 10). The bursal swelling becomes chronic and persistent, leading to conditions such as housemaid knee.

Direct trauma to the skin overlying the bursa can seed the fluid in a swollen bursa with bacteria. The fluid is an excellent medium for bacterial growth, and the infection leads to extensive cellulitis, characterized by heat, swelling, marked local tenderness, and loss of range of motion of the adjacent joint.

Treatment of septic bursitis consists of needle aspiration of the bursa to obtain fluid for culture, administration of appropriate antibiotics, and continuous application of warm, moist compresses to the area of inflammation. If the infected bursa does not respond quickly to such local treatment, it should be incised and drained.

Septic Arthritis

Septic arthritis occurs when a joint is seeded with an infective organism, either by direct contamination through traumatic or operative penetration of the joint, by contiguous spread of infection from osteomyelitis in an adjacent bone, or by hematogenous spread from bacteremia resulting from a distant focus of infection in the body. Hematogenous septic arthritis is particularly common in children, especially in the hip. Because of the unique blood supply to the femoral head, the accumulation of pus under pressure within the hip joint can compress the nutrient vessels to the femoral head. If the pressure persists for more than a few hours, osteonecrosis can develop. Therefore, in a child's hip, the development of pus under pressure as a consequence of septic arthritis must be treated as an emergency. Immediate drainage of the fluid and pus is essential not only to treat the infection but also to avoid the devastating complication of osteonecrosis of the femoral head.

The general principles of the treatment of septic arthritis are similar to those of the treatment of septic bursitis. Aspirated joint fluid is cultured to determine appropriate antibiotics. Aspirations should be repeated as needed to remove the infected and necrotic material from the joint. In most cases, the most effective way to remove the pus is by incision and drainage of the joint, followed by thorough irrigation. Aggressive early treatment usually results in complete resolution of the infection without residual joint problems. Persistent smoldering infections, however, will destroy the articular cartilage, leading to postinfection arthritis and sometimes complete destruction of the joint. □

Septic Joint

Septic bursitis

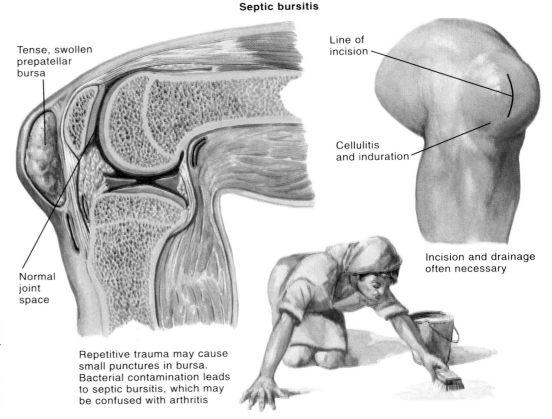

Tense, swollen prepatellar bursa

Normal joint space

Line of incision

Cellulitis and induration

Incision and drainage often necessary

Repetitive trauma may cause small punctures in bursa. Bacterial contamination leads to septic bursitis, which may be confused with arthritis

Septic arthritis

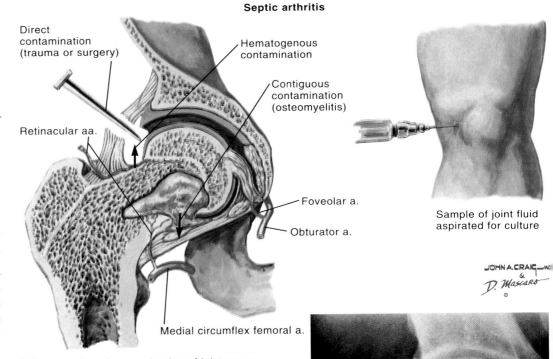

Direct contamination (trauma or surgery)

Retinacular aa.

Hematogenous contamination

Contiguous contamination (osteomyelitis)

Foveolar a.

Obturator a.

Medial circumflex femoral a.

Primary routes of contamination of joint space

Sample of joint fluid aspirated for culture

JOHN A. CRAIG
&
D. Mascaro

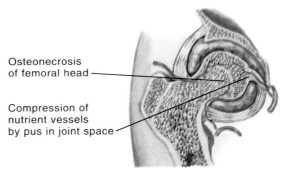

Osteonecrosis of femoral head

Compression of nutrient vessels by pus in joint space

Some joints, such as hip, require prompt surgical decompression to avoid damage to vascular supply

When vascular supply damaged, osteonecrosis occurs, leading to collapse of femoral head

Etiology and Prevalence of Hematogenous Osteomyelitis

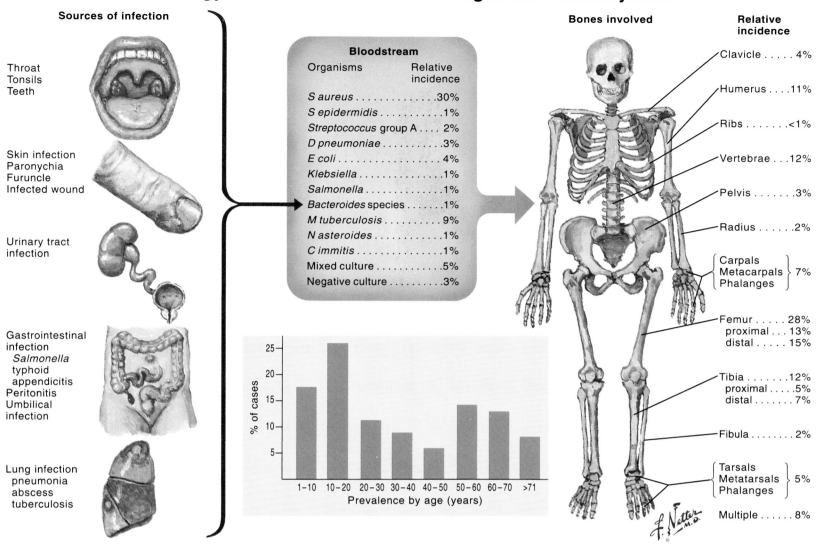

Sources of infection

Throat
Tonsils
Teeth

Skin infection
Paronychia
Furuncle
Infected wound

Urinary tract
infection

Gastrointestinal
infection
Salmonella
typhoid
appendicitis
Peritonitis
Umbilical
infection

Lung infection
pneumonia
abscess
tuberculosis

Bloodstream

Organisms	Relative incidence
S aureus	30%
S epidermidis	1%
Streptococcus group A	2%
D pneumoniae	3%
E coli	4%
Klebsiella	1%
Salmonella	1%
Bacteroides species	1%
M tuberculosis	9%
N asteroides	1%
C immitis	1%
Mixed culture	5%
Negative culture	3%

Prevalence by age (years) — bar chart of % of cases by age group: 1–10, 10–20, 20–30, 30–40, 40–50, 50–60, 60–70, >71

Bones involved

Relative incidence

Clavicle 4%
Humerus 11%
Ribs . . . . <1%
Vertebrae . . . 12%
Pelvis 3%
Radius 2%
Carpals
Metacarpals } 7%
Phalanges
Femur 28%
proximal . . . 13%
distal 15%
Tibia 12%
proximal 5%
distal 7%
Fibula 2%
Tarsals
Metatarsals } 5%
Phalanges
Multiple 8%

Osteomyelitis

An infection of bone, osteomyelitis takes two forms, based on the source of the contamination. Hematogenous osteomyelitis results from an infection carried in the bloodstream. Exogenous (non-hematogenous) osteomyelitis is caused by spread from a nearby infection, open fractures, and surgical procedures in which the bone is penetrated and contaminated.

Etiology and Prevalence of Hematogenous Osteomyelitis

In contrast to direct contamination of the bone from exogenous sources, hematogenous osteomyelitis results when the bone is seeded with bacteria from a distant site of infection in the body (Plate 11). Common sources of infection are the throat, teeth, skin, urinary tract, gastrointestinal tract, and lungs. Infection in these locations can produce showers of bacteria in the bloodstream (bacteremia). Although the reticuloendothelial

system clears most of these bacteria from the bloodstream, occasionally a few settle in the bone, creating a focus of infection. The areas of bone particularly vulnerable to hematogenous infection are the metaphyses of the long bones—especially the humerus, femur, and tibia. The organisms that cause hematogenous osteomyelitis are the same as those responsible for the primary infection; the most common pathogen is *Staphylococcus aureus*. Gram-negative infections are commonly the results of seeding from a primary infection in the urinary tract, usually secondary to medical instrumentation or catheterization.

Hematogenous osteomyelitis is usually seen in children but may develop in adults; a second, fairly high peak in occurrence is seen in persons between 50 and 70 years of age.

Pathogenesis of Hematogenous Osteomyelitis

Hematogenous osteomyelitis is particularly common in growing children for several reasons. Children are especially susceptible to bacterial infections in general and, therefore, are likely to have frequent primary infectious foci and frequent episodes of bacteremia, which can lead to osteomyelitis. In addition, the peculiar anatomy of the growth plate may also play a substantial role in the development of hematogenous osteomyelitis in this age group. Virtually all cases of hematogenous osteomyelitis in children seem to originate

in the metaphyseal bone, just beneath the growth plate. In this region, the terminal branches of the metaphyseal arteries form loops and enter afferent venous sinusoids, which are large and irregular (Plate 12). The size of the vessels increases markedly from the metaphyseal artery to the venous sinusoids, and blood flow slows and becomes turbulent. The abrupt change in the dynamics of blood flow may allow bacteria to sludge and accumulate in this region, creating a focus of infection. Also, the cells in and around the venous sinusoids have little or no phagocytic activity, thus creating an ideal environment for bacterial growth.

After the bone is seeded with bacteria from the bloodstream, rapid bacterial duplication creates a localized abscess just beneath the growth plate. The developing abscess extends along the Volkmann canals to the subperiosteal region, where it elevates the thick periosteum. Elevation of the periosteum eventually stimulates the formation of new bone. Further extension of the abscess may cause it to rupture through the periosteum and extend to the subcutaneous tissue and then through the skin, creating a draining sinus. The infection may extend subperiosteally along the shaft of the bone; this extension strips a portion of the shaft of its blood supply and produces a dense, avascular piece of cortical bone called a sequestrum. The sequestrum, lacking a blood supply to deliver antibiotics or inflammatory cells to fight infection, acts as a nidus for the infection to persist.

Osteomyelitis
(Continued)

Pathogenesis of Hematogenous Osteomyelitis

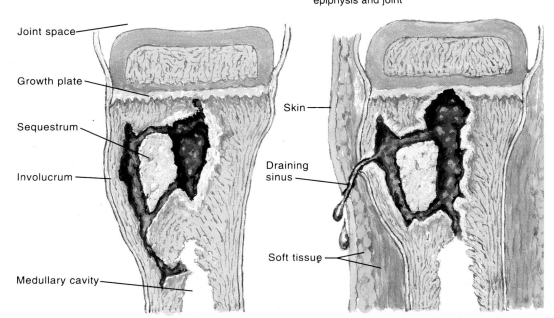

Epiphysis
Looped capillaries
Venous sinusoids
Abscess
Metaphyseal arteries
Nutrient artery

Growth plate
Periosteum

Terminal branches of metaphyseal arteries form loops at growth plate and enter irregular afferent venous sinusoids. Blood flow slowed and turbulent, predisposing to bacterial seeding. In addition, lining cells have little or no phagocytic activity. Area is catch basin for bacteria, and abscess may form

Abscess, limited by growth plate, spreads trans-versely along Volkmann canals and elevates periosteum; extends subperiosteally and may invade shaft. In infants under 1 year of age, some metaphyseal arterial branches pass through growth plate, and infection may invade epiphysis and joint

Joint space
Growth plate
Sequestrum
Involucrum
Medullary cavity

Skin
Draining sinus
Soft tissue

As abscess spreads, segment of devitalized bone (sequestrum) remains within it. Elevated periosteum may also lay down bone to form encasing shell (involucrum). Occasionally, abscess walled off by fibrosis and bone sclerosis to form Brodie abscess

Infectious process may erode periosteum and form sinus through soft tissues and skin to drain externally. Process influenced by virulence of organism, resistance of host, administration of antibiotics, and fibrotic and sclerotic responses

In an attempt to wall off and isolate the infection, the elevated periosteum lays down new bone. This new bone, called an involucrum, is composed of new subperiosteal bone much like that found in a new fracture callus. Thus, histologically acute hematogenous osteomyelitis creates rarefaction in the metaphysis of the long bone due to the destruction of normal cancellous bone, forms sequestra, and creates an involucrum of new bone around the periphery of the infection.

Except in very young children, the infection rarely extends across the physical barrier of the growth plate. In children less than 1 year of age, some branches of the metaphyseal arteries pass through the growth plate to nourish the epiphysis. The passageways for these vessels allow the infection to spread into the epiphysis, then into the adjacent joint space itself.

Occasionally, the body's immune response can effectively eradicate a minor infection in the metaphysis. If the area of infection is walled off and the infecting bacteria are killed, the small, residual abscess cavity may persist indefinitely. The cavity, composed of fibrous tissue but containing no residual viable bacteria, is called a Brodie abscess, even though there is no residual active infection present. In contrast, a more aggressive and virulent infection continues to destroy bone and eventually creates a draining sinus. The sinus will drain until the necrotic and infected tissue is completely removed and replaced with fibrous tissue or noninfected bone.

Early and aggressive diagnosis and treatment of hematogenous osteomyelitis can arrest the destruction of normal, healthy bone by the extending abscess. Treatment includes administration of bacteria-specific antibiotics and surgical drainage of the infectious focus. Therefore, it is especially important to understand the early clinical manifestations of this disease so that appropriate therapy can be initiated promptly.

Clinical Manifestations

Signs and symptoms of hematogenous osteomyelitis are fever, chills, malaise, and pain localized, to some degree, to the area of infection (Plate 13). Fever is present in more than 75% of patients, although it is less common when the infection has been present for a long time. The patient usually reports malaise, decreased appetite, and generalized weakness. Point tenderness can be localized to the tissues around the infected area, and deep palpation also elicits tenderness. Osteomyelitis causes pain when the involved area is moved or used. For example, a child with acute

hematogenous osteomyelitis of the distal femur appears reluctant to stand or walk on the infected limb. Generalized soft tissue swelling develops about the area of infection, and on palpation, the area feels warm to the touch. A so-called sympathetic effusion often develops in an adjacent joint. This reactive swelling of the joint occurs in response to the infection of the nearby bone, but the effusion contains no pathogenic bacteria. Active range of motion of a joint with sympathetic effusion is limited by the pain secondary to the bone infection. Drainage from the abscess is a manifestation of chronic infection only and is not seen in the acute stages of hematogenous osteomyelitis.

Osteomyelitis
(Continued)

Clinical Manifestations of Hematogenous Osteomyelitis

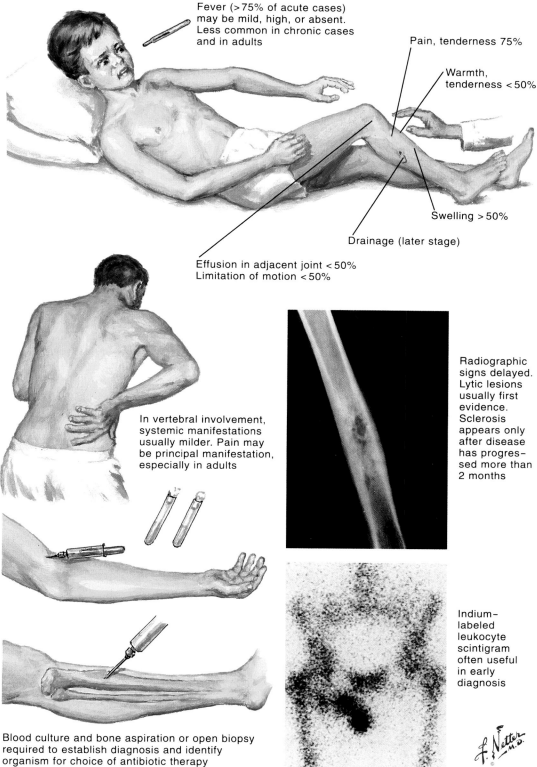

Fever (>75% of acute cases) may be mild, high, or absent. Less common in chronic cases and in adults

Pain, tenderness 75%

Warmth, tenderness <50%

Swelling >50%

Drainage (later stage)

Effusion in adjacent joint <50%
Limitation of motion <50%

In vertebral involvement, systemic manifestations usually milder. Pain may be principal manifestation, especially in adults

Radiographic signs delayed. Lytic lesions usually first evidence. Sclerosis appears only after disease has progressed more than 2 months

Indium-labeled leukocyte scintigram often useful in early diagnosis

Blood culture and bone aspiration or open biopsy required to establish diagnosis and identify organism for choice of antibiotic therapy

Clinical manifestations of acute hematogenous osteomyelitis of the spine are more difficult to define. The patient may complain of a vague backache as well as generalized malaise, decreased appetite, and fever. Pain restricts the active range of motion of the back, and gentle percussion over the spinous processes often causes significant discomfort. This constellation of symptoms is not specific to osteomyelitis, and diagnosis of osteomyelitis may often be overlooked in the many patients who complain of backache. Frequently, osteomyelitis of the spine is secondary to a urinary tract infection. Therefore, a recent history of infection or surgical manipulation of the urinary tract should heighten the clinical suspicion of a secondary infection of the spine.

Diagnosis of hematogenous osteomyelitis requires a careful history, focusing on any recent infection at another site, such as the mouth and teeth, urinary tract, or throat. The physical examination should be thorough enough to identify any primary source of the infection. If the history and physical findings suggest hematogenous osteomyelitis, selected laboratory tests should be performed. A complete blood count often reveals an elevated leukocyte count with a shift to the left in the differential. Frequently, the erythrocyte sedimentation rate is elevated as well.

Radiographs of the painful area should be obtained, although radiographic signs are often

minimal early in the infection. The earliest radiographic evidence of acute hematogenous osteomyelitis is swelling of soft tissue adjacent to the bone; within a few days of onset, lysis in the metaphyseal region becomes visible. Periosteal elevation with its new bone formation and the creation of sequestra become obvious on radiographs after a couple of weeks. A technetium 99m bone scan is an extremely sensitive test for identification of areas of inflammation in the bone. However, the test is not particularly specific to bone infection, because it is also positive after fracture or any other condition that irritates the periosteum and causes new bone formation.

Recently, radioactively labeled leukocytes have been used to diagnose a focus of osteomyelitis. In this technique, a blood sample is drawn from the patient; the leukocyte cells are cultured and labeled with radioactive indium 111 and then reinjected into the patient. As leukocytes tend to accumulate at a focus of infection, the indium-labeled leukocytes also tend to focus in the infected area. The radioactivity can be identified on a scan performed 24 to 72 hours after reinjection.

The specific pathogen responsible for the osteomyelitis must be identified so that appropriate antibiotic therapy can be instituted. Although blood cultures often reveal the infecting organism,

Direct (Nonhematogenous) Causes of Osteomyelitis

Traumatic infections

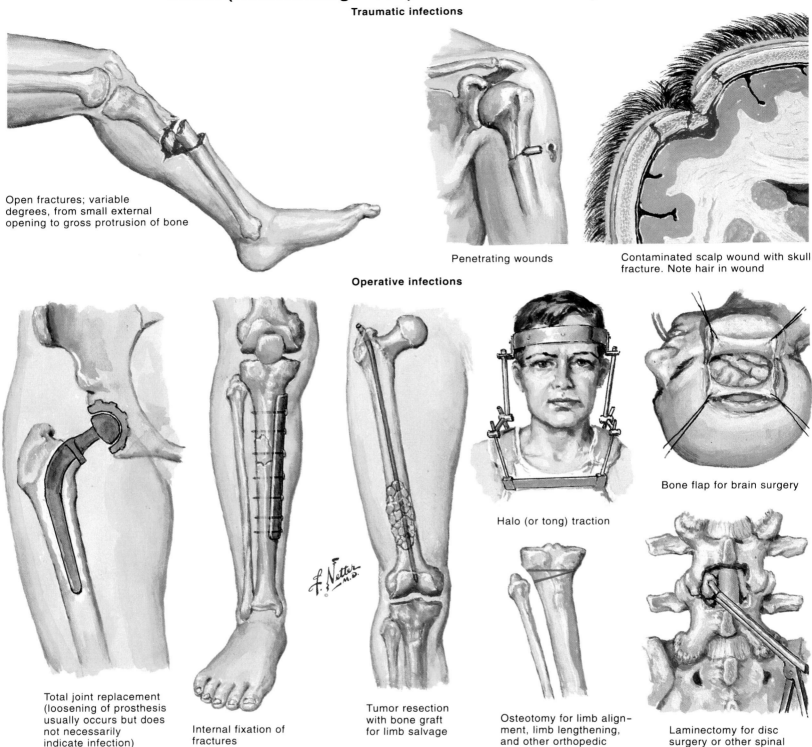

Open fractures; variable degrees, from small external opening to gross protrusion of bone

Penetrating wounds

Contaminated scalp wound with skull fracture. Note hair in wound

Operative infections

Total joint replacement (loosening of prosthesis usually occurs but does not necessarily indicate infection)

Internal fixation of fractures

Tumor resection with bone graft for limb salvage

Halo (or tong) traction

Bone flap for brain surgery

Osteotomy for limb alignment, limb lengthening, and other orthopedic procedures

Laminectomy for disc surgery or other spinal cord compression

Osteomyelitis
(Continued)

the most reliable way to identify the pathogen is direct aspiration of the osteomyelitic focus itself.

Etiology of Exogenous Osteomyelitis

Exogenous (nonhematogenous) osteomyelitis results from the direct contamination of the bone by the infecting organism. The skin, subcutaneous tissue, and periosteum provide a protective barrier to contaminants, and as long as the skin and periosteum remain intact, the bone cannot be contaminated directly. These barriers can be violated by trauma (eg, bullet wound, open fracture, direct blow) or by surgery, or they can be stripped away during displacement of fracture fragments (Plate 14). When the protective skin is penetrated and the bone exposed, bacteria may invade the area, creating a focus of infection. Bone may also be contaminated during total joint replacement, application of traction-fixation devices, and implantation of fracture fixation devices. Even when careful surgical dissection is combined with thorough debridement and prophylactic administration of antibiotics, infection occurs in about 1% of major surgical interventions.

During the implantation of artificial joints and fixation devices, the blood supply is often stripped from the bone, creating areas of dead bone. The dead bone acts as a sequestrum, allowing a bacterial infection to persist. Osteomyelitis may become chronic, persisting until the necrotic sequestrum is completely removed and the foreign body, whether a fracture fixation device or total joint prosthesis, is removed.

Certain soft tissue infections may spread to adjacent bones (Plate 15). For example, large soft tissue abscesses may erode the periosteum to infect the underlying bone. An infection of the pulp of the fingertip, called a felon, frequently extends to

Direct (Nonhematogenous) Causes of Osteomyelitis (continued)
Secondary to contiguous focus of infection

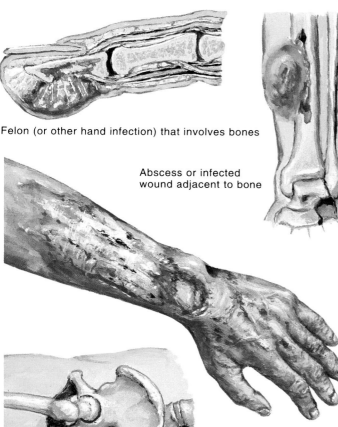

Felon (or other hand infection) that involves bones

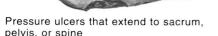

Abscess or infected wound adjacent to bone

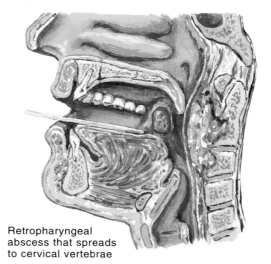

Retropharyngeal abscess that spreads to cervical vertebrae

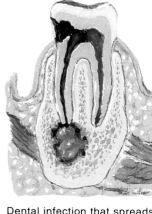

Dental infection that spreads to mandible or maxilla

Infected burns that involve bones

Pressure ulcers that extend to sacrum, pelvis, or spine

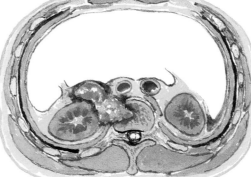

Retroperitoneal abscess that involves vertebrae

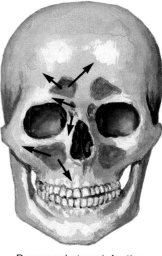

Paranasal sinus infection that spreads to skull bones

Contributory or predisposing factors

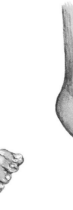

Hematoma

Vascular insufficiency (in diabetes, arteriosclerosis)

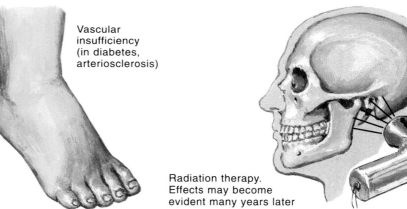

Radiation therapy. Effects may become evident many years later

Osteomyelitis
(Continued)

and infects the distal phalanx, to which the fibrous septa of the pulp of the finger are firmly attached. Retropharyngeal abscesses tend to involve the cervical vertebrae, and periapical infections of the tooth frequently spread to the adjacent mandible or maxilla. Infection in the paranasal sinuses may extend to the adjacent bones of the skull.

Extensive soft tissue injury, such as pressure ulcers and third-degree burns, may erode through the periosteum, exposing the bone and leaving it vulnerable to infection. Similarly, radiation therapy destroys the adjacent soft tissue and damages the periosteum, making the bone and surrounding soft tissues more vulnerable to infection. One of the most common causes of bone infection in adults is the combination of vascular insufficiency and immunocompromise that occurs in diabetes mellitus. In diabetic patients, the foot is particularly susceptible to chronic skin ulcerations and secondary infection of the bone.

Although the many exogenous causes of osteomyelitis vary greatly, the resulting bone infections share some common characteristics. The bone becomes infected because the protective skin and periosteal barriers have been violated, allowing contamination of the bone. The infection usually persists because of the presence of necrotic soft tissue, necrotic bone, or a foreign body that serves as a nidus for continued bacterial proliferation.

Exogenous osteomyelitis can often be prevented immediately after an open fracture with early and thorough debridement of the contaminated bone and administration of broad-spectrum antibiotics. Once established, exogenous osteomyelitis is very difficult to eradicate, and effective treatment requires surgical debridement of the infected necrotic bone, removal of infected foreign bodies (including implants), and long-term intravenous administration of bacteria-specific antibiotics.

Osteomyelitis After Open Fracture

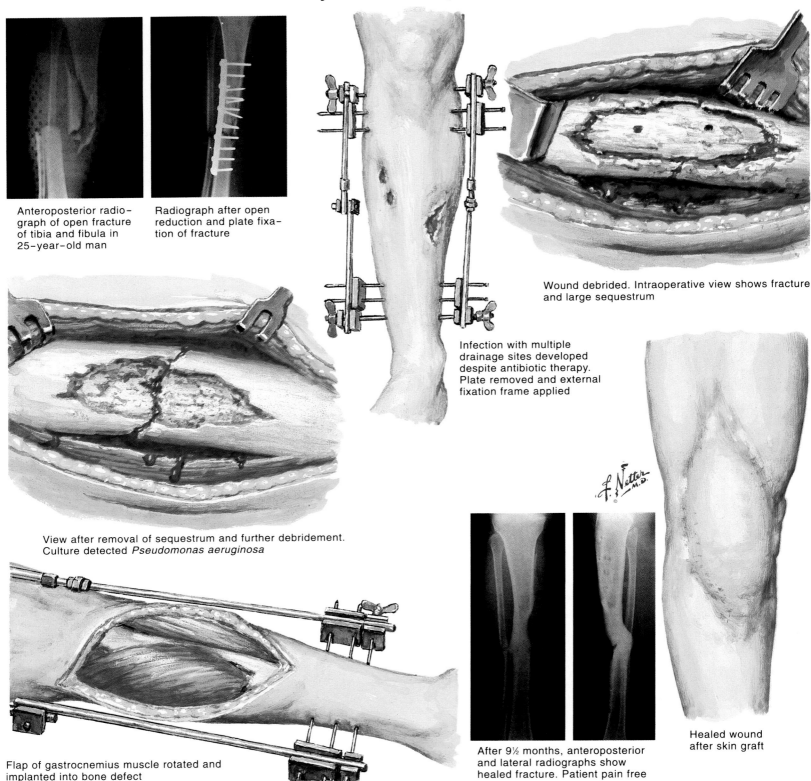

Anteroposterior radio-
graph of open fracture
of tibia and fibula in
25-year-old man

Radiograph after open
reduction and plate fixa-
tion of fracture

Wound debrided. Intraoperative view shows fracture
and large sequestrum

Infection with multiple
drainage sites developed
despite antibiotic therapy.
Plate removed and external
fixation frame applied

View after removal of sequestrum and further debridement.
Culture detected *Pseudomonas aeruginosa*

Flap of gastrocnemius muscle rotated and
implanted into bone defect

After 9½ months, anteroposterior
and lateral radiographs show
healed fracture. Patient pain free

Healed wound
after skin graft

Osteomyelitis

(*Continued*)

Chronic Osteomyelitis

Bone infections are much more difficult to eradicate than soft tissue infections. Soft tissue cellulitis or abscess responds well to surgical drainage
combined with the administration of appropriate
antibiotics. However, simple surgical drainage
combined with the administration of antibiotics
may not eradicate chronic osteomyelitis. Bacteria
become sequestered in the bone in areas where
antibiotics cannot reach them in sufficient concentration. A necrotic bone sequestrum or a fracture fixation device can act as a nidus for continued
bacterial proliferation. Only removal of all of the
necrotic bone and the foreign body can control
the infection. This treatment often necessitates radical surgical debridement with removal of large
segments of bone, creating significant mechanical
instability and loss of function. In some patients,
the infection can be fully eradicated only with
amputation. Plates 16 and 17 depict two cases of
chronic or recurrent osteomyelitis associated with
unsuccessful plating of an open fracture and
intramedullary rod fixation of a closed fracture.

Chronic osteomyelitis frequently manifests as
one or more draining sinuses. The drainage is
green or yellow, often thick, and usually foul
smelling. Radiographs of the infected area show
dense sclerotic bone characteristic of a sequestrum.
Often, the fracture fixation devices loosen.

Treatment of chronic osteomyelitis requires
removal of all infected, necrotic bone and all metal
foreign bodies; debridement of all necrotic soft
tissue; and marsupialization of the necrotic, infected

Recurrent Postoperative Osteomyelitis

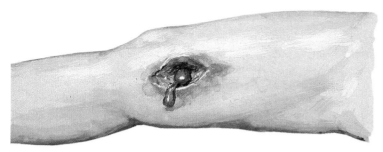

Closed fracture of femur due to skiing accident in 35-year-old woman. Fracture treated with intramedullary rod; drainage on medial side of distal thigh developed about 2 weeks after surgery. Blue staining of drainage fluid and around drainage site due to methylene blue injected into sinus to track course

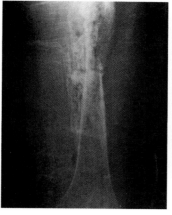

Radiograph reveals callus about fracture with sclerosis and multiple punctate radiolucent areas indicating ongoing infection

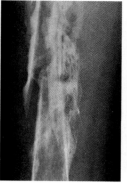

Anteroposterior and lateral tomograms reveal presence of osteomyelitis with formation of sequestra. Intensive antibiotic therapy reinstituted

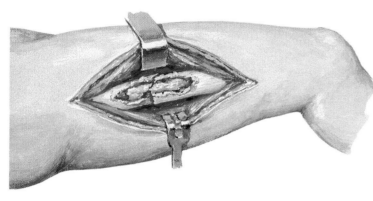

Intraoperative view. Primary problem found to be on lateral thigh even though drainage occurred on medial side. Large sequestrum revealed

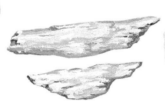

Two sequestra removed

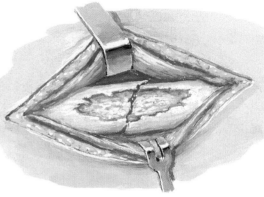

Bone defect after debridement and removal of sequestra. Wound closed

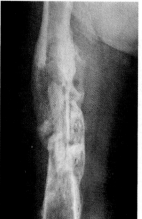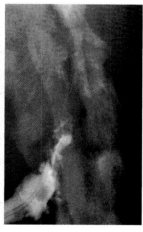

Patient returned 2 months later with drainage from sinus tract. Left: tomogram shows active process and presence of sequestra. Right: sinugram reveals sinus tract extending to site of old fracture

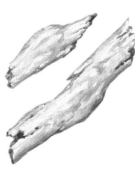

Additional sequestra surgically removed from lesion. Sinus tract excised, and all dead and infected tissue thoroughly debrided

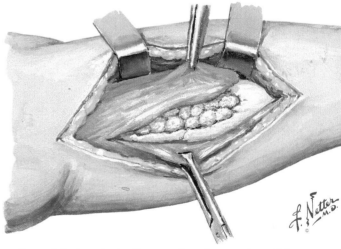

Bone defect packed with cancellous bone autograft from ilium overlaid with muscle flap from vastus lateralis muscle. Patient remained free of pain and drainage

Osteomyelitis
(Continued)

bed. Stability of the limb can often be maintained with the use of an external fixation device that bridges the area of infection (Plate 16). Repeated debridement is often necessary to ensure that all the infected, necrotic tissue is excised. Tissue samples should be obtained from the depths of the wound and cultured to determine the appropriate antibiotics. Antibiotics are then administered intravenously until the wound heals. Between debridements, the wounds are packed open; dressings are changed daily to remove any residual necrotic material while encouraging the development of granulation tissue in the base of the wound. Some researchers recommend the use of hyperbaric oxygen as a supplement to this treatment regimen. Hyperbaric oxygen therapy enhances the function of leukocytes and promotes the growth of granulation tissue.

When the base of the wound is fully covered with granulation tissue, a local muscle flap or a free vascularized myocutaneous flap can be transferred to the defect to provide soft tissue coverage. If the entire underlying bone architecture has been destroyed by the infection, bone grafts are needed to repair the bone after the infection is completely eradicated (Plate 17).

The goal of treatment is to eliminate the draining sinuses and produce a functional limb that is free from pain. The complicated process just described to eradicate a focus of osteomyelitis is very expensive and time-consuming. In some patients, amputation of the infected part may be the most reliable and effective way of restoring a pain-free and productive life.

Osteomyelitis

(Continued)

Delayed Posttraumatic Osteomyelitis in Diabetic Patient

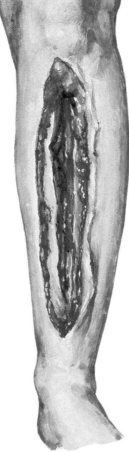

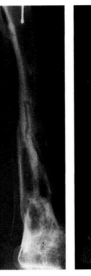

Leg of 19-year-old man with juvenile diabetes who had sustained closed fracture of tibia at age 7. Fracture healed, but hematogenous osteomyelitis later developed in area of decreased resistance. Drainage and tissue breakdown continued for many years, resulting in extensive, oozing wound

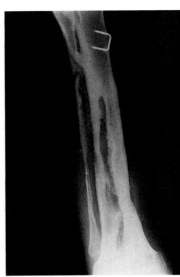

Anteroposterior and lateral radiographs reveal extensive destruction and sclerosis of tibia due to osteomyelitis

Postoperative radiograph following removal of dead and infected bone and sequestra

Delayed Posttraumatic Osteomyelitis in Diabetic Patient

Infection in a diabetic patient can be aggressive and life threatening (Plate 18). Infections often develop around skin ulcerations in the foot. The patient's impaired immune system allows the infection to ascend rapidly into the leg. Even after an aggressive soft tissue infection has been controlled, foot ulcers may persist. The ulcers continue to drain, and the lack of soft tissue coverage over the bone exposes it to chronic irritation and the continued risk of infection. It is therefore important to try to achieve and maintain soft tissue coverage of such ulcerated areas.

The first step in the treatment of osteomyelitis associated with diabetes is extensive debridement of the necrotic tissue and removal of any underlying sequestra. When the necrotic, infected tissue has been removed, wet-to-dry dressings are applied to stimulate the formation of granulation tissue; hyperbaric oxygen therapy can further stimulate the development of a granulation tissue bed. Transplantation of vascularized tissue from other regions of the body (such as a vascularized omental graft) can also be performed to bring additional blood supply to the area to facilitate healing. Once a complete bed of granulation tissue develops, the defect can be covered with a split-thickness skin graft. □

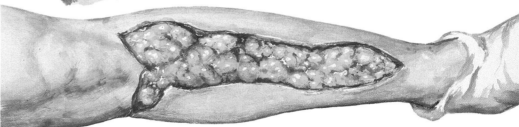

Leg after extensive debridement, removal of sequestra, and packing of cavity with omentum

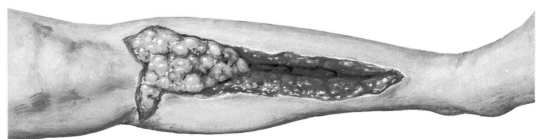

Proximal part of omentum transplant remained viable but distal section died, although good, clean granulation tissue developed there. Distal bone defect filled with cancellous bone graft, and wound healed uneventfully

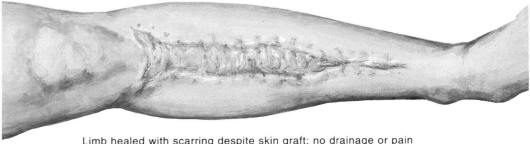

Limb healed with scarring despite skin graft; no drainage or pain

178

Section III
Amputation

Frank H. Netter, M.D.

in collaboration with

James D. Heckman, M.D.   *Plates 1–11*

Amputation

Primary closure

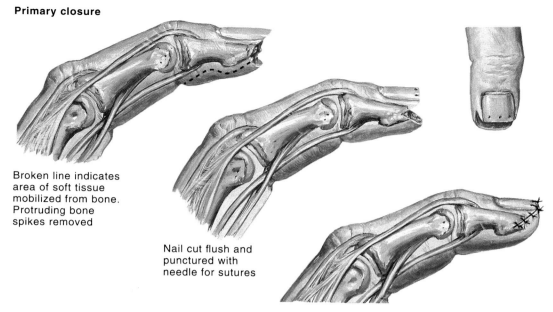

Broken line indicates
area of soft tissue
mobilized from bone.
Protruding bone
spikes removed

Nail cut flush and
punctured with
needle for sutures

Volar skin flap mobilized dorsally and sutured
to fingernail. Closure scar positioned well up
to nail, away from trauma

Amputation refers to the complete separation of a body part from the body. A disarticulation is an amputation that occurs through a joint.

Causes of Amputation

The many different causes of amputation include trauma, vascular disease, infection, tumor, and congenital defect. Injuries frequently lead to the complete separation of a body part (traumatic amputation), and certain diseases and disorders create a situation in which operative amputation becomes necessary. The only reason for operative amputation of a body part is complete loss of the blood supply to that part, rendering it nonviable.

Injury. Obviously, complete traumatic amputation produces a nonviable segment of tissue. Also, extensive injury to blood vessels may destroy the viability of the segment distal to the vessel injury, although the segment may remain attached to the limb. The part without circulation cannot survive unless circulation is restored promptly. If circulation cannot be restored within a few hours, the amputation should be performed.

Vascular Disease. Impaired circulation due to arteriosclerotic vascular disease is one of the more common causes of amputation. Narrowing of the vascular lumen occurs as arteriosclerotic plaques develop in the vessel wall. Eventually, the plaques may completely fill the arterial lumen or form a rough endothelial surface where clots can form and attach, closing off blood flow. Obliteration of the blood supply leads to gangrene of the tissue normally perfused by the affected vessel, and this gangrenous tissue must then be amputated.

Infection. Rarely, an aggressive infection can occur in a limb, causing severe and life-threatening systemic problems. The only effective way to manage the infection and save the patient's life is to amputate the severely infected part. Occasionally, this condition develops in patients with certain life-threatening infections such as gas gangrene and necrotizing fasciitis and in immunocompromised patients with infection. More commonly, infection results in local necrosis of tissue, creating a medium for further bacterial proliferation. Amputation is needed to remove the infected and necrotic tissue and prevent further bacterial spread.

Tumor. Amputation may be necessary to remove an aggressive, malignant tumor, both as a lifesaving procedure and to prevent metastasis of the tumor, and to relieve local symptoms, such as pain, caused by the tumor. In the past decade,

Thick split–thickness skin graft

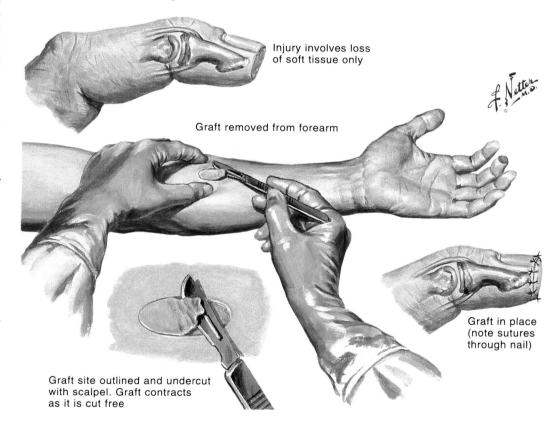

Injury involves loss
of soft tissue only

Graft removed from forearm

Graft site outlined and undercut
with scalpel. Graft contracts
as it is cut free

Graft in place
(note sutures
through nail)

advances in operative techniques for limb salvage and improvements in chemotherapy and radiation therapy have significantly decreased the frequency of amputation for tumors in limbs.

Congenital Defect. Children can be born with partial or complete congenital limb defects; the entire limb, or any portion of it, may be absent. An extensive classification system of congenital limb deficiencies is presented in the CIBA COLLECTION, Volume 8/II, pages 104–116. In most patients, prosthetic devices can be fitted to the affected limb to allow satisfactory function. Only rarely is surgical intervention needed to modify or complete a congenital amputation.

General Principles of Amputation Surgery

Several essential principles must be followed in amputation surgery. The most important goal is to preserve as much of the limb as possible. Preservation of length and—even more important—of as many functional joints as possible should always be the primary considerations. Obviously, gangrene or aggressive infection necessitates the complete removal of affected necrotic or infected tissue; similarly, a malignant tumor must be completely excised. However, radical ablation of healthy, viable, and uninvolved tissue should always be avoided to preserve function of the residual limb.

Amputation of Phalanx

Amputation of distal phalanx

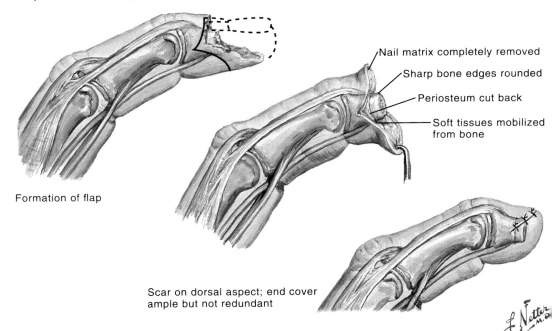

Formation of flap

Nail matrix completely removed

Sharp bone edges rounded

Periosteum cut back

Soft tissues mobilized from bone

Scar on dorsal aspect; end cover ample but not redundant

Amputation
(Continued)

In the nineteenth century, specific levels of amputation were defined and named by famous surgeons. These classic levels of amputation have less significance today, because the quality of prosthetic devices has improved greatly. Modern prostheses can be fabricated and fitted to accommodate virtually any length or shape of a residual limb. Therefore, although the standard techniques of modern surgical practice should be applied during amputation, it is not essential to adhere rigidly to specific amputation levels.

The amputation should produce a residual stump that is covered with a thick layer of healthy skin, because the end of the stump is often required to bear weight or withstand repetitive trauma with use. As a general principle, the skin covering the end of the stump should be full thickness and mobile and have normal protective sensation. The particular shape or contour of the skin flap covering the stump is not so important, as long as the skin is sensate and can tolerate the uses to which it will be put. On the other hand, excessive and redundant skin, muscle, or fat can create problems in fitting the prosthesis; therefore, the skin flap should be just generous enough to cover the underlying bone architecture yet provide a firm, well-contoured amputation stump.

After amputation, the underlying bone architecture continues to provide support for the residual limb. All bony prominences should be covered with full-thickness soft tissue to prevent irritation, particularly from prosthetic devices. At the time of amputation, all sharp bone ends are smoothed and rounded; this helps to prevent painful compression of the skin between bone and prosthesis. The periosteum around the cut end of the bone is removed as well. When the periosteum is stripped from the bone end during fracture or amputation, it is stimulated to produce new bone. Irregular proliferation of this callus may create a painful bone spur in the end of the stump. Excision of the periosteum at the time of amputation decreases the risk of this problem.

During the operation, particular attention must be given to both the blood vessels and the nerves. Because the amputation must be through viable tissue, intact blood vessels will be transected during the procedure. The surgeon must carefully cauterize and ligate the blood vessels to prevent

Amputation of middle phalanx

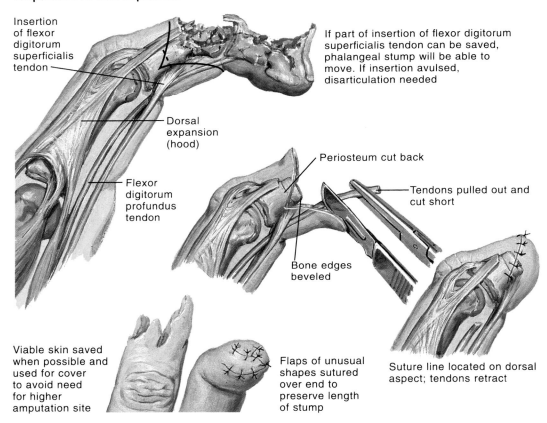

Insertion of flexor digitorum superficialis tendon

Dorsal expansion (hood)

Flexor digitorum profundus tendon

Viable skin saved when possible and used for cover to avoid need for higher amputation site

If part of insertion of flexor digitorum superficialis tendon can be saved, phalangeal stump will be able to move. If insertion avulsed, disarticulation needed

Periosteum cut back

Tendons pulled out and cut short

Bone edges beveled

Flaps of unusual shapes sutured over end to preserve length of stump

Suture line located on dorsal aspect; tendons retract

bleeding following amputation. However, even with vigorous hemostasis at the time of amputation, some further bleeding inevitably occurs in the immediate postoperative period. The formation of a large hematoma under the skin flaps of the amputation stump may, because of excessive pressure, produce necrosis of the skin flaps. In addition, a large hematoma may become infected. Therefore, the amputation stump should be drained with a Penrose or suction drainage system in the immediate postoperative period.

The amputation transects nerves as well as vascular structures, and transected nerves attempt to heal by proliferation of new axonal material at the cut end. This attempt to heal creates a neuroma, a thickened bulbous swelling of the cut nerve end. If the neuroma lies immediately under the skin or adjacent to a bony prominence, it may easily be compressed and irritated, causing persistent symptoms. To minimize the creation of a painful neuroma, the surgeon should carefully identify all nerves at the level of amputation. Gentle traction should be applied to each nerve, and the nerve should be sharply transected and allowed to retract into the muscles of the amputation stump, away from bony prominences. Then, the neuroma that develops is less likely to be compressed with use or by a prosthesis.

Amputation
(Continued)

Amputation of Hand

Amputations of the hand are almost always traumatic in origin; only rarely is amputation required to treat gangrene, infection, or tumor. Traumatic injuries to the hand are quite common, particularly in persons who use power tools in the workplace or the home. The general principles of amputation apply to procedures in the hand, and preservation of length is especially critical. Every effort should be made to salvage as much of each digit as possible.

The most important digit is the thumb, and it is absolutely essential to try to preserve both its length and function following injury. Often, severe injury or amputation of one of the other four fingers is best treated with primary amputation, because the remaining fingers can readily assume most functions. If the other digits are healthy, then prolonged or repeated attempts to reimplant a single finger or restore function to a finger (as distinguished from the thumb) may be time-consuming, costly, and frustrating for the patient. Immediate amputation, combined with an aggressive and immediate rehabilitation program, may often be best for the patient. When multiple fingers are injured, however, the decision to amputate any injured finger must be considered very carefully.

After injury to the hand, amputation should be considered only when three or more of the five tissue areas (skin, tendon, nerve, bone, and joint) require special procedures for salvage. Age is also a factor in the decision to amputate. Amputation is rarely indicated in a child, even after a severe injury. In patients more than 50 years of age, however, removal of a single finger, except the thumb, is often the preferred option, particularly when both the digital nerves and the flexor tendons have been transected.

Amputation of Fingertip. With fingertip amputations, it is also important to preserve as much length as possible (Plate 1). The primary factor influencing the ability to preserve length is the integrity of the volar skin. In fingertip injuries, the volar skin should be preserved, if possible, for use as a flap; this area comprises the best tissue for digital function. If the volar skin has been amputated or destroyed, the finger must be shortened to ensure that the volar surface of the residual digit is covered with full-thickness, sensate skin that will be durable and functional. The digital nerves should be assessed carefully. Each nerve should be transected under gentle traction and allowed to retract deep into the soft tissues to avoid painful neuromas at the end of the

Amputation of Finger and Ray

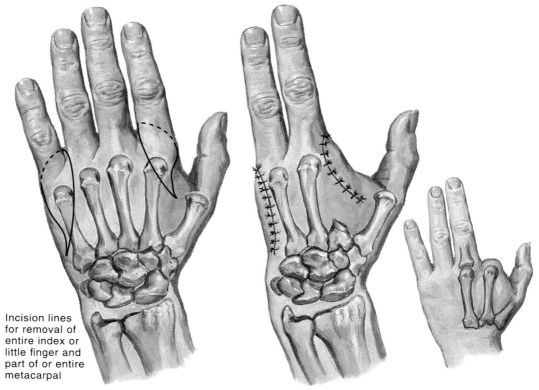

Incision lines for removal of entire index or little finger and part of or entire metacarpal

Final appearance and function improved if head and shaft of metacarpal removed

Deepening of Thenar Web Cleft

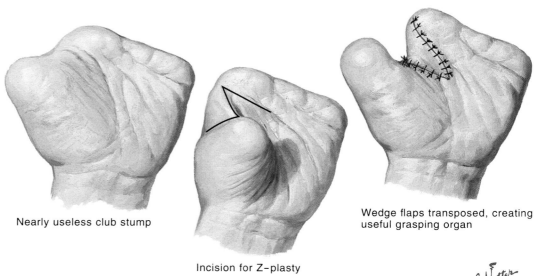

Nearly useless club stump

Incision for Z-plasty

Wedge flaps transposed, creating useful grasping organ

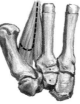

Distal portion of adductor pollicis muscle removed (broken line). Insertion reattached, if necessary

Thenar half of first dorsal interosseous muscle removed

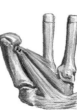

Insertion of flexor pollicis brevis muscle reattached, if necessary

Use of skin graft

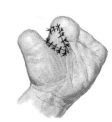

Transverse incision

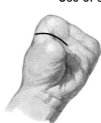

Full-thickness skin graft in place

Skin graft can also be used to deepen cleft

Amputation
(Continued)

Amputation of Forearm and Hand

Lines of incision

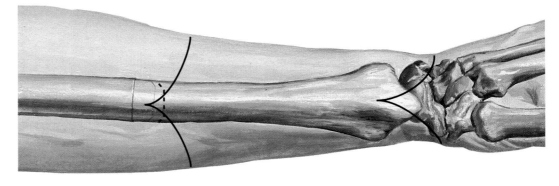

Below–elbow amputation

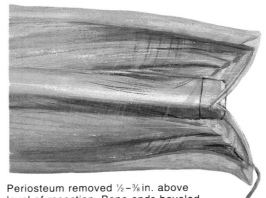

Periosteum removed ½–⅜ in. above
level of resection. Bone ends beveled.
Musculotendinous tissues tapered.
Skin and fascial flaps formed

Disarticulation of wrist

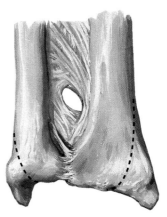

Styloid processes removed
(broken lines) to facilitate
fitting of prosthesis

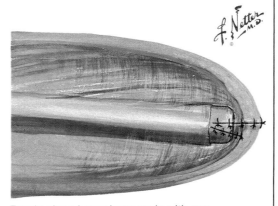

Fascia closed over bone ends with any
adherent muscle. Skin closure slightly
offset from fascial closure

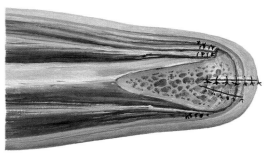

Tendons sutured at resting length to roughened
surface of bones

finger. The end of the bone should be contoured to eliminate bony prominences and a club-shaped stump. The flap should cover the end of the stump securely, but a redundant skin flap should be avoided. Excessive tension on the skin edges must also be avoided to prevent further necrosis of the skin flaps.

When the very tip of the finger has been amputated, the roughened end of the distal phalanx should be smoothed and any protruding bony spikes removed. The volar skin can be mobilized distally by careful dissection along deep tissue planes just superficial to the flexor tendon sheath. The flap is brought up to and sutured to the fingernail, allowing wound closure and the resultant scar to be positioned on the dorsal aspect of the finger, away from the area that will be exposed to repetitive trauma.

When it is essential to preserve length, larger defects that cannot be closed primarily are treated with a thick split-thickness skin graft. The amputation bed is debrided of all necrotic and potentially infected tissue. A thick split-thickness skin graft can be harvested from the volar aspect of the forearm or the medial aspect of the arm just below the axilla. The donor site is closed primarily and the free graft sutured securely over the raw amputation stump. Thin split-thickness skin grafts should be avoided because they are not durable and will break down with repeated use, necessitating later revision of the amputation to a higher level.

Amputation of Distal Phalanx. If the injury damages the distal phalanx—particularly when the damage extends into the nail matrix—the nail will probably be irregular and painful when it grows back. Therefore, in traumatic amputations through the distal phalanx that involve most of the fingernail, the entire nail matrix should be removed (Plate 2). Because the nail matrix extends considerably proximal to the skin fold, extensive dissection may be necessary to remove it completely. The distal portion of the phalanx should be removed as well, but the insertions of the extensor and flexor tendons on the most proximal portion of the distal phalanx should be left intact. The entire nail matrix is identified and sharply excised, and the periosteum overlying the distal phalanx is resected to avoid creating a bone spur. As in fingertip amputations, a volar skin flap is created and the wound closure positioned dorsally. Enough skin should be left to allow closure without tension but also without redundant tissue.

Amputation Through Middle Phalanx. A crushing injury that destroys the distal phalanx and a portion of the middle phalanx necessitates amputation through the middle phalanx (Plate 2). If the insertion of the flexor digitorum superficialis into the base of the middle phalanx can be preserved, some function of the proximal interphalangeal joint may be preserved as well. If the insertion of the tendon has been avulsed, there is little reason to preserve the middle phalanx, and disarticulation through the proximal interphalangeal joint should be considered. The nerves are carefully transected under tension and allowed to retract into the soft tissues. Bony spikes are removed, and the bone ends are smoothed to maximize function of the amputation stump. At this

level, circulation to the residual skin flaps is usually quite good, and if there is any chance of preserving some function of the proximal interphalangeal joint, irregularly shaped flaps may be used to cover the stump to preserve length.

Amputation of Finger and Ray. Occasionally, an entire finger must be amputated because of severe injury, aggressive infection, or malignant tumor. Generally, the distal half of the respective metacarpal is resected as well—a procedure called a ray amputation (Plate 3). When the finger is amputated at the metacarpophalangeal level, leaving the metacarpal intact, a prominent stump persists in the palm. When the patient makes a fist, a hole is created through which objects can fall. The residual metacarpal is a significant problem

Amputation
(Continued)

Amputation of Upper Arm and Shoulder

Above–elbow amputation

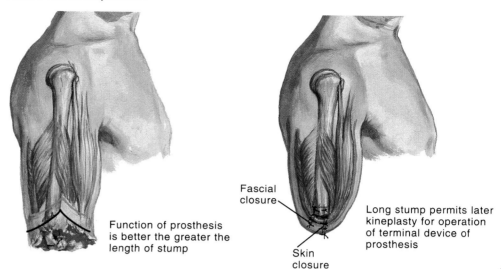

Function of prosthesis is better the greater the length of stump

Fascial closure

Skin closure

Long stump permits later kineplasty for operation of terminal device of prosthesis

Disarticulation of shoulder

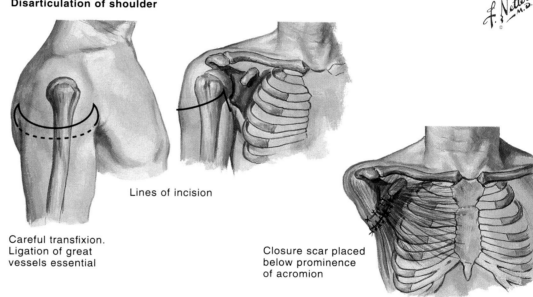

Lines of incision

Careful transfixion. Ligation of great vessels essential

Closure scar placed below prominence of acromion

following injuries of the index finger. If the second metacarpal is left in place, opposition of the thumb to the remaining long finger is difficult. Removal of most of the second metacarpal allows the thumb to lie closer to the middle finger, improving grip and overall function of the hand. Thus, when amputation is necessary at the metacarpophalangeal level, ray resection is often the treatment of choice.

Deepening of Thenar Web Cleft. The most important digit of the hand is the thumb, and all efforts should be made to preserve it and as much of its length as possible. Sometimes, it is even preferable to leave an insensate, motionless stump if the only alternative is complete amputation of the thumb. When all the fingers have been amputated, gross gripping and prehension can be restored to some degree by deepening the thenar web space (Plate 3). Deepening of the web space between the first and second metacarpals is accomplished by resecting a portion of the adductor pollicis muscle and the thenar half of the first dorsal interosseous muscle. A Z-plasty technique is used, and the skin is incised to provide access to the muscles for resection. Then, closure of the Z-plasty flaps creates a cleft in the web space. The residual adductor muscle is used to power the first metacarpal for gross prehension.

Disarticulation of Wrist. When amputation of the hand is needed because of severe injury, infection, or aggressive tumor, a wrist disarticulation is performed (Plate 4). The prominent styloid processes of the ulna and radius are resected to avoid irritation by the prosthesis. Stumps of the flexor tendons sutured to the roughened bone edges at their resting length preserve the muscle mass of the forearm.

Below-Elbow Amputation. Amputation through the forearm, traditionally called a below-elbow amputation, is usually necessitated by severe injury. The bone ends are covered with the fascia of the extensor muscles sutured to the fascia of the flexor muscle groups (Plate 4). Preserving these large muscle groups and suturing their tendons under slight tension facilitate the use of a myoelectric prosthesis at a later stage of rehabilitation. The myoelectric prosthesis powers its terminal device to mimic specific hand functions by using special pads that sense the contraction of these muscle groups.

Forequarter amputation

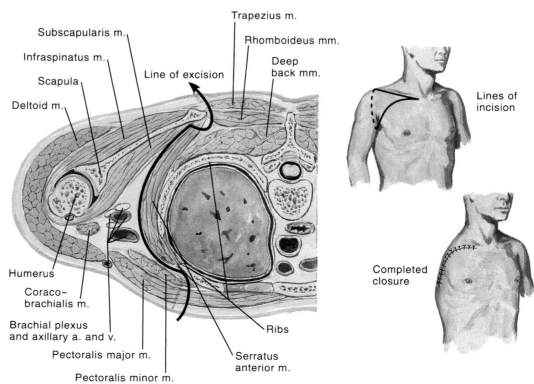

Subscapularis m.

Infraspinatus m.

Scapula

Deltoid m.

Trapezius m.

Rhomboideus mm.

Deep back mm.

Line of excision

Humerus

Coraco-brachialis m.

Brachial plexus and axillary a. and v.

Pectoralis major m.

Pectoralis minor m.

Ribs

Serratus anterior m.

Lines of incision

Completed closure

Amputation of Foot

Amputation

(Continued)

Amputation of toe

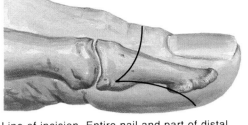

Line of incision. Entire nail and part of distal
phalanx excised

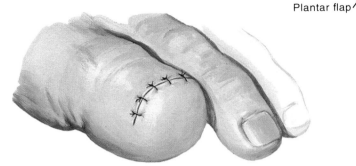

Wound closed without excessive tension

Amputation of 5th ray

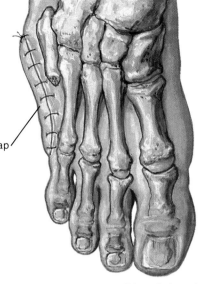

Plantar flap

5th ray removed. Wound closed
with plantar flap

Transmetatarsal amputation

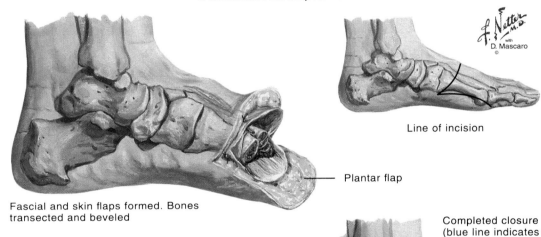

Fascial and skin flaps formed. Bones
transected and beveled

Line of incision

Plantar flap

Completed closure
(blue line indicates
fascial closure)

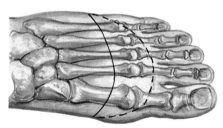

Curve of flaps (broken line indicates
plantar flap)

Amputation of Upper Arm and Shoulder

Above-Elbow Amputation. An amputation
above the elbow should be designed to preserve
as much length of the residual limb as possible.
To function successfully, an artificial upper limb
must have a long lever arm, and as much of the
humerus as possible should be saved to provide
this lever (Plate 5). Even a very short humerus
stump should be retained if possible, because
disarticulation of the shoulder greatly diminishes
the powering of the artificial limb.

Occasionally, a kineplasty technique is used to
enable the patient to operate the terminal device
of an upper limb prosthesis. In this procedure, a
tunnel is made beneath the biceps brachii muscle and the entire tunnel covered with skin, creating a loop of muscle. The cables for the operation
of a terminal device of an upper limb prosthesis
are attached to this muscle loop.

Forequarter Amputation. This radical procedure
is usually reserved for the treatment of aggressive,
malignant tumors. In contrast to the disarticulation of the shoulder joint, a forequarter amputation
removes all of the bone architecture and muscles
of the upper limb (Plate 5). It is a devastating amputation that provides no residual base to support
an artificial limb. Consequently, it is usually
very difficult to obtain a satisfactory fit of the
prosthesis.

Amputation of Foot

Amputation of Toe. Frequently, a portion of
the distal phalanx of the toe must be amputated
because of injury or chronic infection. The appropriate procedure is a terminal Syme amputation
(Plate 6). A long plantar skin flap is used, as in
the classic Syme ankle-level amputation. The entire
nail and its germinal matrix are removed to prevent the regrowth of irregular nail fragments, and
a part of the distal phalanx is excised. The long
plantar skin flap is brought up dorsally and
approximated to the dorsal skin flap without
excessive tension. The long plantar flap is usually
better vascularized than the dorsal skin; it is also
more durable and tolerates weight-bearing pressures better than the thinner dorsal skin.

Amputation of Ray. When injury or infection
involves an entire toe, resection of a single ray
(the digit plus the head and shaft of the corresponding metatarsal) can preserve foot function,
particularly in amputation of one of the lateral
four toes (Plate 6). Resection of the first ray can
also result in good function, although the power
in push-off is significantly impaired. The plantar
skin should be preserved and the wound closed
on the dorsum of the foot, if possible.

Transmetatarsal Amputation. One of the most
common amputations for forefoot infections in
diabetic patients and for severe forefoot trauma
involves removal of the forefoot by transecting the

metatarsals (Plate 6). The line of skin incision is
positioned more distally on the plantar than on
the dorsal aspect of the foot. This approach allows
the wound closure to be placed on the dorsum of
the foot so that it will not break down with weight
bearing.

Usually, transection of the metatarsal is through
the necks, although more proximal levels of transection can be used to allow wound closure without excessive tension. The metatarsals are transected
in a smooth parabola, with the shaft of the second
metatarsal remaining the longest. In addition, the
bones are beveled plantarly so that no bone spikes
stick down into the plantar aspect of the foot.

Amputation
(Continued)

Closure of the deep fascia over the end of the bone provides a supportive pad for weight bearing.

The major advantage of this level of amputation is that it preserves enough length to allow the patient to wear a normal lace-up shoe, using a foam filler in the toe box. Most patients with transmetatarsal amputation are able to walk without a special prosthesis.

Syme Amputation (Wagner Modification). Syme described a technique for disarticulation of the ankle that preserves the heel pad. Wagner devised a two-stage modification of this technique that is commonly used today (Plate 7). In the first stage, the bones of the foot are resected. Transverse incisions are made across the dorsum of the foot at the level of the talar neck and on the plantar aspect of the foot at about the level of the calcaneocuboid joint. Particular care must be taken to avoid laceration of the posterior tibial artery because it supplies the plantar skin and heel pad. With forcible plantar flexion of the ankle, the surgeon exposes the talus by transecting the extensor tendons and incising the anterior capsule of the ankle joint. The talus is disarticulated from the ankle joint; further plantar flexion exposes the attachment of the Achilles tendon to the posterior tuberosity of the calcaneus. Using very sharp and careful dissection, the surgeon shells the calcaneus out of the plantar fat pad, which is preserved along with the posterior tibial neurovascular bundle. After all the bones of the foot have been shelled out of the amputation stump, the plantar flap, including the retained plantar heel pad, is loosely approximated to the anterior skin flap over a drain.

The second stage of the procedure is performed after the flaps have healed, usually in 6 to 10 weeks. The medial and lateral aspects of the ankle

Syme Amputation (Wagner Modification)
Stage I

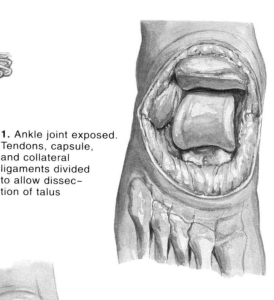

1. Ankle joint exposed. Tendons, capsule, and collateral ligaments divided to allow dissection of talus

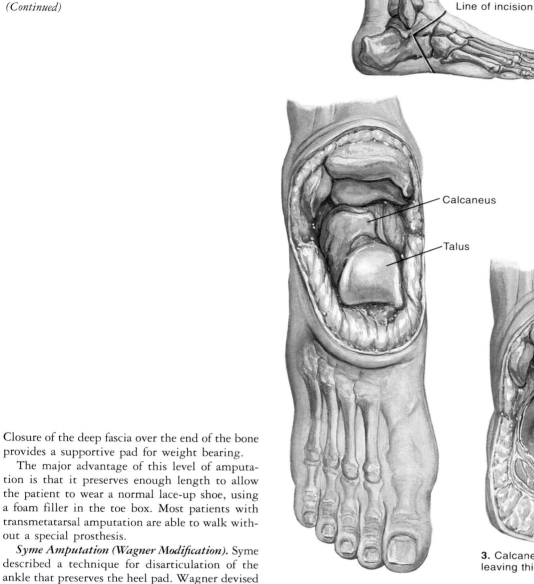

Calcaneus

Talus

2. Talus dislocated and foot placed in plantar flexion to allow dissection of calcaneus

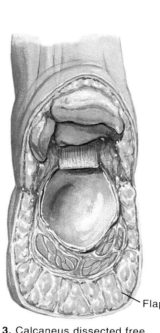

Flap

3. Calcaneus dissected free, leaving thick plantar pad flap

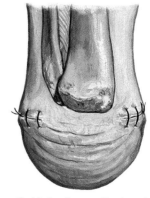

Flap

4. Heel pad flap rotated up over distal tibia and fibula and closed in layers over drain

JOHN A. CRAIG—AD
&
D. Mascaro

Stage II (delayed)

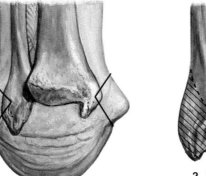

1. "Dog ears" elliptically excised, exposing malleoli

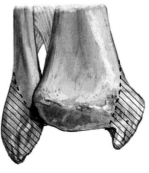

2. Medial and lateral malleoli and flares (shaded area) resected flush with joint

3. Malleoli smoothed and wounds closed

are exposed and the prominent malleoli removed. When the bones heal, the plantar fat pad and intact plantar heel skin adhere to the distal end of the tibia. The chief advantage of the Syme amputation is that the plantar skin and the heel pad are retained. The integrity of these structures allows full, unprotected weight bearing on the amputation stump. Although the residual limb is short, the patient can walk for short distances without using an artificial limb.

Below–Knee Amputation

Amputation
(Continued)

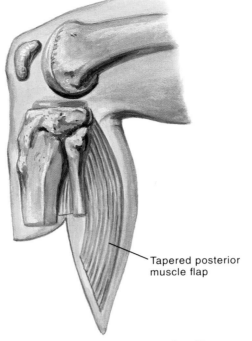

Tapered posterior
muscle flap

1. Short anterior and long posterior skin
flaps created. Tibia and fibula resected

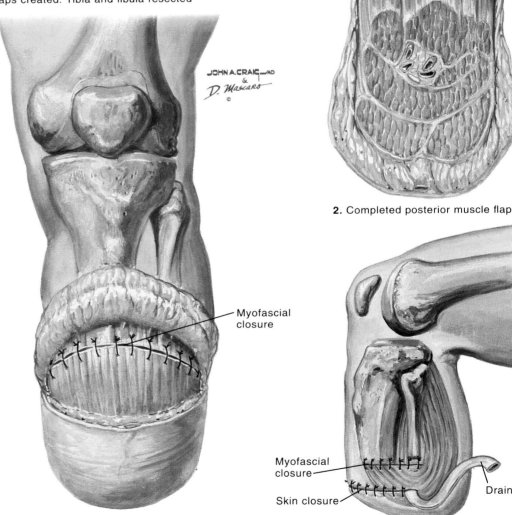

JOHN A. CRAIG—AD
&
D. Mascaro

2. Completed posterior muscle flap

Myofascial
closure

3. Muscle flap folded anteriorly and sutured
to fascia and periosteum

Myofascial
closure

Skin closure

Drain

4. Completed closure

Amputation of Lower Limb and Hip

Below-Knee Amputation. The most common amputation performed in patients with diabetic foot infections and gangrene of the foot resulting from peripheral vascular disease is a below-knee amputation (Plate 8). Both conditions usually involve most of the foot, preventing successful amputation at a more distal level. Because the blood supply to the posterior muscles of the leg is usually better than that to the anterior musculature, the most common method for a below-knee amputation involves the creation of a long posterior muscle and skin flap. Usually, a below-knee amputation is performed about 10 cm below the level of the knee joint. The anterior skin incision is made at this level and the tibia transected; the anterior tibial crest is carefully beveled. The fibula is usually transected about 1 cm shorter than the tibia. The posterior muscle mass is preserved 8 to 10 cm longer, along with the posterior skin and subcutaneous tissue. The posterior muscle mass is tapered with a sharp knife, and the long posterior flap is folded forward. The superficial fascia of the posterior muscle flap is sutured to the superficial fascia of the anterior compartment muscles to create a deep myofascial closure. The skin is closed over a drain.

The knee joint should be preserved whenever possible. Even a below-knee amputation with a short stump of only 4 or 5 cm may permit some knee joint function, greatly facilitating the fitting of a prosthetic limb. The knee joint also allows the patient to walk more efficiently. This efficiency is best demonstrated by measuring the oxygen demands of patients with lower limb amputations. When walking on a level surface, patients with a unilateral above-knee amputation

use twice as much oxygen as patients with a unilateral below-knee amputation.

Disarticulation of Knee. This procedure may be chosen when it is not possible to preserve the limb below the level of the knee (Plate 9). Anterior and

posterior skin flaps of equal length are fashioned, preserving the patellar ligament and patella. The patellar ligament is sutured into the stumps of the cruciate ligaments to provide a stable point of fixation for the quadriceps femoris muscle.

Amputation
(Continued)

Disarticulation of Knee

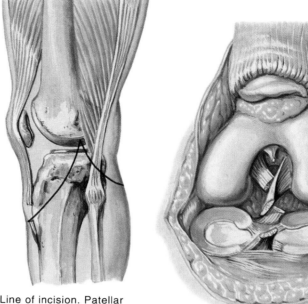

Line of incision. Patellar ligament and pes anserinus included in anterior flap

Capsular structures divided and knee disarticulated

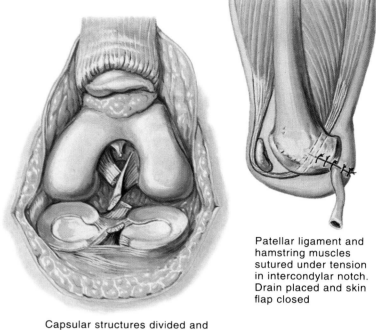

Patellar ligament and hamstring muscles sutured under tension in intercondylar notch. Drain placed and skin flap closed

Above–Knee Amputation

Above-Knee Amputation. Amputation above the knee is frequently required for severe vascular insufficiency after attempts to reconstruct the vascular tree have failed. The amputation is usually performed through the midportion of the femur (Plate 9). At this level, the blood supply to the muscles of the lower limb improves significantly; very often, viable muscle is encountered. The muscle must be closed securely over the end of the femur by suturing the fascia of the hamstring muscles to that of the quadriceps femoris muscle. The skin is always closed over a drain.

Disarticulation of Hip. Aggressive tumors, infection, and necrosis may necessitate a disarticulation of the hip or a hindquarter amputation (Plate 10). With hip disarticulation, the entire femur is removed, and a large posterior skin flap is preserved and brought forward. The surgeon should attempt to preserve the gluteus muscles, which can serve as a cushion for sitting and for supporting a lower limb prosthesis.

Hindquarter Amputation. Hindquarter amputation, or hemipelvectomy, includes removal of the entire lower limb and the entire innominate bone of the pelvis (Plate 10). Three levels of resection have been described. The standard approach is a disarticulation through the sacroiliac joint. In a modified, or conservative, approach, the line of resection is just lateral to the sacroiliac joint, preserving a small rim of the ilium. When the tumor extends across the sacroiliac joint, an extended resection through the sacral foramina may be necessary. Regardless of the level of ilium resection posteriorly, the surgeon tries to preserve some

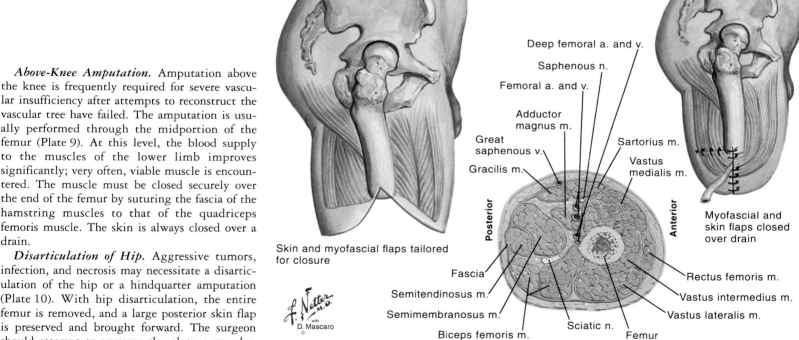

Skin and myofascial flaps tailored for closure

Deep femoral a. and v.
Saphenous n.
Femoral a. and v.
Adductor magnus m.
Great saphenous v.
Gracilis m.
Sartorius m.
Vastus medialis m.
Posterior
Anterior
Fascia
Semitendinosus m.
Semimembranosus m.
Biceps femoris m.
Sciatic n.
Femur
Rectus femoris m.
Vastus intermedius m.
Vastus lateralis m.
Myofascial and skin flaps closed over drain

gluteus muscles to provide coverage of the abdominal organs, which will otherwise be vulnerable to injury following resection of the ilium.

Complications After Amputation

Many complications can result from the traumatic or operative amputation of a limb (Plate 11). Use of careful operative techniques prevents many of these problems. Wound necrosis, excessive bleeding, and infection are problems that can arise in the immediate postoperative period.

The most common cause of wound necrosis is excessively tight closure of the skin over an amputation stump. Therefore, the skin edges should always be closed loosely. An adequate amount of bone should be resected to allow closure of the skin without excessive tension.

Bleeding is also a common problem following amputation. During the operation, all large vessels must be ligated, and every small vessel that is bleeding must be cauterized. A tourniquet is rarely needed in an amputation unless excessive blood loss threatens the stability of the patient's circulatory system. If a tourniquet is required, it should be deflated before wound closure so that the surgeon can ascertain that all bleeding sites are completely controlled. In addition, all amputation wounds should be drained postoperatively.

Amputation
(Continued)

In small amputation sites such as a fingertip or ray resection, a Penrose drain is placed in the depths of the wound. In larger amputation sites, a suction drain is placed to evacuate any hematoma that may form. The amount of blood loss following amputation must be monitored closely to maintain hemodynamic stability.

Inadequate resection of necrotic, gangrenous, or infected tissue leads to failure of the amputation. If the viability of the soft tissues at the level of amputation is questionable, the amputation stump is left open and a compression dressing applied to the stump. The patient is returned to the operating room in 24 to 48 hours for reinspection of the soft tissues. If the soft tissues are found to be viable, secondary closure is carried out at that time. The finding of further necrotic or infected tissue, however, necessitates amputation at a higher level. Careful handling of the tissues with minimal trauma and exclusive use of simple sutures to loosely approximate the skin edges minimize the risk of causing further necrosis of the skin edges.

Late complications of amputations include bone overgrowth, joint contractures, phantom limb pain, and formation of neuromas. At the site of amputation through a bone, disruption of the periosteum stimulates new bone formation, similar to the formation of callus during the fracture repair process. The formation of an exuberant amount of callus over the end of the bone creates irregular, protuberant osteophytes. These osteophytes may erode through the skin, particularly when they press on the inner surface of a prosthesis. The presence of a large osteophyte may prevent effective fitting of a prosthesis and necessitate operative revision of the strip to avoid skin ulceration.

Disarticulation of Hip

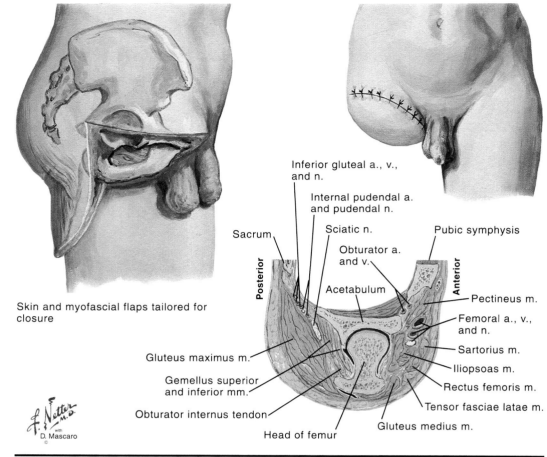

Skin and myofascial flaps tailored for closure

Inferior gluteal a., v., and n.

Internal pudendal a. and pudendal n.

Sacrum

Sciatic n.

Pubic symphysis

Obturator a. and v.

Acetabulum

Posterior

Anterior

Pectineus m.

Femoral a., v., and n.

Sartorius m.

Iliopsoas m.

Rectus femoris m.

Tensor fasciae latae m.

Gluteus medius m.

Gluteus maximus m.

Gemellus superior and inferior mm.

Obturator internus tendon

Head of femur

Hindquarter Amputation (Hemipelvectomy)

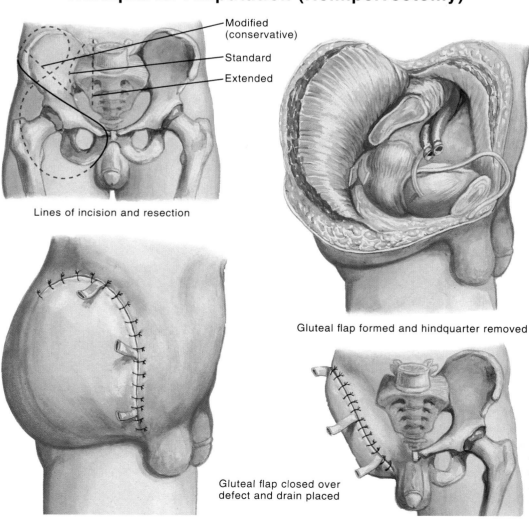

Modified (conservative)

Standard

Extended

Lines of incision and resection

Gluteal flap formed and hindquarter removed

Gluteal flap closed over defect and drain placed

Complications of Amputation

Amputation
(Continued)

Necrosis of wound edges caused by excessively tight sutures

Necrotic wound edges in immediate postoperative period

Osteophyte

Ulceration

Pressure necrosis and ulceration of overlying skin caused by formation of osteophytes

Flexion contracture of knee in below–knee amputation prevents full extension of limb

Phantom limb pain

Nerve cut under gentle traction and allowed to retract into soft tissues

Joint contracture is one of the most common problems following amputation. In the immediate postoperative period, a physical therapy program must be instituted to prevent the development of joint contractures proximal to the level of amputation. Contractures can be prevented with an aggressive program of passive stretching conducted by a physical or occupational therapist trained in the management of patients with amputations (see Section IV, Plate 2). The passive stretching program must be performed daily, and the patient must avoid positions that promote the development of contractures. In particular, patients with a below-knee amputation must never sleep with a pillow beneath the knee, because that posture promotes flexion contractures of both knee and hip. One of the most effective ways of avoiding knee flexion contracture following below-knee amputation is with the use of rigid surgical dressing in the immediate postoperative period. This plaster cast (developed by Burgess) performs many functions: it holds the knee in full extension; protects the soft tissues and facilitates healing of the amputation stump; prevents the formation of edema, which frequently leads to skin breakdown; accommodates a pylon that will be used to permit weight bearing in the early healing phases; and accelerates the rehabilitation process.

Persistent pain following an amputation has many causes. Osteophytes may produce a pressure point, leading to irritation of the overlying skin. Transected nerves may also be a source of persistent pain. Following transection of a nerve, the normal reparative processes form a neuroma at the cut nerve end in an attempt to regenerate axons and restore nerve function. The neuroma that forms at the cut surface of any nerve is sensitive and easily irritated, particularly by direct pressure from a prosthetic limb. A neuroma is embedded in the

amputation scar is especially vulnerable to pressure and irritation. The best way to avoid this problem is to apply gentle traction to the nerve, cut it sharply, and allow it to retract proximally into the soft tissues of the limb.

Following amputation, patients usually experience the phantom limb phenomenon, which occurs because the proximal portions of the nerves to the amputated part are still present and because the image of the amputated part remains imprinted in the cerebral cortex. The patient experiences the sensation that the limb is still present after amputation. All patients experience this sensation to some degree, although usually it gradually subsides in

several months. The use of a rigid dressing seems to facilitate the resolution of these symptoms. Rarely, the phantom limb phenomenon persists and becomes very painful, producing a chronic and intractable set of symptoms called phantom limb pain. Once established, phantom limb pain is extremely difficult to eradicate.

An early, aggressive, and well-organized rehabilitation program helps to minimize many of the complications of amputation. A successful program requires a team of therapists and physicians well schooled in the principles of rehabilitation after amputation, as presented in Section IV, Plates 1–5. □

Section IV
Rehabilitation

Frank H. Netter, M.D.

in collaboration with

Daniel Dumitru, M.D.   *Plates 6 – 12*
Leslie D. Porter, M.D.   *Plates 13 – 15*
Nicolas E. Walsh, M.D.   *Plates 1 – 5, 16 – 17*

Rehabilitation

Rehabilitation focuses on restorating function and on helping patients to adapt to their environment. The rehabilitation team is coordinated by a physician who specializes in physical medicine and rehabilitation, and comprises physical and occupational therapists, nurses, and other health care professionals. The goals of rehabilitation are (1) to restore functional capacity of the affected systems, (2) to prevent additional disability, (3) to enhance unaffected systems to improve functional capabilities, (4) to use adaptive and supportive equipment to promote function, and (5) to modify the environment to increase the patient's functional independence.

Immobilization

Prolonged immobilization can be devastating to all the systems of the body (Plate 1). Because immobility frequently prolongs and complicates the rehabilitation process, the duration of immobilization should be minimized and the immobility limited to the involved area. Most adversely affected are the musculoskeletal, cardiovascular, nervous, and integumentary systems.

Preservation of range of joint motion and muscle strength is essential to the rehabilitation of any patient. Joint contractures limit the patient's mobility and performance of daily activities and impede general nursing care. Immobilization for even 24 hours initiates contractures of capsule, soft tissue, and muscle. Two weeks of immobilization may result in a contracture that may take months of exercises to correct, and after 2 months of immobilization, the contracture may require surgical correction.

Contractures can be prevented by proper positioning, early mobilization, and active or passive range-of-motion exercises for each joint performed at least every 8 hours. Bed rest and immobility should be minimized with active physical therapy, self-care activities, and recreational diversion, which significantly reduce the risk of disuse atrophy. Contractures that do occur are treated with passive range-of-motion exercises with terminal stretch, prolonged stretch with heat modalities, progressive dynamic orthoses, and surgical release.

Immobility also decreases muscle strength and reduces endurance and aerobic function. Altered muscle function may also manifest in poor coordination and functional movement. Decreased muscle strength due to disuse or immobilization may be prevented with a program of daily muscle contractions, electric stimulation (for muscle immobilized in a cast), and isometric exercises.

The stresses of weight bearing and muscle pull maintain the normal calcium content of bones. With immobility or nonweight bearing, this stress is reduced significantly, and osteoclastic activity exceeds osteoblastic activity. Within days, increases in urinary loss of calcium can be documented. The resulting osteopenia weakens the bone, predisposing to pathologic fractures. Calcium loss may be prevented by immobilization in the antigravity position. When only a limb is immobilized, low-level electric stimulation can be used to increase bone deposition.

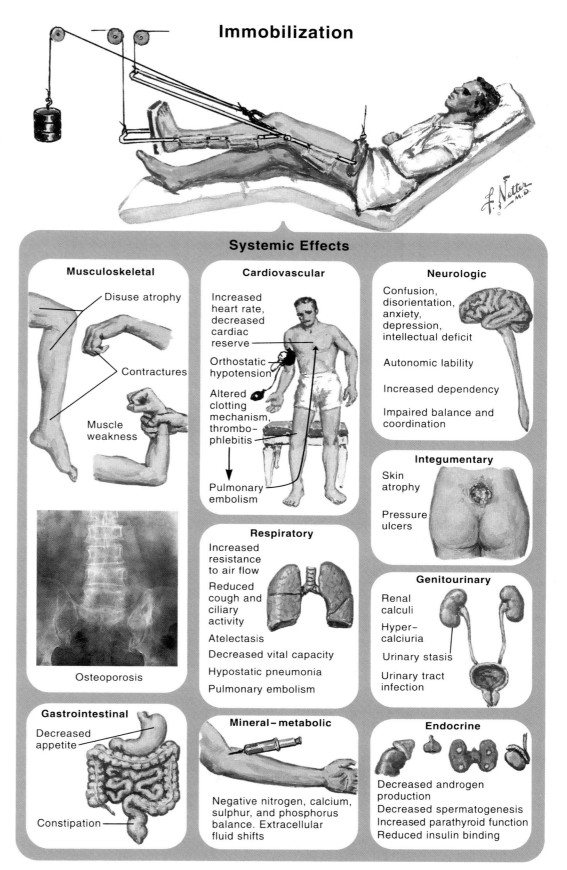

Immobilization

Systemic Effects

Musculoskeletal
- Disuse atrophy
- Contractures
- Muscle weakness
- Osteoporosis

Cardiovascular
- Increased heart rate, decreased cardiac reserve
- Orthostatic hypotension
- Altered clotting mechanism, thrombophlebitis
- Pulmonary embolism

Neurologic
- Confusion, disorientation, anxiety, depression, intellectual deficit
- Autonomic lability
- Increased dependency
- Impaired balance and coordination

Integumentary
- Skin atrophy
- Pressure ulcers

Respiratory
- Increased resistance to air flow
- Reduced cough and ciliary activity
- Atelectasis
- Decreased vital capacity
- Hypostatic pneumonia
- Pulmonary embolism

Genitourinary
- Renal calculi
- Hyper-calciuria
- Urinary stasis
- Urinary tract infection

Gastrointestinal
- Decreased appetite
- Constipation

Mineral–metabolic
- Negative nitrogen, calcium, sulphur, and phosphorus balance. Extracellular fluid shifts

Endocrine
- Decreased androgen production
- Decreased spermatogenesis
- Increased parathyroid function
- Reduced insulin binding

The cardiovascular system responds to prolonged immobility with postural hypotension, impaired exercise tolerance, and thrombophlebitis. Each of these complications may be prevented with early mobilization and physical therapy. Bed rest and the resulting sensory deprivation adversely affect the nervous system, impairing balance and coordination and decreasing intellectual capacity. Sensory deprivation leads to confusion and disorientation, which contribute to anxiety and depression. Immobilization also tends to promote helplessness and dependency, and the longer a patient is immobilized, the more difficult the rehabilitation and return to independence may become.

Decubitus ulcers are common, expensive, and preventable complications of bed rest. Prolonged pressure is the principal cause, and patients immobilized in a bed, wheelchair, or cast need to be moved frequently from one position to another. Careful observation of skin areas where pressure necrosis usually occurs is essential. □

Rehabilitation After Amputation

Approximately 150,000 surgical amputations are performed in the United States every year. Many times, only a stump remains, extending a few inches beyond the proximal joint. A prosthetic limb allows amputees to lead a near-normal life by providing a mechanical extension to the residual limb. Whereas surgical amputation is often lifesaving, it produces major physical changes and emotional consequences that require functional and psychologic rehabilitation. Ideally, rehabilitation of the amputee begins with physical intervention to increase strength in the sound limbs and maximize range of motion in the primary joints.

Preprosthetic Rehabilitation

The preprosthetic phase of the rehabilitation program focuses on educating the patient in coping with operative losses and with care of the residual limb. Often, the initial evaluation of the patient is completed before surgery; functional capability, limitations in range of motion, and strength in both the involved and uninvolved limbs are identified. Information about the patient's level of independence in activities of daily living, social support, and postoperative expectations should also be obtained. The anticipated level of amputation and the prognosis for the ultimate functional outcome are discussed with the patient and family. Instruction is given in range-of-motion and strengthening activities, correct positioning of the residual limb, and postoperative therapies.

During surgery, the surgeon determines the optimal level of amputation that will leave a functional residual limb. The residual limb may be fitted with an immediate postoperative prosthesis in the operating room; this procedure helps to control edema and promotes healing. Alternatively, air splints, controlled environment treatment dressings, and figure-of-8 elastic bandage can be used.

Postoperatively, prevention of joint contractions is of major importance. The residual limb must be positioned in proper alignment, and all joints proximal to the amputation should be moved through full range of motion three times a day.

The postoperative rehabilitation program prepares the patient and the residual limb for prosthesis fitting (Plate 2). The incision is allowed to heal, and the patient participates in a physical therapy program to maintain range of motion and strength in the remaining limbs. The stump is kept wrapped in an elastic compression bandage to decrease edema and protect the wound. In addition to shrinking the stump and protecting the wound, the elastic compression bandage helps to mold the residual limb. In patients who are unable to use elastic compression bandages, a stump shrinker, a removable or nonremovable rigid dressing, or an Unna paste cast (Unna boot) may be used. Activities are designed to allow the new

Rehabilitation After Amputation

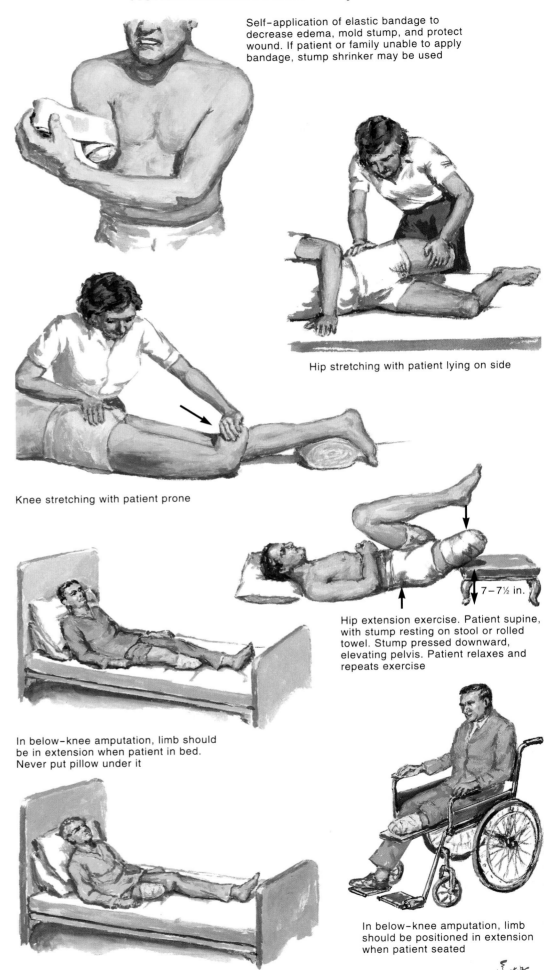

Self-application of elastic bandage to decrease edema, mold stump, and protect wound. If patient or family unable to apply bandage, stump shrinker may be used

Hip stretching with patient lying on side

Knee stretching with patient prone

Hip extension exercise. Patient supine, with stump resting on stool or rolled towel. Stump pressed downward, elevating pelvis. Patient relaxes and repeats exercise

7–7½ in.

In below-knee amputation, limb should be in extension when patient in bed. Never put pillow under it

In above-knee amputation, limb should be maintained in adduction when patient in bed

In below-knee amputation, limb should be positioned in extension when patient seated

Prosthetic Rehabilitation After Amputation

Rehabilitation After Amputation

(Continued)

amputee to successfully demonstrate independence in mobility and tasks of daily living. Psychologic support is important, because the loss of a limb has significant impact on the patient's self-image and induces a feeling of loss.

The preprosthetic phase of rehabilitation is often completed in 3 to 6 weeks for upper limb amputation, 4 to 7 weeks for lower limb amputation resulting from trauma, and 6 to 10 weeks for lower limb amputation resulting from vascular disorders.

Prosthetic Rehabilitation

More than 70% of amputees are fitted with a prosthesis (Plate 3). Candidates for prosthetic rehabilitation should demonstrate adequate wound healing, range of motion, muscle strength, motor control, and cognitive ability to learn to use the prosthesis. Owing to the increased metabolic demands of prosthesis use, these patients should also have adequate pulmonary and cardiovascular reserves. Factors that suggest a patient is a poor candidate for a functional prosthesis include lack of motivation, severe neurologic problems, inadequate wound healing of the residual limb, above-knee amputation with a 45° flexion contracture at the hip, below-elbow amputation with a flail elbow or shoulder, and multiple major physical impairments. Although clearly defined criteria are not available, the patient with a lower limb amputation who can walk with a walker or crutches without a prosthesis will usually be able to ambulate with a prosthesis. Patients whose potential for functional use of a prosthesis is questionable are first fitted with a trial prosthesis and evaluated.

The fabricated prosthesis is assessed for fit and function. The patient with an upper limb prosthesis is taught to don and doff the prosthesis in a manner similar to slipping a shirt on and off. The patient learns to control each mechanism of the prosthetic limb, first using isolated movements of each control mechanism and then integrating these movements into complete actions. Occupational therapy trains the patient to use the limb in activities of daily living and work.

The patient with a lower limb amputation is taught to apply and remove the prosthesis and begins standing between parallel bars, shifting weight from the sound leg to the limb with the prosthesis. The patient learns to ambulate by placing the sound foot forward and letting the momentum of the body swing the prosthesis through. Emphasis is placed on maintaining an even gait pattern. Then, functional activities such as rising from and sitting in a chair, climbing steps, and negotiating curbs are initiated. The final test of functional capability is ambulation over grass and rough ground. Young, athletic amputees are taught to run, pivot, and traverse obstacles. Most amputees are trained on an outpatient basis, attending therapy three times a week for 4 to 10 weeks.

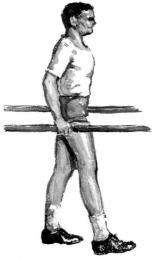

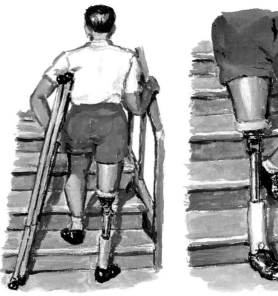

Patient learns to walk with prosthesis using parallel bars

Patient practices going up and down stairs with lower limb prosthesis

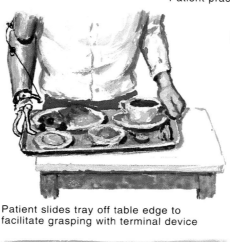

Patient slides tray off table edge to facilitate grasping with terminal device

Patient learns shop work with prosthesis

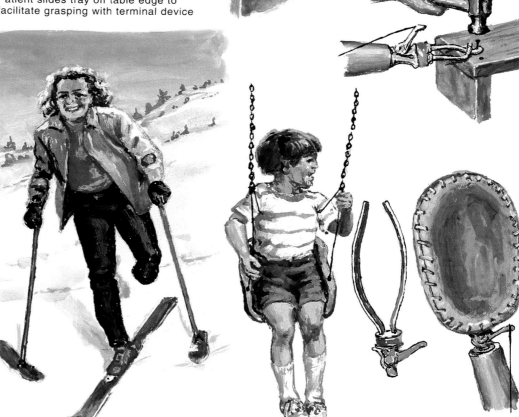

Patient with lower limb amputation enjoys winter sports

Child with myoelectric prosthesis on right upper limb participates in playground activities

Special terminal device and glove for playing baseball

Prostheses for Lower Limb

Rehabilitation After Amputation

(Continued)

Follow-up Care

Routine follow-up evaluations should occur at 2-month intervals for the first 6 months, then at yearly intervals. The residual and contralateral limbs are examined for weakness, decreased range of motion, tenderness, ulceration, ischemia, irritation, and infection, the prosthesis is inspected for fit and breakdown.

Special problems of the amputee include phantom limb pain, dermatologic disorders, socket fit, and altered biomechanics. After amputation of a limb, the patient usually has a phantom limb sensation—a feeling that the most distal and highly innervated part of the severed limb, usually the foot or hand, is still attached (see Section III, Plate 11). Some patients experience pain in the phantom limb, which may be due to the phantom limb phenomenon or to a neuroma of the transected nerves. Neuromas are most successfully treated with neurolysis; phantom limb pain responds best to tricyclic antidepressants. Other treatments include phantom limb exercises and therapeutic modalities. Phantom limb sensation and pain usually resolve with the successful fitting of the prosthesis.

Dermatologic disorders in amputees may be minimized by washing and drying the residual limb daily and using clean, dry, absorbent stump socks to minimize skin maceration. Hyperhidrosis is controlled with application of concentrated antiperspirants. Folliculitis may require antibiotics, and allergic dermatitis is controlled by eliminating the cause of the irritation.

Another chronic problem for the amputee is socket fit. Significant changes in weight or limb topography necessitate fabrication of a new socket for the prosthesis. Significant tissue atrophy occurs in the first 12 to 18 months after amputation, often necessitating replacement of the socket. During the first 5 years, a patient with a lower limb amputation typically requires three to five new sockets. The average prosthesis lasts 3 to 5 years.

The patient with a lower limb prosthesis uses more energy to walk at the same velocity as a normal person and adapts to these increased energy requirements by reducing walking speed. Although loss of a limb restricts some activities, amputees adapt to most vocational and recreational activities, and many continue to work. The loss of a limb rarely prevents a person from finding recreational endeavors that are challenging and satisfying.

Prosthetic Design

The components of a prosthesis include a socket, a suspension mechanism, a joint unit, a terminal device for the hand or an artificial foot, and a skeleton to connect these parts. The most important aspect of a prosthesis is the socket. Ultimately, the design and fit of a socket determine patient acceptance, comfort, suspension, and energy expenditure.

The exoskeletal and endoskeletal constructions provide strength and stability to the prosthesis. The

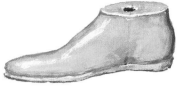

SACH foot. Used in conjunction with most lower limb prostheses

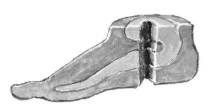

Seattle foot (sagittal section). May be used as alternative to SACH foot. Note flexible plastic keel

Flexfoot with cosmetic cover

SACH foot applied directly to end of Syme amputation, held by socket that conforms to bulbous end of stump

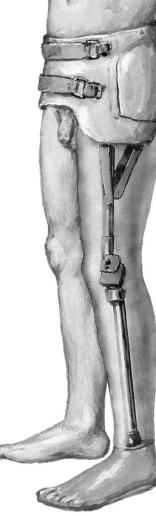

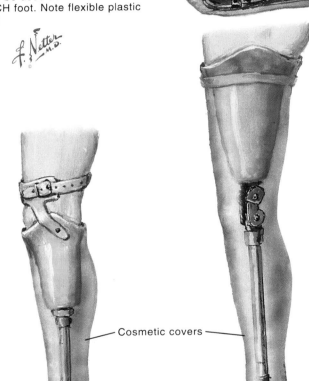

Cosmetic covers

Below-knee endoskeletal prosthesis held with strap; includes SACH foot

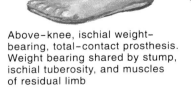

Above-knee, ischial weight-bearing, total-contact prosthesis. Weight bearing shared by stump, ischial tuberosity, and muscles of residual limb

Hip disarticulation or hemipelvectomy prosthesis with pelvic socket

exoskeletal system is composed of a rigid plastic lamination over wood or foam; the endoskeletal system comprises internal modular components connected by tubing. Although exoskeletal prostheses are more durable and less expensive, they are heavier, more difficult to adjust, and less cosmetically acceptable.

Prostheses for Lower Limb. The functions replicated by the lower limb prosthesis are weight bearing, ambulation, and cosmesis (Plate 4). To optimize function, the physician must consider the patient's limitations and needs.

The socket is designed to provide a close fit with the residual limb and distribute weight over pressure-tolerant areas. In the Syme amputation, body weight is transmitted to the socket directly from the end of the stump with some weight bearing at the patellar tendon (see Section III, Plate 7). A total-contact patellar tendon–bearing (PTB) socket is routinely used for patients with a transtibial below-knee amputation. Weight is distributed primarily over the patellar tendon and tibial flare, with weight bearing reduced over pressure-sensitive areas at the bony prominences. The patient with an above-knee amputation is usually fitted with a total-contact quadrilateral socket or a narrow medial-lateral (ML) socket that stabilizes the prosthesis and the residual limb

Rehabilitation After Amputation

(Continued)

during gait. Weight bearing occurs primarily over the ischial tuberosity and gluteal surface, minimizing pressure over the residual limb.

The socket of the Syme prosthesis is shaped to the lower leg over the bulbous end, and no straps are necessary for suspension. The below-knee prosthesis is usually attached by a suprapatellar strap or a neoprene sleeve; a patellar tendon/supracondylar suspension (PTSC) may be used for more stability. Some prostheses are held in place with a rubber sleeve to maintain skin traction. Suction suspension for an above-knee prosthesis is accomplished with a one-way valve near the end of the socket. In patients who are not able to use suction suspension, a Silesian belt, a pelvic band, or a total elastic suspension (TES) belt is added.

The solid ankle cushion heel (SACH) is the most widely prescribed ankle-foot for all lower limb prostheses because of its cushioned heel strike and enhanced push-off during ambulation. The newest ankle-foot units are constructed of resilient, flexible, and energy-storing materials that improve the push-off stage of ambulation. These new designs may lower energy consumption and increase efficiency in ambulation. These and other feet, such as the Flex Foot, carbon copy, and Seattle Foot, have been extensively used by athletes with excellent results.

A variety of joints provide knee stability for above-knee prostheses. In lower limb joints, stability must always be weighed against flexibility. The most commonly used knee joint has a single axis and constant friction. Young and very active patients can use hydraulic knee units, which provide a much more normal gait. Older patients often require a safety (limited slip) knee to inhibit buckling. Other knee joints provide increased flexibility at the expense of stability.

Prostheses for Upper Limb. The levels of upper limb amputation are designated as partial hand, wrist disarticulation, below elbow, elbow disarticulation, above elbow, shoulder disarticulation, and forequarter. The upper limb prosthesis replicates complex motions that involve positioning the hand in space for specific grasping and manipulating maneuvers (Plate 5). The prosthesis does not adequately reproduce the tactile sensation provided by the fingers.

The socket for the upper limb prosthesis is custom-made to provide total contact, and it allows the involved joint a maximum range of motion. Suspension is achieved with suction or with a harness; the harness also provides an anchor point for the cable that controls the terminal device. The harness must be comfortable to wear. A shoulder saddle harness is the best suspension for persons who carry heavy loads with the prosthesis.

The prosthetic wrist joint may provide some degree of supination/pronation and flexion/extension as well as providing the socket for interchangeable terminal devices. The elbow joint for the below-elbow prosthesis is often made up of flexible hinges attached to the triceps brachii cuff.

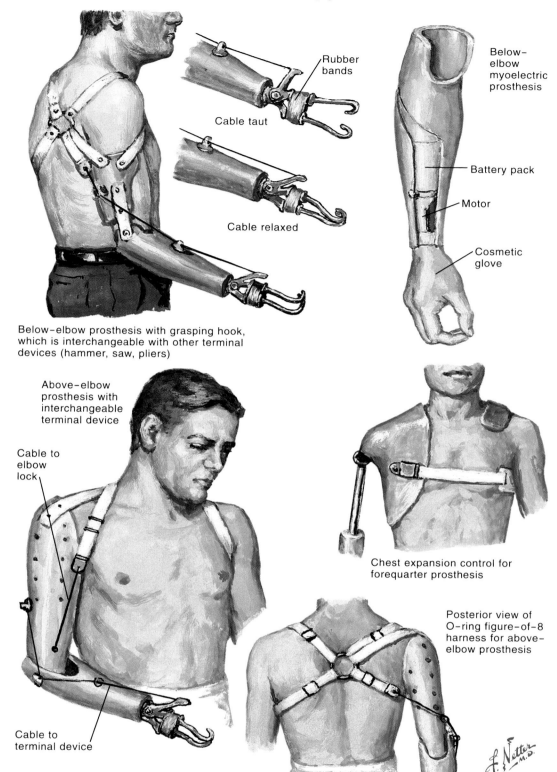

Rubber bands

Cable taut

Cable relaxed

Below-elbow prosthesis with grasping hook, which is interchangeable with other terminal devices (hammer, saw, pliers)

Below-elbow myoelectric prosthesis

Battery pack

Motor

Cosmetic glove

Above-elbow prosthesis with interchangeable terminal device

Cable to elbow lock

Cable to terminal device

Chest expansion control for forequarter prosthesis

Posterior view of O-ring figure-of-8 harness for above-elbow prosthesis

In below-elbow amputations with decreased range of motion at the elbow, a polycentric elbow joint or a split socket with step-up hinges is used to provide increased range of motion. The above-elbow prosthesis requires an elbow unit that can be locked in various positions of flexion and allows for passive positioning of humeral rotation.

Terminal devices for the upper limb prosthesis replicate some of the grasping functions of the hand. The most common devices are hooks and functional hands with voluntary opening; others include saws, hammers, pliers, and other tools. Functional prosthetic hands are covered with a cosmetic glove that gives a skinlike appearance.

An upper limb prosthesis is controlled with body-powered control cables and harness, external battery-supplied electricity with myoelectric controls, or electric switches. The conventional control cables are attached to the harness, and the patient operates the terminal device with movement of the scapula and shoulder. The elbow joint has one cable to activate the elbow lock and one to control elbow flexion when the elbow joint is unlocked and the terminal device when the elbow joint is locked. The myoelectric control system uses surface electrodes on the inner wall of the socket over appropriate muscles. When the muscles contract, the motor drives the device. □

Rehabilitation After Stroke

Every year, approximately 500,000 persons suffer a stroke in the United States, and 40% of them die. Many who survive experience cognitive and physical deficits as a result of the stroke and require some form of rehabilitation. For successful rehabilitation, the stroke victim must be able to learn and retain information and physically tolerate the demands of therapy. A person who has intellectual and physical dysfunction but is still capable of following commands and participating in therapy is a candidate for rehabilitation. The patient with no residual deficits may not require rehabilitation. However, the primary care physician must ensure that the stroke patient with no obvious impairments is truly free of subtle cognitive or self-care deficits. If there is any doubt, an evaluation should be performed by a physiatrist—a physician trained in all aspects of acute and chronic rehabilitative care.

The patient's medical and psychosocial status is evaluated, and a progressive interdisciplinary program for rehabilitation is designed while the patient is still on the acute medical service. The physical and occupational therapist and nurses, under the direction of the physiatrist and the primary care physician, plan a program to increase the patient's level of independence. A speech pathologist can often help patients with dysphasia or dysarthria to solve problems with swallowing or to improve communication.

Improving the patient's self-concept and diminishing dependency are major goals of rehabilitation. It is important to remember that the stroke patient is often fearful and unsure and may have difficulty with communication, spatial perception, vision, motor planning, memory, and sensation. All team members must keep these potential deficits in mind and offer communication that is simple, repetitive, and supportive. The patient must experience a sense of accomplishment in the first attempts at self-care activities.

Provided there are no medical contraindications, rehabilitation efforts should begin immediately following a stroke. The patient with deficits in the distribution of the middle cerebral artery is used here as a model: a lesion affecting the left cerebral hemisphere produces a right hemiparesis associated with a possible communication difficulty (dysphasia) or visual field deficit or both; damage to the right cerebral hemisphere causes left hemiparesis and possibly perceptual impairment with left-sided neglect and visual field loss. Persons with sroke damage in the distribution of the posterior cerebral artery, basilar artery, and other regions may also benefit from rehabilitation.

Positioning in Bed

During the early phase after a stroke, frequent changes of position in bed are essential. Proper positioning in bed is depicted on Plate 6. Immobility can cause excessive pressure over bony prominences, and the development of even one pressure

Positioning in Bed After Stroke

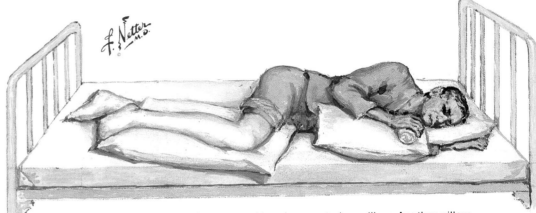

Supine position. Mattress firm, left flat. To avoid dependent edema, affected upper limb supported on pillow with shoulder abducted, hand slightly higher than elbow, and elbow slightly higher than shoulder. Small towel roll or orthosis used to maintain hand in functional position and minimize contractures of finger or wrist. Towel roll alongside trochanteric region and thigh (extending slightly under body to secure it) prevents external rotation of paretic limb. Foot board deters contracture of Achilles tendon and equinus of foot. Pressure stockings prevent deep vein thrombosis and thrombophlebitis, which may result in pulmonary embolism. Patient's position must be changed frequently because total immobility with continuous pressure over bony prominences may lead to pressure ulcers

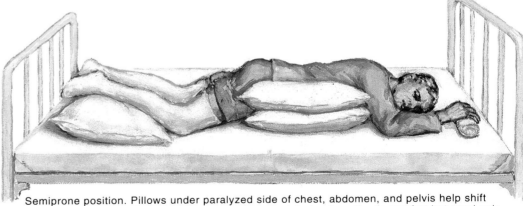

Side–lying position. Patient's forearm and hand supported on pillow. Another pillow placed under paretic lower limb, between knees and ankles. Note towel roll in hand and pressure stockings

Semiprone position. Pillows under paralyzed side of chest, abdomen, and pelvis help shift weight to good side. Optional pillow under legs contributes to patient's comfort but used only for short periods to avoid flexion contractures in knees

ulcer increases hospital stay and expenses significantly. As alertness and strength improve, the patient is taught to change position unaided. Pressure stockings may prevent deep venous thrombosis and pulmonary embolism in the lower limbs; thigh-high stockings must be maximally extended to avoid creases that may act as a tourniquet and impede venous flow.

The development of contractures significantly impedes subsequent rehabilitation efforts. The mattress should provide firm support and be left flat to avoid promoting flexion contractures. Proper positioning, combined with gentle and passive range-of-motion exercises for the dysfunctional

limbs are simple but highly effective methods of avoiding contractures and pain resulting from tight joint capsules.

Passive Range-of-Motion Exercises

After a stroke, all affected joints should be moved gently and passively through a complete range of motion at least twice a day (Plate 7). Range-of-motion exercises help to prevent contractures and muscle shortening, decrease muscle and joint pain caused by stiffness and disuse, and increase sensory input through the affected limb. The paretic limbs must always be moved slowly and gently to avoid injury to the nerve structures.

Passive Range–of–Motion Exercises After Stroke

Rehabilitation After Stroke
(Continued)

Common and often neglected complications of stroke are intellectual regression and depression associated with sensory deprivation. Usually, the patient cannot move in bed and is often left alone, unable to see anything but the ceiling or wall. Medical personnel may speak of the patient in the third person, even in the patient's presence. These factors can aggravate depression, which is often ascribed exclusively to the stroke and not to the environment. Frequent turning, range-of-motion exercises, and speaking directly to the patient help prevent sensory deprivation.

Bladder and Bowel Training

Indwelling catheters should be removed as soon as possible and replaced with intermittent catheterization, if medically warranted. Periodic catheterization, although more time-consuming, reduces the chance of urinary tract infection while allowing documentation of fluid output. This regimen should be followed by a bladder-training program. A bowel program should also be established to avoid constipation, impaction, and straining with defecation.

Transfer From Bed to Wheelchair

As soon as the patient is medically stable and sufficiently alert, every effort should be made to gradually increase mobility, which often represents a very important physical and psychological milestone. The nursing and physical therapy staffs work together to achieve safe transfers between the bed and a wheelchair or commode, with the patient helping in the transfer. The procedures for transferring from bed to wheelchair and from wheelchair to bed are depicted on Plates 8 and 9. Verbal assurance and encouragement throughout the process help allay the patient's fears. Safety is continually emphasized, and the wheelchair brakes must be locked every time a transfer is attempted.

Comprehensive Rehabilitation

Patients who are physically too ill or cognitively incapable of participating in therapy or who lack family support may require a prolonged convalescence in an extended care facility. Other patients qualify for transfer to a comprehensive rehabilitation unit. Spontaneous neurologic recovery is usually complete 3 to 6 months after the stroke. The patient is taught to use the remaining functional capabilities to compensate for the residual deficits of stroke.

The patient's medical condition is monitored closely, and the primary care physician is usually encouraged to continue follow-up of the patient. At weekly or biweekly conferences, the rehabilitation team discusses all aspects of the patient's performance and goals of rehabilitation. Emphasis is on range-of-motion exercises and transfers. As strength, confidence, and skill are regained, the patient gradually assumes responsibility for these activities.

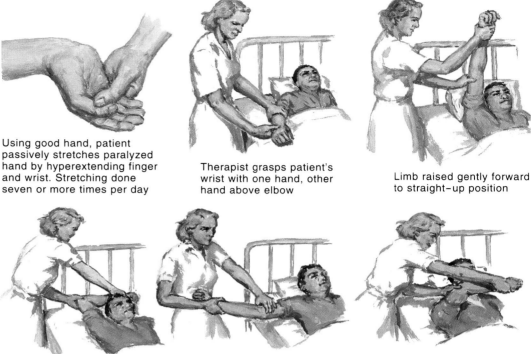

Using good hand, patient passively stretches paralyzed hand by hyperextending finger and wrist. Stretching done seven or more times per day

Therapist grasps patient's wrist with one hand, other hand above elbow

Limb raised gently forward to straight–up position

Elbow flexed; forearm moved above head as far as pain permits

Limb swung gently outward instead of upward

Limb carried across chest instead of above head

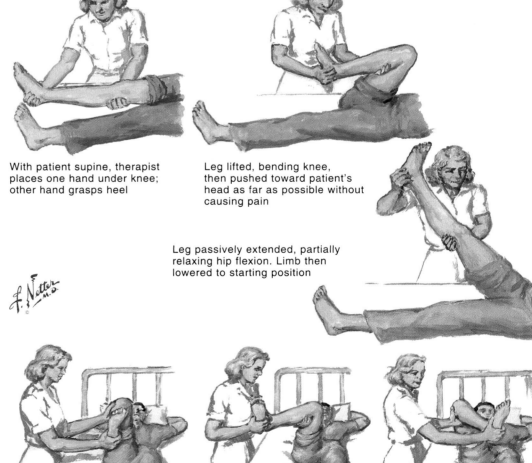

With patient supine, therapist places one hand under knee; other hand grasps heel

Leg lifted, bending knee, then pushed toward patient's head as far as possible without causing pain

Leg passively extended, partially relaxing hip flexion. Limb then lowered to starting position

Hip flexion–rotation exercises with patient supine. Hip and knee passively flexed, then limb rotated laterally and medially as pain permits

Transfer From Bed to Wheelchair After Stroke

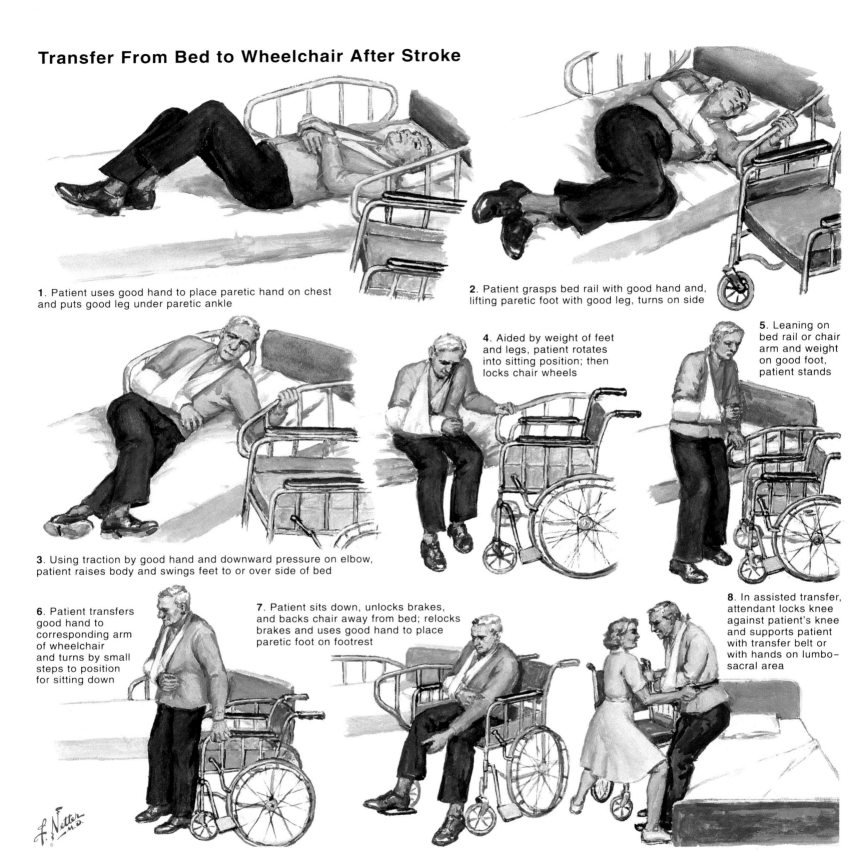

1. Patient uses good hand to place paretic hand on chest and puts good leg under paretic ankle

2. Patient grasps bed rail with good hand and, lifting paretic foot with good leg, turns on side

3. Using traction by good hand and downward pressure on elbow, patient raises body and swings feet to or over side of bed

4. Aided by weight of feet and legs, patient rotates into sitting position; then locks chair wheels

5. Leaning on bed rail or chair arm and weight on good foot, patient stands

6. Patient transfers good hand to corresponding arm of wheelchair and turns by small steps to position for sitting down

7. Patient sits down, unlocks brakes, and backs chair away from bed; relocks brakes and uses good hand to place paretic foot on footrest

8. In assisted transfer, attendant locks knee against patient's knee and supports patient with transfer belt or with hands on lumbo-sacral area

SECTION IV PLATE 8 Slide 4968

Rehabilitation After Stroke
(Continued)

The rehabilitation program is individualized, based on the patient's residual strengths and weaknesses. Exercises are continued to retard contracture formation and minimize soft tissue pain. Mobility in a wheelchair, using the functional lower and upper limbs, is taught first. Then, a graduated progressive resistance exercise program is prescribed. The unaffected limbs must be strengthened to compensate for the paretic arm and leg. Strength, endurance, and balance activities are emphasized to prepare the patient for possible ambulation.

Ambulation

Approximately 80% of stroke patients eventually relearn to walk. The patient must be able to follow instructions (verbal or nonverbal) and to maintain standing balance; have no contractures of the hip, knee, or ankle; have some position sense of the affected lower limb; and have enough voluntary motor function to stabilize the hip and, to a lesser degree, the knee. The patient has already learned the basics of gait training with standing balance and weight shifting during transfer activities. An ambulation program usually begins in the parallel bars and gradually progresses until the patient can walk on a flat surface, using an ankle-foot brace and canes with decreasing bases of support (Plate 10). Patients who do not completely regain function often ambulate with a gait pattern influenced by spasticity. Many patients, however, do eventually walk with an ankle-foot orthosis and single-tip cane or without any supportive device.

Transfer From Wheelchair to Bed After Stroke

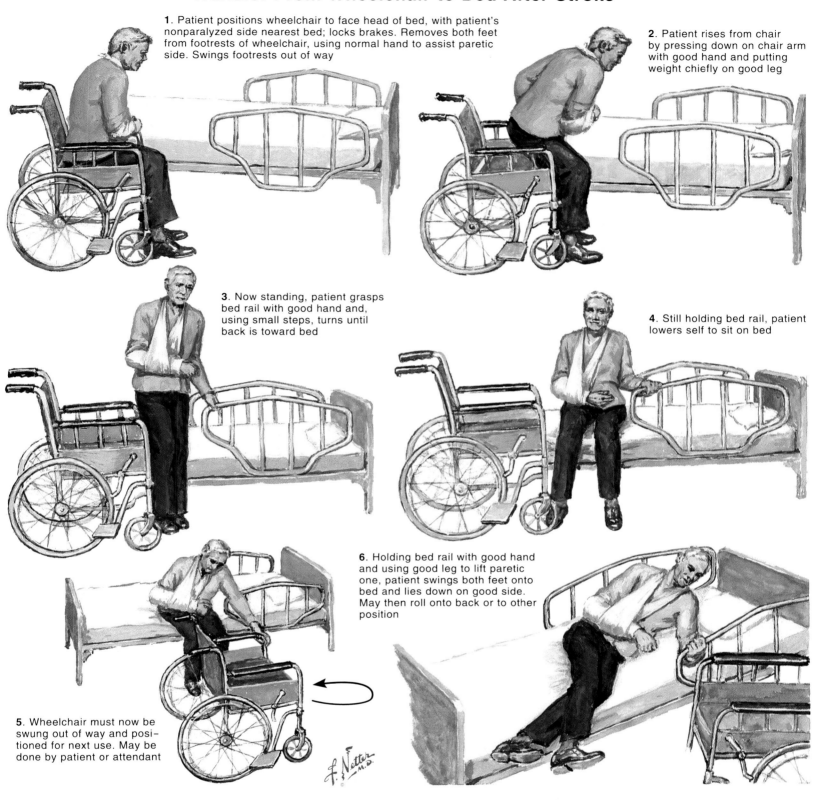

1. Patient positions wheelchair to face head of bed, with patient's nonparalyzed side nearest bed; locks brakes. Removes both feet from footrests of wheelchair, using normal hand to assist paretic side. Swings footrests out of way

2. Patient rises from chair by pressing down on chair arm with good hand and putting weight chiefly on good leg

3. Now standing, patient grasps bed rail with good hand and, using small steps, turns until back is toward bed

4. Still holding bed rail, patient lowers self to sit on bed

5. Wheelchair must now be swung out of way and positioned for next use. May be done by patient or attendant

6. Holding bed rail with good hand and using good leg to lift paretic one, patient swings both feet onto bed and lies down on good side. May then roll onto back or to other position

Rehabilitation After Stroke
(Continued)

Function of Upper Limb

After the patient's abilities to perform the activities of daily living are evaluated, the focus is on the improvement of specific tasks and spatial orientation, visual perception, and motor planning. Mastering personal hygiene and dressing improves the patient's sense of independence and self-worth. Approximately 90% of stroke patients do not regain fine motor control in the affected hand. The patient is given continually increasing responsibilities, and the family is taught how to assist the patient when necessary without impeding the growth of independence.

When the patient is discharged from the hospital, a social worker provides the patient and family with a list of community resources that help fund environmental alterations to the home, sponsor stroke support groups, or arrange continued outpatient rehabilitation services. A vocational counselor may also assist the family.

Special Problems

Cognitive Dysfunction. A stroke can result in a wide range of cognitive and visual impairments: confusion, disorientation, depression, language impairment (aphasia), altered judgment, decreased ability to learn, and visual field deficits.

A lesion affecting the right cortical hemisphere may result in left-sided neglect. Patients do not acknowledge any object, including their own body, to the left of midline. This is a difficult problem to deal with, and overcoming it depends largely on the patient's inherent ability to compensate and learn new material.

Rehabilitation After Stroke
(Continued)

Cortical lesions in the dominant hemisphere can result in aphasia, a communications disorder that crosses all aspects of language with impairment of symbolization and association. Lesions in the superior-posterior portion of the temporal lobe and the inferior portion of the parietal lobe (the Wernicke area) create deficits associated with all aspects of language comprehension. Injury to the posterior-inferior region of the frontal lobe (the Broca area) results in deficits of speech production. Severe strokes producing lesions of both brain areas lead to global aphasia—the patient is unable to comprehend or produce speech. The speech pathologist can identify the remaining avenues of communication (eg, nonverbal forms) and assist patients with swallowing problems or dysarthria.

Spasticity. Immediately following a stroke, the affected limb is usually flaccid, but within 48 hours, spasticity usually emerges. Spasticity is characterized by increased tone reflexes and resistance to quick passive stretch. In the lower limb, mild-to-moderate spasticity of the extensor muscles when the patient is in the upright position may be used to assist in ambulation when voluntary motor control is partially present.

Spasticity should be treated only if it interferes with ambulation or activities of daily living. To reduce spasticity, all factors that may enhance it must be eliminated, such as tight-fitting shoes, pressure ulcers, fecal impaction, infection, ingrown toenails, and contractures. Mobile joints must be maintained with a good stretching program to minimize spasticity. Application of ice to the muscle often provides temporary relief. Treatments with medications may also be effective. Administration of local anesthetics and, if effective, a dilute phenol solution may also provide relief from spasticity. Precautions must be taken to not remove all the spasticity, because a flaccid leg is unable to bear weight.

Initially, poor or absent muscle tone about the shoulder girdle permits depression and inferior rotation of the scapula, elongation of the supraspinatus and deltoid muscles, and overstretching of the superior part of the shoulder joint capsule. There may be mild superior and anterior subluxation of the shoulder, causing pain, decreasing the range of motion, and applying a traction force to the brachial plexus. The flaccid musculature and absence of a muscle pump may allow dependent edema and swelling to occur in the affected hand. Swelling decreases range of motion and encourages the formation of contractures in the hand. Judicious use of arm slings, overhead slings, well-padded troughs in the wheelchair arm, and snug-fitting gloves helps reduce soft tissue injuries of the shoulder and dependent edema. Range-of-motion exercises should be performed to prevent tightness.

Shoulder-Hand Syndrome. This form of reflex sympathetic dystrophy may occur in the stroke patient. Usually, the disorder begins insidiously with mild swelling of the paretic hand and

Ambulation After Stroke

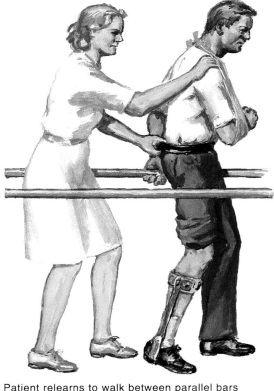

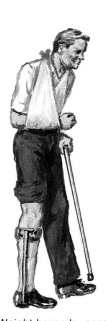

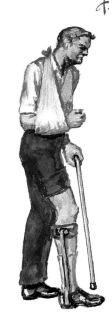

Double upright ankle–foot orthosis

Lightweight plastic orthosis for weakness of ankle dorsiflexion; fits easily into most shoes

Patient relearns to walk between parallel bars wearing ankle–foot brace or orthosis. Support by attendant usually necessary at first

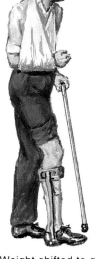

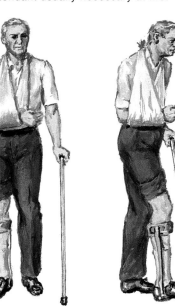

Patient may progress to walking with cane. Tip of cane ~6 in. in front and ~4 in. to side of toes

Weight shifted to good leg and cane. Patient swings paretic foot forward about 6 in.

Weight borne by paretic limb and cane. Patient moves good foot forward about 6 in.

Weight shifted back to good leg. Paretic leg moved forward again; process repeated

shoulder discomfort. Passive flexion of the metacarpophalangeal and proximal and distal interphalangeal joints is painful. If these findings are ignored, the pain and swelling progress rapidly. The patient often refuses to have the affected limb touched or put through range-of-motion exercises, preferring to keep it immobile. Soft tissue contractures quickly develop. The skin may become atrophic, cold and sweaty, or warm and dry. Osteoporosis may be quite marked.

Aggressive intervention is mandatory. The first goal is to reduce pain with sympathetic blockade, if symptoms are severe. Transcutaneous electrical nerve stimulation (TENS) may be administered.

In severe cases, TENS may also be used as an adjunct to sympathetic blockade. A rapidly tapering oral corticosteroid is an option if there are contraindications to a stellate ganglion block and no contraindications to the corticosteroid therapy. When the pain is tolerable, a program to mobilize and desensitize the hand is instituted; ultrasound and range-of-motion exercises are prescribed for shoulder joint tightness. Intraarticular or periarticular injection of a corticosteroid compound may also help resolve pain and tightness of soft tissues. When the shoulder-hand syndrome is controlled, the rehabilitation program for the upper limb may resume. □

Prevention of Contractures After Burn Injury

Rehabilitation After Burn Injury

Advances in medical technology and resuscitation continue to improve the survival of burn patients. As a result, a growing number of patients require rehabilitative efforts to prevent the potentially devastating and deforming sequelae of thermal injury—profound edema, joint contractures, loss of conditioning resulting from immobilization, and hypertrophic scarring.

Rehabilitation of the burn patient to thwart the formation of edema and joint contractures is begun immediately following the lifesaving measures of fluid replacement and removal of constricting eschars. Following debridement, a burned limb is usually elevated to control swelling. Proper positioning of the patient—the cornerstone in the rehabilitation of acute burns—should be done by persons experienced in preventing the formation of contractures. A joint that is improperly positioned may sustain brachial plexus or lumbosacral plexus injuries, peripheral nerve compression, or intrinsic joint damage.

The patient with an acute burn usually experiences significant pain and attempts to find the most comfortable position. Unfortunately, the body posture often chosen is flexion, which leads to joint contractures with resultant limited mobility. A burn scar continues to contract until it meets an opposing force; this opposing protective force is provided by positioning, splinting, and exercise.

Prevention of Contractures

Significant burns of the neck region may contract until the mandible is fixed to the chest wall and the lower lip is severely everted. This complication is avoided by positioning the neck in slight extension (Plate 11). A formfitting neck splint keeps the mandible from retracting and limits neck flexion. Patients with neck burns should not use pillows under the head, because pillows promote flexion contractures of the neck. Thermal injury of the anterior thorax often accompanies neck injury. A towel roll placed between the shoulder blades counters a forward inclination of the shoulders that could lead to decreased expansion of the chest wall and ventilatory compromise. Microstomia is a frequent complication of mouth burns. A mouth splint or an orthodontic appliance that conforms to the teeth keeps the mouth free of contractures and permits the intake of nutrition, communication, and oral hygiene. Treatment of contractures of the axilla is especially difficult. The challenge is to apply continuous and sufficient pressure to the hollow of the axilla. The shoulders should be abducted approximately 90° with 10° flexion.

In the elbow, a slight amount of flexion and cubital padding and close observation are necessary to determine the development of heterotopic ossification and avoid compression of the ulnar nerve. A burned wrist and hand are splinted to maintain the wrist in slight extension, the metacarpophalangeal joints in 70° to 90° flexion, the interphalangeal joints in extension, and the thumb in abduction, opposition, and flexion.

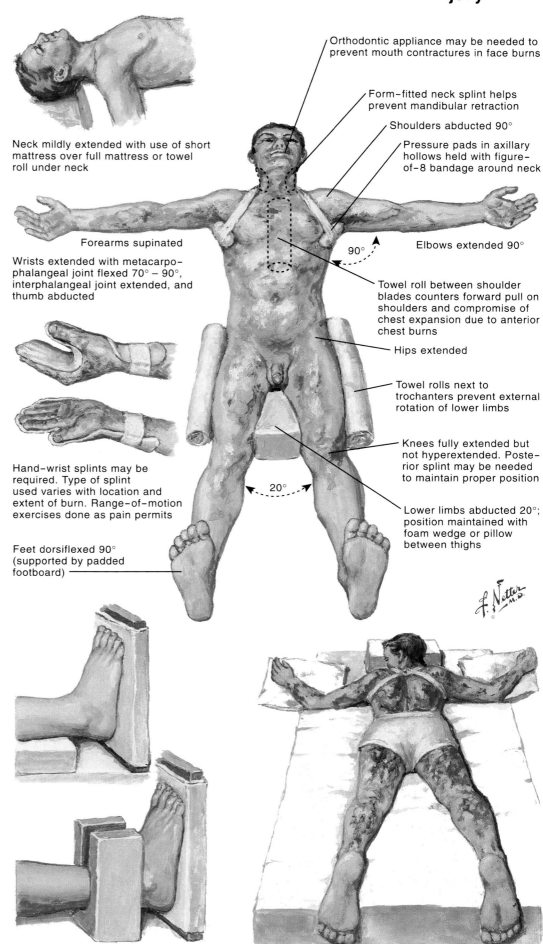

Neck mildly extended with use of short mattress over full mattress or towel roll under neck

Orthodontic appliance may be needed to prevent mouth contractures in face burns

Form-fitted neck splint helps prevent mandibular retraction

Shoulders abducted 90°

Pressure pads in axillary hollows held with figure-of-8 bandage around neck

Forearms supinated

Wrists extended with metacarpophalangeal joint flexed 70° – 90°, interphalangeal joint extended, and thumb abducted

90°

Elbows extended 90°

Towel roll between shoulder blades counters forward pull on shoulders and compromise of chest expansion due to anterior chest burns

Hips extended

Towel rolls next to trochanters prevent external rotation of lower limbs

Hand-wrist splints may be required. Type of splint used varies with location and extent of burn. Range-of-motion exercises done as pain permits

20°

Knees fully extended but not hyperextended. Posterior splint may be needed to maintain proper position

Lower limbs abducted 20°; position maintained with foam wedge or pillow between thighs

Feet dorsiflexed 90° (supported by padded footboard)

Short mattress or foam ankle collar used to avoid decubitus ulcers on heel as feet held at right angles by padded footboard

Patient in prone position on foam mattress cut to allow arms to drop forward slightly and feet to hang over end. Head supported with foam pad

Pressure Garments and Devices in Burn Rehabilitation

Rehabilitation After Burn Injury
(Continued)

In the lower limb, the hip should be maintained in neutral rotation and 20° abduction to prohibit hip flexion and adduction, which may predispose to hip dislocation and lumbosacral plexus injury. Foam wedges or pillows may be used to maintain the hip in proper alignment. Placing the patient in the prone position also prevents hip contractures, provided the patient can tolerate the position and there are no medical contraindications. In addition, hip flexion and external rotation commonly cause knee flexion and excessive pressure on the head of the fibula, which may injure the peroneal nerve, resulting in foot drop. Involved knees must be kept extended, with use of a posterior knee splint if appropriate; care must be taken not to hyperextend the knee and damage its internal structures. The ankle is difficult to position because the strength of the gastrocnemius and soleus muscles combines with gravity to plantar flex the foot. Plantar flexion may be prevented by using dorsiflexion splints that keep the ankle dorsiflexed 5°.

Splints require frequent observation. A tight-fitting splint may lead to compression of vital structures such as arteries or nerves, and a well-fitting orthosis may loosen when the edema resolves.

Exercise and Ambulation

Therapeutic exercise is essential to the restoration of the patient's physical and psychological health. The exercise program must be supervised by the attending physician to ensure that the patient can tolerate the increased metabolic demand. Areas of the body that are not burned should be exercised regularly to avoid the consequences of immobilization. Burned areas must be exercised frequently by a physical therapist or a trained nurse. Passive exercises are carried out by the therapist to maintain normal range of motion in the joint. Active-assisted exercises are begun when the patient is able to start but not complete the desired movement. A gentle stretching program is also instituted for all involved joints to prevent contractures.

Ambulation should begin as soon as the patient is medically stable and can bear weight on the lower limbs. However, exercise of grafted limbs should be avoided for 7 to 14 days. Exercise may also be contraindicated for critically ill patients and those with unstable fractures or dislocations.

Pressure Garments and Devices

The potential for contractures and unsightly hypertrophic scars may last as long as 3 years after the successful grafting and healing of burn wounds. During this phase, the primary therapy consists of constant pressure and splinting (Plate 12). The force exerted on the burn scar must exceed a capillary pressure of 25 mmHg.

To help prevent hypertrophic scarring of the face and neck, a transparent plastic mask is used at night, and a custom-fitted elastic hood cover-

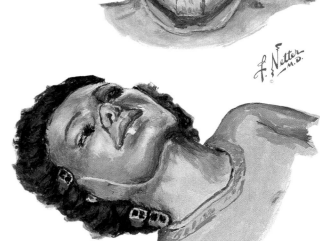

Custom-fitted elastic stocking for head and face. Inserts may be added to conform to facial contours

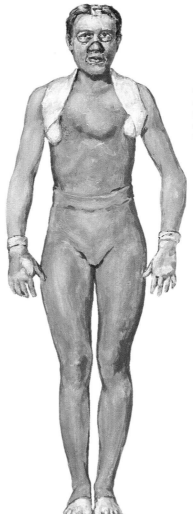

Total-body elastic garment used in entirety or in part, depending on extent and location of burn eschar. Note lamb's wool inserts for breast cleavage and axilla pads held by clavicular figure-of-8 bandage

Extension and compression orthosis for face and neck made of heat-malleable transparent plastic and held with elastic straps. Applies pressure and blanches hyperemic scars. Worn primarily at night. Head and neck pieces usually made as separate pieces and worn together

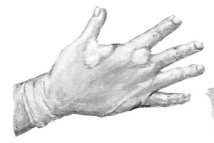

Elastic glove applied over lamb's wool inserts in thumb web and between 2nd and 3rd fingers

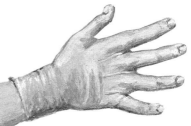

Custom-fitted elastic glove. Series of gloves of increasing tightness used and applied carefully to avoid skin shearing

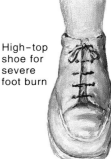

High-top shoe for severe foot burn

ing the entire head is used during the day. Scarring and contractures of the axilla are difficult to manage but may be controlled with a figure-of-8 clavicle strap and crescent-shaped axilla pads. Tubular pressure garments successfully prevent deformities of the arms and legs, and pressure gloves with an expanded thumb are used on the hands. High-top shoes and shoe inserts are used for foot burns. Elastic garments are fitted to the trunk, with padded inserts to protect buttock creases, breast cleavage, and the interscapular region. To control the formation of hypertrophic scarring in the genital region, the patient must wear the pressure garment or conforming splints

23 hours every day until the scar matures, which may take 3 years. A mature burn scar is no longer red, raised, and sensitive; it lightens in color, flattens out, and blends with the normal tissue.

Patient compliance is often a major problem in dealing with scars and contractures. It may be difficult to convince the patient and family of the need for continued stretching exercises and wearing of pressure garments. Regular visits to the clinic are important, and detailed descriptions of scars and measurements of range of motion in the joint must be recorded. The patient may require counseling in coping with pain, deformity, and developing a new concept of self. □

Rehabilitation After Sports Injury

Injury to Ankle Ligaments

Ankle sprains occur frequently in sports activities as well as in daily activities. In addition, a previously sprained ankle is at significant risk for reinjury. Ankle sprains usually occur in persons less than 35 years of age, most commonly in teenagers 15 to 19 years of age.

Nonoperative management of a medial ligament injury requires a prolonged healing period. Initially, the ankle should be treated with rest, ice (applied for 30 minutes every 4 hours), compression, and elevation for the first 48 hours (Plate 13). Subsequently, the injured ankle should be immobilized in a cast for 6 weeks to allow the torn deltoid ligament to heal.

The initial management of a lateral ligament injury should also include rest, ice, compression, and elevation, followed by 4 to 6 weeks of immobilization with the ankle positioned in as much dorsiflexion as possible. Cast immobilization, fracture brace, or daily taping may be used to maintain this position. The fracture brace or taping allows the patient to maintain a normal range of motion and minimizes muscular atrophy. After surgical repair of the medial or lateral ligament complex, a 6-week period of immobilization may be required before rehabilitation can begin.

During the immobilization period, the patient should practice isometric exercises in all directions of ankle motion. After the cast or brace is removed, the patient should ambulate with crutches using partial weight bearing until the ankle is free of pain.

Once the patient resumes full weight bearing, the emphasis of rehabilitation becomes isometric strengthening exercises for the peroneal muscles and ankle dorsiflexors. Strengthening these muscles helps to prevent a recurrence of the ankle sprain. After the patient becomes proficient in isometric exercises, a concentric and eccentric exercise program for the ankle dorsiflexors and everters is initiated. Surgical tubing or elastic bands are used for resistance. Three sets of 10 exercises are done for each muscle group with the muscles held at maximal contraction for 10 seconds. The patient may also begin to use a balance board, initially using both feet, then advancing to single-foot exercises; the ankles should be dorsiflexed, plantar flexed, inverted, everted, and rotated in circles. When the patient can walk without pain, running is introduced, finally followed by running and cutting.

Rehabilitation of a lateral ankle injury usually takes 4 to 6 weeks, with the patient returning to a normal level of activity. An injury to the medial ankle structures heals much more slowly.

Injury to Knee Ligaments

The goal of conservative management of ligament injuries of the knee is to stabilize the action of the knee with the remaining uninjured, supportive structures (Plate 14). Rehabilitation must begin as soon as possible after injury, because

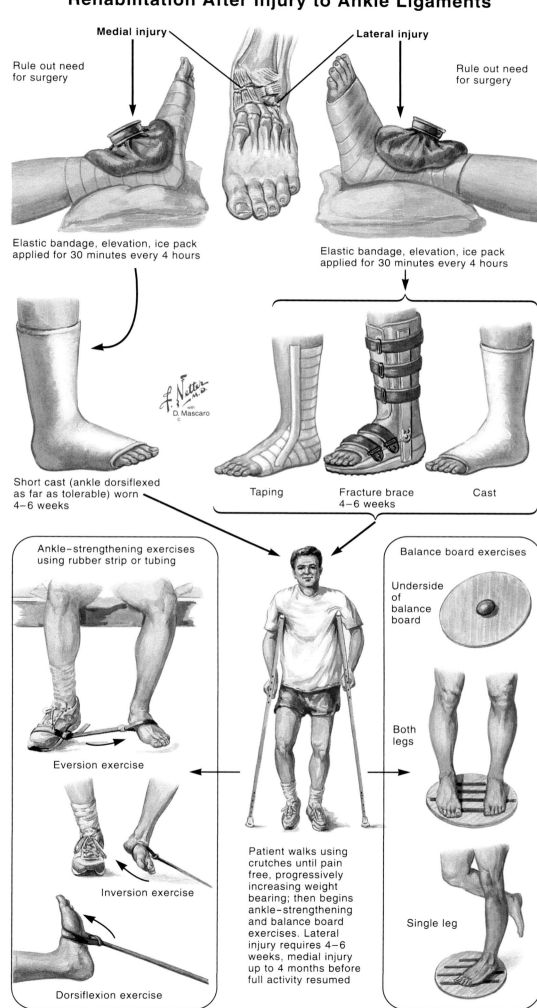

Rehabilitation After Injury to Ankle Ligaments

Medial injury

Lateral injury

Rule out need for surgery

Rule out need for surgery

Elastic bandage, elevation, ice pack applied for 30 minutes every 4 hours

Elastic bandage, elevation, ice pack applied for 30 minutes every 4 hours

Short cast (ankle dorsiflexed as far as tolerable) worn 4–6 weeks

Taping

Fracture brace 4–6 weeks

Cast

Ankle-strengthening exercises using rubber strip or tubing

Eversion exercise

Inversion exercise

Dorsiflexion exercise

Balance board exercises

Underside of balance board

Both legs

Single leg

Patient walks using crutches until pain free, progressively increasing weight bearing; then begins ankle-strengthening and balance board exercises. Lateral injury requires 4–6 weeks, medial injury up to 4 months before full activity resumed

Rehabilitation After Injury to Knee Ligaments

Rehabilitation After Sports Injury
(Continued)

disuse atrophy of the muscles occurs rapidly. Rehabilitation focuses on muscle strengthening, particularly strengthening of the extensor (quadriceps) muscles and the flexor (medial and lateral hamstring) muscles.

The knee is flexed in an arc of motion between 30° and 90°, avoiding full extension. Resistance is applied in the pain-free portion of the range of motion, with the tibia internally and externally rotated to strengthen the hamstring muscles. The exercises can be done with the patient prone or standing.

Isokinetic resistance is also initiated, starting at slow speeds and gradually increasing. Isotonic, isometric, or isokinetic extension of the knee may also be initiated. The knee should remain pain free through the entire arc of motion. End-arc discomfort may occur. Extension exercises are begun with the starting position at less than 90° flexion and termination at less than full extension. Hip flexion and abduction exercises can be isometric or isotonic. Double-foot raises (raising both heels off the floor simultaneously) in sets of 50, done with the knee slightly bent, strengthen the gastrocnemius muscles that help stabilize the knee.

Endurance training should be added to initiate cardiovascular conditioning. Use of a stationary bicycle, with the resistance set at zero, is effective and also improves the range of motion in the knee. Once the knee is pain free, the resistance can be increased for further cardiovascular benefits.

Postoperative rehabilitation following surgical reconstruction of the knee consists of a progressive program that is conducted in stages. Immediately after surgery, the knee is typically placed in a hinged fracture brace to allow controlled motion, unless the patient is in a continuous passive motion machine. The benefits of an early, passive range-of-motion program are controlled mobilization, decrease of pain, reduction of swelling, prevention of adhesions, improvement of proprioceptive function, and more rapid return of joint range of motion.

When the patient can be mobilized from bed, the hinged fracture brace can be locked to restrict the extent of both passive flexion and passive extension. The patient is taught to use crutches with progressive weight bearing on the affected side. This protected weight bearing is continued until the surgeon is confident that the ligaments have healed. During the healing phase, passive range-of-motion exercises should be supervised, with extension being passively assisted by gravity pulling the leg toward an exercise mat and limited by the extension stop of the brace. Active flexion exercises can be started with the patient using the hamstring muscles. Straight-leg raises, flexion-to-extension exercises within the safe range of limited motion, cocontractions, hip flexion exercises, and leg curls are also started to maintain muscle tone and strength. The amount of resistance and the number of sets or repetitions are gradually increased as tolerated.

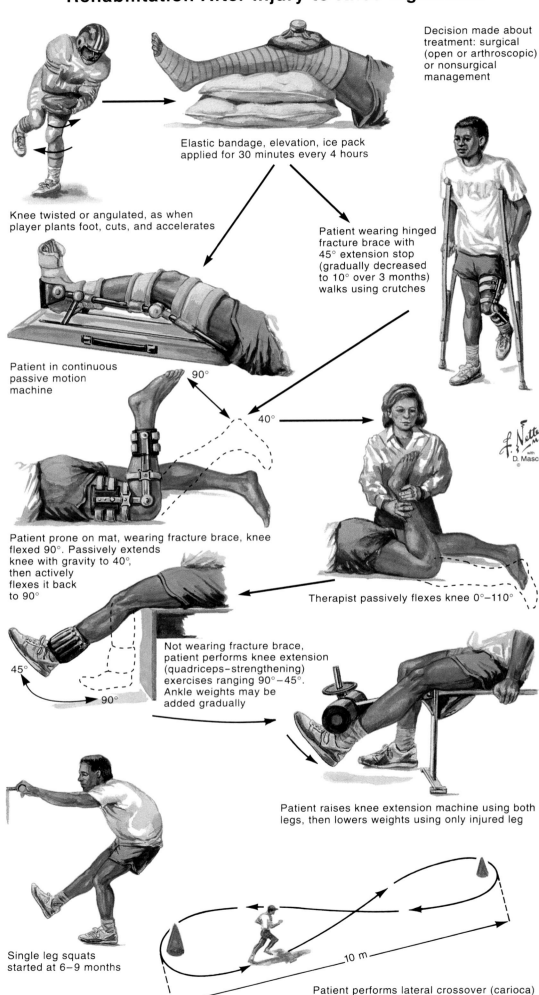

Knee twisted or angulated, as when player plants foot, cuts, and accelerates

Elastic bandage, elevation, ice pack applied for 30 minutes every 4 hours

Decision made about treatment: surgical (open or arthroscopic) or nonsurgical management

Patient wearing hinged fracture brace with 45° extension stop (gradually decreased to 10° over 3 months) walks using crutches

Patient in continuous passive motion machine

Patient prone on mat, wearing fracture brace, knee flexed 90°. Passively extends knee with gravity to 40°, then actively flexes it back to 90°

Therapist passively flexes knee 0°–110°

Not wearing fracture brace, patient performs knee extension (quadriceps–strengthening) exercises ranging 90°–45°. Ankle weights may be added gradually

Patient raises knee extension machine using both legs, then lowers weights using only injured leg

Single leg squats started at 6–9 months

Patient performs lateral crossover (carioca) run to regain athletic conditioning

10 m

Rehabilitation After Injury to Hand and Fingers

Rehabilitation After Sports Injury

(Continued)

Usually, the brace can be discarded within 3 months after surgery, and the program for strengthening knee flexion and extension accelerated. By 6 months, a program to achieve full extension should have begun with slow, progressive resistance exercises, such as light squatting with the thighs parallel with the floor. Swimming is encouraged to increase endurance. The patient should avoid running until the injured limb has regained 80% of the strength of the normal limb.

Subluxation or dislocation of the patella typically occurs in adolescents or young adults and is classified as either acute or chronic (see Section I, Plate 98). Conservative management focuses on strengthening the vastus medialis muscle to minimize lateral displacement. The vastus medialis muscle is active throughout the entire range of knee motion and is principally responsible for stabilizing lateral movement of the patella during the terminal phase of extension. In addition to muscle strengthening, bracing the patella with circumferential strapping may minimize lateral subluxation or dislocation of the patella during intense physical activity. If instability persists after maximal rehabilitation and strengthening of the quadriceps mechanism, surgical intervention should be considered.

Injury to Hand and Fingers

Failure to identify a significant hand injury may result in prolonged disability due to excessive scarring, which can significantly reduce hand and finger motion. Early diagnosis and treatment and proper rehabilitation are needed to establish full function (Plate 15). The goal of treatment of hand and finger injuries is to promote healing of the injured structures while maintaining a functional range of motion and preventing the formation of joint contractures. Because certain structures of the hand are fragile, the rehabilitation team must clearly understand the extent and severity of the injury and take appropriate precautions, as identified by the attending hand surgeon, before initiating rehabilitation therapy.

The first step in hand and finger rehabilitation consists of assessment of muscle strength and restriction of range of motion, with formal measurement of the motion of each involved joint. After the baseline factors are established, progress should be monitored at weekly or biweekly intervals. During passive range-of-motion exercises, the range of motion should be increased to the point of discomfort, but not beyond. As the injury heals, a more aggressive program can be adopted, including active and active-assisted range-of-motion exercises of the affected joints. If possible, the hand should be warmed in a paraffin bath before or during the range-of-motion activity. The hand should then be kept in the stretched position until it has cooled to normal temperatures. Exercises can be performed by the patient at home, with weekly monitoring by the physical therapist. □

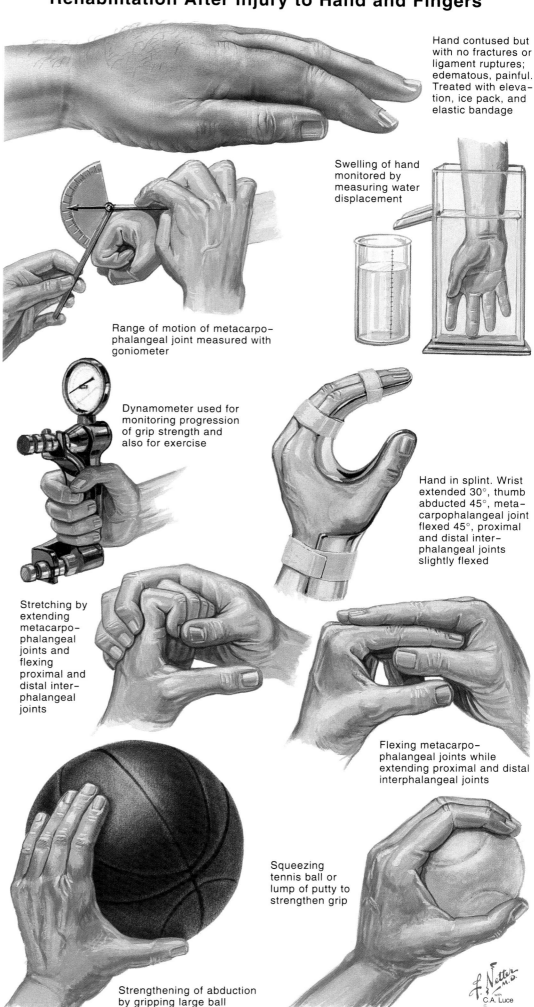

Hand contused but with no fractures or ligament ruptures; edematous, painful. Treated with elevation, ice pack, and elastic bandage

Swelling of hand monitored by measuring water displacement

Range of motion of metacarpo-phalangeal joint measured with goniometer

Dynamometer used for monitoring progression of grip strength and also for exercise

Hand in splint. Wrist extended 30°, thumb abducted 45°, meta-carpophalangeal joint flexed 45°, proximal and distal inter-phalangeal joints slightly flexed

Stretching by extending metacarpo-phalangeal joints and flexing proximal and distal inter-phalangeal joints

Flexing metacarpo-phalangeal joints while extending proximal and distal interphalangeal joints

Squeezing tennis ball or lump of putty to strengthen grip

Strengthening of abduction by gripping large ball

Rehabilitation After Joint Replacement

Before joint replacement, the rehabilitation team should evaluate the patient for muscle strength in all limbs, ability to perform transfers, ambulatory status, and range of motion in the lower limbs. The aim of this preoperative phase of rehabilitation is to educate the patient in all exercise protocols, postoperative precautions, deep breathing and coughing, gait training, and proper use of walking aids. The patient practices with a walker, using a three-point gait with partial weight bearing on the entire plantar aspect of the foot rather than on just the toes. In addition to learning short-arc quadriceps-strengthening, calf-pumping, and heel-sliding exercises, the patient learns isometric exercises for the quadriceps and gluteus muscles. The patient should also receive instruction in the correct postoperative position of the limb when the patient is both in and out of bed.

Postoperative rehabilitation includes optimizing musculoskeletal function and educating the patient to avoid overstressing the prosthetic joint.

Total Hip Replacement

On the first and second postoperative days, the patient performs deep-breathing and coughing exercises and isometric gluteus and quadriceps-setting exercises (Plate 16). Calf-pumping exercises are initiated to decrease the risk of thrombophlebitis. Lower limbs are maintained in position with an abduction splint. Active-assisted to mild resistive exercises are prescribed for unaffected joints and limbs. On the third postoperative day, the patient begins active-assisted range of motion of the affected hip and knee in all planes, with hip flexion limited to 80° and extension limited to neutral. The patient is instructed in proper transfer techniques and is assisted in getting out of bed to stand for 15-minute periods.

On the fourth and fifth postoperative days, the patient adds short-arc quadriceps-strengthening exercises and begins progressive standing, transfers, and ambulation. Initial gait training in the parallel bars provides proprioceptive feedback with partial weight bearing. During ambulation, the patient is evaluated for limb length discrepancy. The patient advances from partial weight bearing to full weight bearing as tolerated. The abduction wedge is removed for ambulation if the patient demonstrates good lower limb control, but it is used at night for 6 weeks after surgery.

During the sixth through tenth postoperative days, active hip flexion, extension, and abduction are added. Progressive ambulation continues until the patient achieves independent ambulation with assistive devices. Then, the patient may use supportive devices to walk without supervision.

From the tenth postoperative day until discharge from the hospital, the patient continues the strengthening and range-of-motion exercises

Rehabilitation After Total Hip Replacement

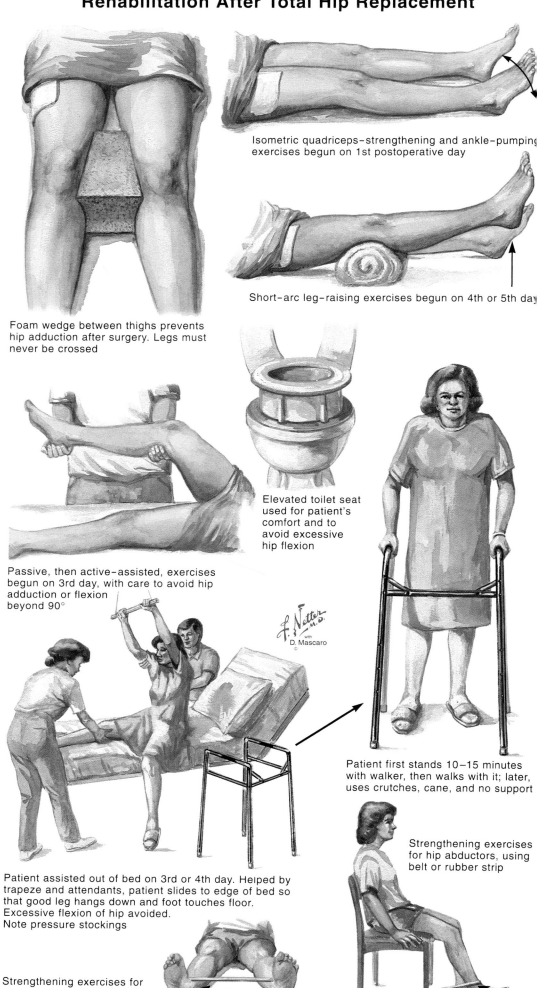

Foam wedge between thighs prevents hip adduction after surgery. Legs must never be crossed

Isometric quadriceps-strengthening and ankle-pumping exercises begun on 1st postoperative day

Short-arc leg-raising exercises begun on 4th or 5th day

Passive, then active-assisted, exercises begun on 3rd day, with care to avoid hip adduction or flexion beyond 90°

Elevated toilet seat used for patient's comfort and to avoid excessive hip flexion

Patient assisted out of bed on 3rd or 4th day. Helped by trapeze and attendants, patient slides to edge of bed so that good leg hangs down and foot touches floor. Excessive flexion of hip avoided. Note pressure stockings

Patient first stands 10–15 minutes with walker, then walks with it; later, uses crutches, cane, and no support

Strengthening exercises for hip abductors, using belt or rubber strip

Strengthening exercises for hip abductors, using belt or elastic loop

Rehabilitation After Joint Replacement

(Continued)

and learns to negotiate steps and curbs. Hip abductor and quadriceps femoris exercises are advanced to progressive resistive exercises. Instruction is given in the use of assistive devices for dressing. At the time of discharge, the patient is provided with written instructions to be followed at home, and with adaptive equipment to compensate for the limited hip flexion (bathtub seat, elevated toilet seat, long shoehorn). When the patient is pain free, isometric exercises to increase hip muscle strength are added. The only proscribed activities are extreme hip flexion, internal rotation, adduction past neutral, and lifting weights more than 50 lbs. However, excessive athletic stress to the prosthesis is not recommended. During the first 6 to 8 weeks after discharge, the patient normally uses a cane in the opposite hand to protect the joint. Active hip extension exercises are added after 6 to 8 weeks.

Total Knee Replacement

After total knee replacement, pain is usually a significant limiting factor in the initial rehabilitation program. On the first postoperative day, limited exercises are performed—calf pumping to promote circulation, and deep-breathing and coughing exercises to prevent pulmonary complications (Plate 17). On the second postoperative day, isometric gluteus and quadriceps-setting exercises and straight-leg raises are added. The patient is taught to transfer into a chair a few days after surgery.

Active-assisted range-of-motion exercises usually begin on the third day, after the surgical dressings and splints have been replaced with a knee immobilizer brace. Use of a continuous passive motion machine increases the range of motion, reduces postoperative pain, and helps to avoid the need for orthopedic manipulation.

On the fourth and fifth postoperative days, active-assisted range-of-motion exercises are continued in the physical therapy section. The patient starts standing for longer periods, performs transfers, and ambulates in the parallel bars, advancing from partial weight bearing to full weight bearing as tolerated. If the terminal knee extension is no greater than 10°, ambulation is done wearing a knee immobilizer brace using toe-touch weight bearing only. On the sixth to fourteenth postoperative days, the patient performs active range-of-motion exercises, continuing to work toward regaining full extension by achieving 90° or greater knee flexion. Forcible passive exercises or manipulation is avoided. The patient progresses to ambulating independently with a walker, crutches, or cane.

The knee immobilizer brace is discontinued as soon as the patient attains adequate control of the quadriceps muscles; it is worn at night, however, for 6 to 8 weeks to maintain knee extension. Once adequate knee flexion has been achieved, maintenance of a normal gait pattern is essential. At this

Rehabilitation After Total Knee Replacement

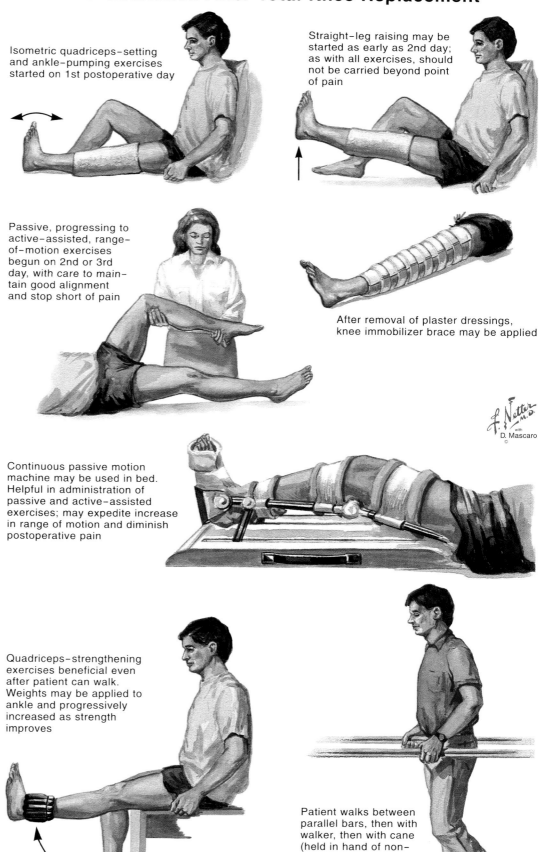

Isometric quadriceps-setting and ankle-pumping exercises started on 1st postoperative day

Straight-leg raising may be started as early as 2nd day; as with all exercises, should not be carried beyond point of pain

Passive, progressing to active-assisted, range-of-motion exercises begun on 2nd or 3rd day, with care to maintain good alignment and stop short of pain

After removal of plaster dressings, knee immobilizer brace may be applied

Continuous passive motion machine may be used in bed. Helpful in administration of passive and active-assisted exercises; may expedite increase in range of motion and diminish postoperative pain

Quadriceps-strengthening exercises beneficial even after patient can walk. Weights may be applied to ankle and progressively increased as strength improves

Patient walks between parallel bars, then with walker, then with cane (held in hand of non-operated side), and finally with no support

point, strengthening of the quadriceps and hamstring muscles can advance with supervision. The patient is ready for discharge when the knee can be flexed at least 90°. If the patient has not achieved at least 70° knee flexion by the tenth

postoperative day, the joint is manipulated under anesthesia.

The rate of progress in rehabilitation depends largely on the determination of the patient and the degree of preoperative impairment. □

Selected References

Section I

General References

CHARNLEY J: *Closed Treatment of Common Fractures*. Baltimore, Williams & Wilkins, 1961

DEPALMA AF: *The Management of Fractures and Dislocations*. Philadelphia, WB Saunders, 1970

ROCKWOOD CA JR, WILKINS KE, KING RE (eds): *Fractures in Children*, ed 2. Philadelphia, JB Lippincott, 1984

ROCKWOOD CA JR, GREEN DP, BUCHOLZ RW (eds): *Rockwood and Green's Fractures in Adults*, ed 3. Philadelphia, JB Lippincott, 1992

	Plates
ACLAND RD: *Manual of Microvascular Surgery*. St Louis, CV Mosby, 1988	117, 120
AKBARNIA B, TORG JS, KIRKPATRICK J, et al: *Manifestations of the battered child syndrome*. J Bone Joint Surg 1974, 56A:1159–1166	135
AMERICAN MEDICAL ASSOCIATION: *Standard Nomenclature of Athletic Injuries*. Chicago, AMA, 1966	99–101
ANDERSON D: *Fractures of the odontoid process of the axis*. J Bone Joint Surg 1974, 56A:1663–1674	69–78
ARNOCZKY SP, WARREN RF: *The microvasculature of the meniscus and its response to injury. An experimental study in the dog*. Am J Sports Med 1983, 11(3):131–141	95
ARNOLD JA, COKER TP, HEATON LM, et al: *Natural history of anterior cruciate tears*. Am J Sports Med 1979, 7:305–313	99–101
BADO JL: *The Monteggia lesion*. Clin Orthop 1967, 50:71–86	47–60
BALFOUR GW, MOONEY V, ASHBY ME: *Diaphyseal fractures of the humerus treated with a ready-made fracture brace*. J Bone Joint Surg 1982, 64A:11–13	33–40
BARDENHEUER L: *Die entstehung und behandlung der ischämischen muskelkontractur und gangrän*. Dtsch Z Chir 1911, 108:44	15
BARWICK WJ, GOODKIND DJ, SERAFIN D: *The free scapular flap*. Plast Reconstr Surg 1982, 69:779–787	124
BASSETT FH III: *Acute dislocation of the patella, osteochondral fractures, and injuries to the extensor mechanism of the knee*. Instr Course Lect 1976, 25:40–49	96–98

Section I *(continued)*

	Plates
BLICK SS, BRUMBACK RJ, POKA A, et al: *Compartment syndrome in open tibial fractures*. J Bone Joint Surg 1986, 68:1348–1353	11
BRIGHTON CT: *Principles of fracture healing. Part I. The biology of fracture repair*. Instr Course Lect 1984, 33:60–82	23–25
BRIGHTON CT, HUNT RM: *Early histological and ultrastructural changes in medullary fracture callus*. J Bone Joint Surg 1991, 73A:832–847	23–25
BUTMAN AM, PATURAS JL: *Pre-Hospital Trauma Life Support*. Akron OH, Emergency Training, 1986	26–32
BYWATERS EGL, BEALL D: *Crush injuries with impairment of renal function*. Br Med J 1941, 1:427–432	12
CAMPBELL JT, KAPLAN FS: *The role of morphogens in endochondral ossification*. Calcif Tissue Int 1992, 50:283–289	23–25
CANALE ST, KELLY FB JR: *Fractures of the neck of the talus. Long-term evaluation of seventy-one cases*. J Bone Joint Surg 1978, 60A:143–156	107–116
CAPLAN AI: *Mesenchymal stem cells*. J Orthop Res 1991, 9:641–650	23–25
CARROLL RE, MATCH RM: *Avulsion of the flexor profundus tendon insertion*. J Trauma 1970, 10:1109–1118	61–68
CASSEBAUM WH: *Open reduction of T & Y fractures of the lower end of the humerus*. J Trauma 1969, 9:915–925	41–46
CHESHER SP, SCHWARTZ KS, KLEINERT HE: *A new early-mobilization splint for proximal interphalangeal joint replacements*. J Hand Therapy 1988, 1:200–203	123
CLANCY WG, SHELBOURNE KD, ZOELLNER GB, et al: *Treatment of knee joint instability secondary to rupture of the posterior cruciate ligament. Report of a new procedure*. J Bone Joint Surg 1983, 65A:310–322	103
COTLER HB, KULKARNI MV, BONDURANT FJ: *Magnetic resonance imaging of acute spinal cord trauma: preliminary report*. J Orthop Trauma 1988, 2:1–4	69–78
CRENSHAW RP, VISTNES LM: *A decade of pressure sore research: 1977–1987*. J Rehabil Res Dev 1989, 26:63–74	3–4
CROSS MJ, POWELL JF: *Long-term follow-up of posterior cruciate ligament rupture: a study of 116 cases*. Am J Sports Med 1984, 12:292–297	103
CRUESS RL: *Healing of bone, tendon, and ligament*. In ROCKWOOD CA JR, GREEN DP (eds): *Fractures in Adults*, ed 2. Philadelphia, JB Lippincott, 1984, pp 147–167	23–25
D'AMBROSIA R, DREZ D JR (eds): *Prevention and Treatment of Running Injuries*. Thorofare NJ, Slack Inc, 1982	136–137
DANIEL D, DANIELS E, ARONSON D: *The diagnosis of meniscus pathology*. Clin Orthop 1982, 163:218–224	95
DELEE JC, GREEN, DP, WILKINS KE: *Fractures and dislocations of the elbow*. In ROCKWOOD CA JR, GREEN DP (eds): *Fractures in Adults*, ed 2. Philadelphia, JB Lippincott, 1984, pp 559–652	41–46
DENIS F: *Spinal instability as defined by the three-column spine concept in acute spinal trauma*. Clin Orthop 1984, 189:65–76	69–78
DENIS F: *The three-column spine and its significance in the classification of acute thoracolumbar spinal injuries*. Spine 1983, 8:817–831	69–78
EATON RG: *Joint Injuries of the Hand*, ed 2. Springfield IL, Charles C Thomas, 1971	61–68

Section I *(continued)*

	Plates
ENGRAV LH, HEIMBACH DM, REUS JL, et al: *Early excision and grafting vs. nonoperative treatment of burns of indeterminate depth: a randomized prospective study*. J Trauma 1983, 23:1001–1004	10
ENNEKING WF: *A system of staging musculoskeletal neoplasms*. Instr Course Lect 1988, 37:3–10	138–139
EPPS CH JR: *Complications of Orthopedic Surgery*, ed 2. Philadelphia, JB Lippincott, 1986	140–151
FAHMY NR, WILLIAMS EA, NOBLE J: *Meniscal pathology and osteoarthritis of the knee*. J Bone Joint Surg 1983, 65B:24–28	95
FALSTIE-JENSEN S, SONDERGARD PETERSEN PE: *Incarceration of the meniscus in fractures of the intercondylar eminence of the tibia in children*. Injury 1984, 15:236–238	102
FEAGIN JOHN A JR: *The Cruciate Ligaments*. New York, Churchill Livingstone, 1988	99
FROST HM: *The biology of fracture healing. An overview for clinicians. Part I*. Clin Orthop 1989, 248:283–293	23–25
GALWAY HR, MACINTOSH DL: *The lateral pivot shift: a symptom and sign of anterior cruciate ligament insufficiency*. Clin Orthop 1980, 147:45–50	99–101
GARFIN SR, MUBARAK SJ, EVANS KL, et al: *Quantification of intracompartmental pressure and volume under plaster casts*. J Bone Joint Surg 1981, 63A:449–453	15
GELBERMAN RH, URBANIAK JR, BRIGHT DS, et al: *Digital sensibility following replantation*. J Hand Surg 1978, 3:313–319	122–123, 125
GELBERMAN RH, ZAKAIB GS, MUBARAK SJ, et al: *Decompression of forearm compartment syndromes*. Clin Orthop 1978, 134:225–229	15
GOLDNER RD: *Postoperative management*. Hand Clinics 1985, 1:205–215	121, 123
GOLLEHON DL, TORZILLI PA, WARREN RF: *The role of the posterolateral and cruciate ligaments in the stability of the human knee*. J Bone Joint Surg 1987, 69A:233–242	103
GOODE PS, ALLMAN RM: *The prevention and management of pressure ulcers*. Med Clin North Am 1989, 73:1511–1524	3–4
GREEN DP, O'BRIEN ET: *Fractures of the thumb metacarpal*. South Med J 1972, 65:807–814	61–68
GREEN DP, ROWLAND SA: *Fractures and dislocations in the hand*. In ROCKWOOD CA JR, GREEN DP (eds): *Fractures and Dislocations in Adults*, ed 2. Philadelphia, JB Lippincott, 1984	61–68
GUSTILO RB, MERKOW RL, TEMPLEMAN D: *The management of open fractures*. Bone Joint Surg 1990, 72A:299–304	140–151
HAMBERG P, GILLQUIST J, LYSHOLM J: *Suture of new and old peripheral meniscus tears*. J Bone Joint Surg 1983, 65A:193–197	95
HAMILTON RB, O'BRIEN BM, MORRISON A, et al: *Survival factors in replantation and revascularization of the amputated thumb—10 years experience*. Scand J Plast Reconstr Surg 1984, 18:163–173	117–122, 124–125
HARTY M, JOYCE JJ III: *Surgical approaches to the elbow*. J Bone Joint Surg 1964, 46A:1598–1606	41–46
HECKMAN JD: *Emergency Care and Transportation of the Sick and Injured*, ed 4. Park Ridge IL, AAOS, 1987	26–32
HECKMAN JD: *Fractures and dislocations of the foot*. In ROCKWOOD CA JR, GREEN DP (eds): *Fractures in Adults*, ed 2. Philadelphia, JB Lippincott 1984	107–116

Section I (continued)

Plates

HEIM U, PFEIFFER KM: *Small Fragment Set Manual. Technique Recommended by the ASIF Group,* ed 2. New York, Springer-Verlag, 1982   107–116

HELFET DL: *Bicondylar intraarticular fractures of the distal humerus in adults: their assessment, classification and operative management.* Adv Orthop Surg 1985, 9:223–235   41–46

HEPPENSTALL RB: *Fracture healing.* In HEPPENSTALL RB (ed): *Fracture Treatment and Healing.* Philadelphia, WB Saunders, 1980, pp 35–64   23–25

HEPPENSTALL RB: *Fracture Treatment and Healing.* Philadelphia, WB Saunders, 1980   138–139

HERBERT TJ: *The Herbert Scaphoid Screw Bone System.* Warsaw IN, Zimmer Inc, 1982   47–60

HERBERT TJ, FISHER WE: *Management of the fractured scaphoid using a new bone screw.* J Bone Joint Surg 1984, 66B:114–123   59–60

HOLDSWORTH F: *Fractures, dislocations, and fracture-dislocations of the spine.* J Bone Joint Surg 1970, 52A:1534–1551   69–78

HOWE J, JOHNSON RJ: *Knee injuries in skiing.* Orthop Clin North Am 1985, 16:303–314   99–101

HUGHSTON JC: *Fracture of the distal radial shaft: mistakes in management.* J Bone Joint Surg 1957, 39A:249–264   47–60

HUGHSTON JC, BARRETT GR: *Acute anteromedial rotatory instability. Long-term results of surgical repair.* J Bone Joint Surg 1983, 65A:145–153   99–101

HULTH A: *Current concepts in fracture healing.* Clin Orthop 1989, 249:265–284   23–25

INSALL JN, HOOD RW: *Bone block transfer of the medial head of the gastrocnemius for posterior cruciate insufficiency.* J Bone Joint Surg 1982, 64A:691–699   103

INSALL J, JOSEPH DM, AGLIETTI P, et al: *Bone-block iliotibial-band transfer for anterior cruciate insufficiency.* J Bone Joint Surg 1981, 63A:560–569   102

JACKSON DM: *Second thoughts on the burn wound.* J Trauma 1969, 9:839–862   5

JAMES JIP, WRIGHT TA: *Fractures of the metacarpals and proximal and middle phalanges of the finger. In proceedings of the British Orthopaedic Association.* J Bone Joint Surg 1966, 48B:181–182   61–68

JANZEROVIC Z: *The burn wound from the surgical point of view.* J Trauma 1975, 15:42–62   10

KANE WJ: *Fractures of the pelvis. In* ROCKWOOD CA JR, GREEN DP (eds): *Fractures in Adults,* ed 2. Philadelphia, JB Lippincott 1984, pp 1093–1209   79–83

KAPLAN EB: *Functional and Surgical Anatomy of the Hand,* ed 2. Philadelphia, JB Lippincott, 1965   61–68

KAPLAN EB: *Anatomy, injuries, and treatment of the extensor apparatus of the hand and the digits.* Clin Orthop 1959, 13:24–41   61–68

KATSAROS J, SCHUSTERMAN M, BEPPU M, et al: *The lateral upper arm flap: anatomy and clinical applications.* Ann Plast Surg 1984, 12:489–500   125

KAUFER H: *Mechanical function of the patella.* J Bone Joint Surg 1971, 53A:1551–1560   96–98

KELLY RP, WHITESIDES TE JR: *Transfibular route for fasciotomy of the leg.* J Bone Joint Surg 1967, 49A:1022–1026   16

KLEINERT HE, JUHALA CA, TSAI TM, et al: *Digital replantation–selection, technique, and results.* Orthop Clin North Am 1977, 8:309–318   117–122, 124, 126

KLEINERT HE, KUTZ JE, ASHBELL TS, et al:

Section I (continued)

Plates

Primary repair of lacerated flexor tendons in "no-man's land." J Bone Joint Surg 1967, 49:577   119

KOMATSU S, TAMAI S: *Successful replantation of a completely cut-off thumb. Case report.* Plast Reconstr Surg 1968, 42:374–377   117–126

KUCZYNSKI K: *The proximal interphalangeal joint. Anatomy and causes of stiffness in the fingers.* J Bone Joint Surg 1968, 50B:656–663   61–68

LETOURNEL E, JUDET R: *Fractures of the Acetabulum.* New York, Springer-Verlag, 1981   84–85

LISTER GD: *Intraosseous wiring of the digital skeleton.* J Hand Surg 1978, 3:427–435   118

LISTER GD, KLEINERT HE: *Replantation.* In GRABB WX, SMITH JW (eds): *Plastic Surgery,* ed 3. Boston, Little, Brown, 1980, pp 697–715   117–126

LISTER GD, SCHEKER LR: *Emergency free flaps to the upper extremity.* J Hand Surg 1988, 13:22–28   124

LODER RT: *The influence of diabetes mellitus on the healing of closed fractures.* Clin Orthop 1988, 232:210–216   23–25

LOSEE RE, JOHNSON TR, SOUTHWICK WO: *Anterior subluxation of the lateral tibial plateau. A diagnostic test and operative repair.* J Bone Joint Surg 1978, 60A:1015–1030   99–101

MALT RA, MCKHANN C: *Replantation of severed arms.* JAMA 1964, 189:716–722   117, 120–121, 123–124

MARIANI PP, PUDDU G, FERRETTI A: *Hemarthrosis treated by aspiration and casting. How to condemn the knee.* Am J Sports Med 1982, 10:343–345   95

MAST JW, SPIEGEL PG: *Complex ankle fractures.* In MEYERS MH (ed): *The Multiply Injured Patient With Complex Fractures.* Philadelphia, Lea & Febiger, 1984, p 304   107–116

MATSEN FA: *Compartment Syndromes.* New York, Grune & Stratton, 1980   11–16

MAYFIELD JK, JOHNSON RP, KILCOYNE RK: *Carpal dislocations: pathomechanics and progressive perilunar instability.* J Hand Surg 1980, 5:226–241   47–60

MCCUE FC, HAKALA MW, ANDREWS JR, et al: *Ulnar collateral ligament injuries of the thumb in athletes.* J Sports Med 1974, 2:70–80   61–68

MCELFRESH EC, DOBYNS JH, O'BRIEN ET: *Management of fracture dislocation of the proximal interphalangeal joints by extension block splinting.* J Bone Joint Surg 1972, 54A:1705–1711   61–68

MCKIBBIN B: *The biology of fracture healing in long bones.* J Bone Joint Surg 1978, 60B:150–162   23–25

MCMANUS AT, KIM SH, MCMANUS WF, et al: *Comparison of quantitative microbiology and histopathology in divided burn-wound biopsy specimens.* Arch Surg 1987, 122:74–76   8

MCMANUS WF, GOODWIN CW JR, PRUITT BA JR: *Subeschar treatment of burn-wound infection.* Arch Surg 1983, 118:291–294   8

MCMANUS WF, MASON AD JR, PRUITT BA JR: *Excision of the burn wound in patients with large burns.* Arch Surg 1989, 124:718–720   10

MEURMAN KO, ELFVING S: *Stress fracture in soldiers: a multifocal bone disorder. A comparative radiological and scintigraphic study.* Radiology 1980, 134:483–487   136–137

MEYERS MH, MCKEEVER FM: *Fracture of the intercondylar eminence of the tibia.* J Bone Joint Surg 1970, 52A:1677–1684   102

MORRISON WA, O'BRIEN BM, MACLEOD AM: *Digital replantation and revascularization. A*

Section I (continued)

Plates

long term review of one hundred cases. Hand 1978, 10:125–134   117–122

MOYLAN JA JR, INGE WW JR, PRUITT BA JR: *Circulatory changes following circumferential extremity burns evaluated by the ultrasonic flowmeter: an analysis of 60 thermally injured limbs.* J Trauma 1971, 11:763–770   7

MOZINGO DW, SMITH AA, MCMANUS WF, et al: *Chemical burns.* J Trauma 1988, 28:642–647   6

MUBARAK SJ: *Etiologies of compartment syndromes.* In MUBARAK SJ, HARGENS AR (eds): *Compartment Syndromes and Volkmann's Contracture.* Philadelphia, WB Saunders, 1981   11

MUBARAK SJ, CARROLL NC: *Volkmann's contracture in children: aetiology and prevention.* J Bone Joint Surg 1979, 61B:285–293   16

MUBARAK SJ, HARGENS AR (eds): *Compartment Syndromes and Volkmann's Contracture.* Philadelphia, WB Saunders, 1981   11–16

MUBARAK SJ, HARGENS AR, OWEN CA, et al: *The wick catheter technique for measurement of intramuscular pressure. A new research and clinical tool.* J Bone Joint Surg 1976, 58:1016–1020   14

MUBARAK SJ, OWEN CA: *Double incision fasciotomy of the leg for decompression in compartment syndromes.* J Bone Joint Surg 1977, 59A:184–187   16

MUBARAK SJ, OWEN CA, HARGENS AR, et al: *Acute compartment syndromes: diagnosis and treatment with the aid of the wick catheter.* J Bone Joint Surg 1978, 60A:1091–1095   15

MULLER ME, ALLGOWER M, SCHNEIDER R, et al (eds): *Manual of Internal Fixation,* ed 2. New York, Springer-Verlag, 1979   84–93, 105–106

NEER CS II: *Fractures of the distal third of the clavicle.* Clin Orthop 1968, 58:43–50   33–40

O'BRIEN BMcC: *Microvascular Reconstructive Surgery.* London, Churchill Livingstone, 1977   117, 120

O'BRIEN ET: *Fractures of the metacarpals and phalanges.* In DP GREEN (ed): *Operative Hand Surgery,* ed 2. New York, Churchill Livingstone, 1988   61–68

ODENSTEIN M, GILLQUIST J: *Functional anatomy of the anterior cruciate ligament and a rationale for reconstruction.* J Bone Joint Surg 1985, 67A:257–262   99–101

OGDEN JA: *Skeletal Injury in the Child,* ed 2. Philadelphia, Lea & Febiger, 1990   140–151

OGDEN JA: *Injury to the growth mechanisms of the immature skeleton.* Skeletal Radiol 1981, 6:237–253   127–134

OWEN CA, MUBARAK SJ, HARGENS AR, et al: *Intramuscular pressures with limb compression: clarification of the pathogenesis of the drug-induced muscle-compartment syndrome.* N Engl J Med 1979, 300:1169–1172   11–12

PEACOCK EE JR: *Wound Repair,* ed 3. Philadelphia, WB Saunders, 1984   17–18

PETROFF PA, PRUITT BA JR: *Pulmonary disease in the burn patient.* In ARTZ CP, MONCRIEF JA, PRUITT BA JR (eds): *Burns.* Philadelphia, WB Saunders, 1979, pp 95–106   7

PITT RM, PARKER JC, JURKOVICH GJ, et al: *Analysis of altered capillary pressure and permeability after thermal injury.* J Surg Res 1987, 42:693–702   6

PRUITT BA JR: *Electric injury.* In WYNGAARDEN JB, SMITH LH JR (eds): *Cecil Textbook of Medicine.* Philadelphia, WB Saunders, 1988, pp 2380–2382   6

Section II (continued)

Plates

COOMBS RRH, FITZGERALD RH (eds): *Infections in the Orthopaedic Patient.* London, Butterworth, 1987 — 11–18

FITZGERALD RH JR, COONEY WP 3RD, WASHINGTON JA 2ND, et al: *Bacterial colonization of mutilating hand injuries and its treatment.* J Hand Surg 1977, 2:85–89 — 1

GOLDSTEIN EJ, BARONES MF, MILLER TA: *Eikenella corrodens in hand infections.* J Hand Surg 1983, 8:563–567 — 4

GUNTHER SF, ELLIOTT RC, BRAND RL, et al: *Experience with atypical mycobacterial infection in the deep structures of the hand.* J Hand Surg 1977, 2:90–96 — 3

HUGHES SDF, FITZGERALD RH (eds): *Musculoskeletal Infections.* Chicago, Year Book Med Pub, 1986 — 11–18

KANAVEL AB: *Infections of the Hand: A Guide to the Surgical Treatment of Acute and Chronic Suppurative Processes in the Fingers, Hand, and Forearm,* ed 5. Philadelphia, Lea & Febiger, 1925 — 1

KILGORE ES JR: *Hand infections.* J Hand Surg 1983, 8:723–726 — 3

KILGORE ES JR, BROWN LG, NEWMEYER WL, et al: *Treatment of felons.* Am P Surg 1975, 130:194–198 — 2

LEDDY JP: *Infections of the upper extremity.* J Hand Surg 1986, 11A:294–297 — 5

LEVIN ME, O'NEAL LW (eds): *The Diabetic Foot,* ed 4. St Louis, CV Mosby Year Book Inc, 1988 — 7–9

LINSCHEID RL, DOBYNS JH: *Bone and soft tissue infections of the hand and wrist.* In EVARTS CM (ed): *Surgery of the Musculoskeletal System,* Vol 2, ed 2. New York, Churchill Livingstone, 1989, pp 1159–1195 — 1

MANN RJ, HOFFELD TA, FARMER CB: *Human bites of the hand: twenty years of experience.* J Hand Surg 1977, 2:97–104 — 3

MASON ML, KOCH SL: *Human bite infections of the hand, with a study of the routes of extension of infection from the dorsum of the hand.* Surg Gynec Obst 1930, 51:591–625 — 3

MCKAY D, PASCARELLI EF, EATON RG: *Infections and sloughs in the hands of drug addicts.* J Bone Joint Surg 1973, 55A:741–745 — 3

MELENY FL: *Hemolytic streptococcus gangrene.* Arch Surg 1924, 9:317 — 5

NELSON C. *Infections.* In EVARTS CM (ed): *Surgery of the Musculoskeletal System,* ed 2. New York, Churchill Livingstone, 1990, pp 4299–4592 — 11–18

NORTH HH, ZIMMERMANN B, HO G JR: *Septic bursitis: confirming the diagnosis and treating appropriately.* J Musculoskel Med 1992, 9:52–64 — 10

PETRIE PW, LAMB DW: *Severe hand problems in drug addicts following self-administered injections.* Hand 1973, 5:130–134 — 5

ROWE JG, AMADIO PC, EDSON RS: *Sporotrichosis.* Orthopedics 1989, 12:981–985 — 3

SAMMARCO GJ: *The Foot in Diabetes.* Philadelphia, Lea & Febiger, 1991 — 7–9

SHAW BA, KASSER JR: *Acute septic arthritis in infancy and childhood.* Clin Orthop 1990, 257:212–225 — 10

SPIEGEL JD, SZABO RM: *A protocol for the treatment of severe infections of the hand.* J Hand Surg 1988, 13A:254–259 — 2

STEIN PJ, STANECK JL, MCDONOUGH JJ, et al: *Established hand infections: a controlled, prospective study.* J Hand Surg 1983, 8:553–557 — 2

Section II (continued)

Plates

WALDVOGEL FA, MEDOFF G, SWARTZ MN: *Treatment of osteomyelitis.* N Engl J Med 1970, 283:822 — 11–18

Section III

AMERICAN ACADEMY OF ORTHOPAEDIC SURGEONS STAFF: *Atlas of Limb Prosthetics: Surgical and Prosthetic Principles.* St Louis, Mosby-Year Book Inc, 1981 — 11–21

BEASLEY RW: *General considerations in managing upper limb amputations.* Orthop Clin North Am 1981, 12:743–749 — 11–21

BROWN PW: *The rational selection of treatment for upper extremity amputations.* Orthop Clin North Am 1981, 12:843–848 — 11–21

BURGESS EM, MATSEN FA III: *Determining amputation levels in peripheral vascular disease.* J Bone Joint Surg 1981, 63A:1493–1497 — 11–21

BURGESS EM, ROMANO RL, ZETTL JH: *The Management of Lower Extremity Amputations, TR 10-6.* Washington, Veterans Administration, 1969 — 11–21

GONZALEZ EG, CORCORAN PJ, REYES RL: *Energy expenditure in below-knee amputees: correlation with stump length.* Arch Phys Med Rehabil 1974, 55:111–119 — 11–21

MOONEY V, HARVEY JP JR, MCBRIDE E, et al: *Comparison of postoperative stump management: plaster vs soft dressings.* J Bone Joint Surg 1971, 53A:241–249 — 11–21

MOONEY V, WAGNER W JR, WADDELL J, et al: *The below-the-knee amputation for vascular disease.* J Bone Joint Surg 1976, 58A:365–368 — 11–21

OMER GE JR: *Nerve, neuroma, and pain problems related to upper limb amputations.* Orthop Clin North Am 1981, 12:751–762 — 11–21

SHERMAN R, SHERMAN C, GALL N: *A survey of current phantom limb pain treatments in the United States.* Pain 1980, 8:85–90 — 11–21

TOOMS RE: *General principles of amputations.* In CRENSHAW AH (ed): *Campbell's Operative Orthopaedics,* ed 8. St Louis, CV Mosby, 1992, pp 677–686 — 11–21

Section IV

AMERICAN ACADEMY OF ORTHOPAEDIC SURGEONS STAFF: *Atlas of Limb Prosthetics: Surgical and Prosthetic Principles.* St Louis, Mosby-Yearbook Inc, 1981 — 5

BENDER LF: *Upper extremity prosthetics.* In KOTTKE FJ, STILLWELL GK, LEHMANN JF (eds): *Krusen's Handbook of Physical Medicine and Rehabilitation,* ed 3. Philadelphia, WB Saunders, 1982 — 5

BLACKBURN TA JR: *Rehabilitation of anterior cruciate ligament injuries.* Orthop Clin North Am 1985, 16:241–269 — 14–15

BURGESS EM: *Amputation surgery and postoperative care.* In BANERJEE SN (ed): *Rehabilitation Management of Amputees.* Baltimore, Williams & Wilkins, 1982 — 2

Section IV (continued)

Plates

CAVANAGH T: *General deconditioning.* In BASMAJIAN JV, KIRBY RL: *Medical Rehabilitation.* Baltimore, Williams & Wilkins, 1984 — 1

CORCORAN PJ: *Disability consequences of bed rest.* In STOLOV WC, CLOWERS MR: *Handbook of Severe Disability.* Washington, US Department of Education, Rehabilitation Services Administration, 1981 — 1

DELISA JA, MIKULIC MA, MELNICK RR, et al: *Stroke rehabilitation. Part II. Recovery and complications.* Am Fam Physician 1982, 26:143–151 — 6–10

DELISA JA, MILLER RM, MELNICK RR, et al: *Stroke rehabilitation. Part I. Cognitive deficits and prediction of outcome.* Am Fam Physician 1982, 26:207–214 — 6–10

FISHER SV, HELM PA: *Comprehensive Rehabilitation of Burns.* Baltimore, Williams & Wilkins, 1984 — 11–12

FORTUNE WP: *Lower limb joint replacement.* In NICKEL VL (ed): *Orthopaedic Rehabilitation.* New York, Churchill Livingstone, 1982 — 16–17

FRIEDMANN LW: *Amputation.* In STOLOV WC, CLOWERS MR (eds): *Handbook of Severe Disability.* Washington, US Department of Education, Rehabilitation Services Administration, 1981 — 3

GARRISON SJ, ROLAK LA, DODARO RR, et al: *Rehabilitation of the stroke patient.* In DELISA JA, CURRIE DM, GANS BM, et al (eds): *Rehabilitation Medicine–Principles and Practice.* Philadelphia, JB Lippincott, 1988, pp 565–584 — 6–10

GERBER LH, HURWITZ SR: *Biomechanical principles pertinent to rehabilitation of patients with rheumatic disease.* In EHRLICH GE (ed): *Rehabilitation Management of Rheumatic Conditions,* ed 2. Baltimore, Williams & Wilkins, 1986 — 16–17

HALAR EM, BELL KR: *Contracture and other deleterious effects of immobility.* In DELISA JA, CURRIE DM, GANS BM, et al (eds): *Rehabilitation Medicine–Principles and Practice.* Philadelphia, JB Lippincott, 1988 — 1

HELM PA, KEVORKIAN CG, LUSHBAUGH M, et al: *Burn injury: rehabilitation management in 1982.* Arch Phys Med Rehabil 1982, 63:6–16 — 11–12

HICKS JE, GERBER LH: *Rehabilitation of the patient with arthritis and connective tissue disease.* In DELISA JA, CURRIE DM, GANS BM, et al (eds): *Rehabilitation Medicine–Principles and Practice.* Philadelphia, JP Lippincott, 1988 — 16–17

HOLLIDAY PJ: *Early postoperative care of the amputee.* In KOSTUIK JP (ed): *Amputation Surgery and Rehabilitation.* New York, Churchill Livingstone, 1982 — 2

KISNER C, COLBY LA: *Therapeutic Exercise: Foundations and Techniques.* Philadelphia, FA Davis, 1985 — 16–17

KRIEGSMAN J, BERG D, SMITH M: *Conservative treatment of the torn anterior cruciate ligament.* Contemp Orthop 1988, 16:35–42 — 14

LANDON GC, RICHTSMEIER K: *Restoring function to the hip and knee.* Geriatrics 1981, 36:125–136 — 16–17

LEONARD JA, MEIER RH: *Prosthetics.* In DELISA JA, CURRIE DM, GANS BM, et al (eds): *Rehabilitation Medicine–Principles and Practice.* Philadelphia, JB Lippincott, 1988 — 2–5

MAEHLUM S, DALJORD OA: *Acute sports injuries in Oslo–A one-year study.* Br J Sports Med 1984, 18:181–185 — 13

Section IV *(continued)* — Plates

MAY BJ: *Postoperative management.* In SANDERS GT (ed): *Lower Limb Amputations: A Guide to Rehabilitation.* Philadelphia, FA Davis, 1986 — 2

Mensch G, Ellis PM: *Physical Therapy Management of Lower Extremity Amputations.* Rockville MD, Aspen Publishers, 1986 — 2–3

OKAMOTO GA, PHILLIPS TJ: *Physical Medicine and Rehabilitation.* Philadelphia, WB Saunders, 1984 — 5

PAULOS L, NOYES FR, GROOD E, et al: *Knee rehabilitation after anterior cruciate ligament reconstruction and repair.* Am J Sports Med 1981, 9:140–149 — 14

PELLICCI P, SALVATI E: *Complications of hip surgery.* Contemp Orthop 1985, 10:27–39 — 16–17

Section IV *(continued)* — Plates

SANDERS GT: *Lower Limb Amputations: A Guide to Rehabilitation.* Philadelphia, FA Davis, 1986 — 3

SHARPLESS JW: *Mossman's A Problem-Oriented Approach to Stroke Rehabilitation,* ed 2. Springfield IL, Charles C Thomas, 1982 — 6–10

SMITH RW, REISCHL SF: *Treatment of ankle sprains in young athletes.* Am J Sports Med 1986, 14:465–471 — 13

STEADMAN JR: *Rehabilitation of acute injuries of the anterior cruciate ligament.* Clin Orthop 1983, 172:129–132 — 14

STONER EK: *Management of the lower extremity amputee.* In KOTTKE FJ, STILLWELL GK, LEHMANN JF (eds): *Krusen's Handbook of Physical Medicine and Rehabilitation,* ed 3.

Section IV *(continued)* — Plates

Philadelphia, WB Saunders, 1982 — 4

VALLBONA C: *Bodily responses to immobilization.* In KOTTKE FJ, STILLWELL GK, LEHMANN JF (eds): *Krusen's Handbook of Physical Medicine and Rehabilitation.* Philadelphia, WB Saunders, 1982 — 1

ZIMBLER S, SMITH J, SCHELLER A, et al: *Recurrent subluxation and dislocation of the patella in association with athletic injuries.* Orthop Clin North Am 1980, 11:755–770 — 14

VARGHESE G, REDFORD JB: *Preoperative assessment in management of amputees.* In BANERJEE SN (ed): *Rehabilitation Management of Amputees.* Baltimore, Williams & Wilkins, 1982 — 2

Subject Index

Boldface numbers refer to terms that appear on plates

THE NETTER COLLECTION OF MEDICAL ILLUSTRATIONS

The NETTER COLLECTION OF MEDICAL ILLUSTRATIONS has enjoyed an enthusiastic reception from the medical community since the publication of its first volume. The remarkable illustrations by Frank H. Netter, M.D., and text by leading specialists make these books unprecedented in their educational and clinical value.